Health Care: Systems and Practices

Health Care: Systems and Practices

Edited by Neil Perry

hayle
medical

New York

Hayle Medical,
750 Third Avenue, 9th Floor,
New York, NY 10017, USA

Visit us on the World Wide Web at:
www.haylemedical.com

ISBN: 978-1-63241-625-4

Cataloging-in-Publication Data

Health care : systems and practices / edited by Neil Perry.
    p. cm.
Includes bibliographical references and index.
ISBN 978-1-63241-625-4
1. Medical care. 2. Public health. 3. Health services administration.
4. Health planning. I. Perry, Neil.
RA776 .H43 2019
613--dc23

Table of Contents

Preface

Every book is a source of knowledge and this one is no exception. The idea that led to the conceptualization of this book was the fact that the world is advancing rapidly; which makes it crucial to document the progress in every field. I am aware that a lot of data is already available, yet, there is a lot more to learn. Hence, I accepted the responsibility of editing this book and contributing my knowledge to the community.

The diagnosis, prevention, and treatment of illnesses, injuries and diseases for the purpose of maintaining and improving health is known as health care. It is provided by health professionals. It plays a crucial role in the promotion of physical health, mental health and the wellbeing of people. Some of the common fields which fall under health care include physical therapy, pharmacy, optometry, dentistry, audiology, psychology, midwifery and occupational therapy. An organization of people, institutions and resources meant to deliver health care services to fulfil the health needs of people is called a health care system. This book is a compilation of chapters that discuss the most vital concepts and emerging trends in the field of health care. The various advancements in health care are glanced at and their applications as well as ramifications are looked at in detail. For all those who are interested in health care, this book can prove to be an essential guide.

While editing this book, I had multiple visions for it. Then I finally narrowed down to make every chapter a sole standing text explaining a particular topic, so that they can be used independently. However, the umbrella subject sinews them into a common theme. This makes the book a unique platform of knowledge.

I would like to give the major credit of this book to the experts from every corner of the world, who took the time to share their expertise with us. Also, I owe the completion of this book to the never-ending support of my family, who supported me throughout the project.

Editor

The Financial Implications of a Well-Hidden and Ignored Chronic Lyme Disease Pandemic

The Financial Implications of a Well-Hidden and Ignored Chronic Lyme Disease Pandemic

Marcus Davidsson

Economist and Independent Researcher, https://papers.ssrn.com/sol3/cf_dev/AbsByAuth.cfm?per_id=895329; davidsson_marcus@hotmail.com

Abstract: 1 million people are predicted to get infected with Lyme disease in the USA in 2018. Given the same incidence rate of Lyme disease in Europe as in the USA, then 2.4 million people will get infected with Lyme disease in Europe in 2018. In the USA by 2050, 55.7 million people (12% of the population) will have been infected with Lyme disease. In Europe by 2050, 134.9 million people (17% of the population) will have been infected with Lyme disease. Most of these infections will, unfortunately, become chronic. The estimated treatment cost for acute and chronic Lyme disease for 2018 for the USA is somewhere between 4.8 billion USD and 9.6 billion USD and for Europe somewhere between 10.1 billion EUR and 20.1 billion EUR. If governments do not finance IV treatment with antibiotics for chronic Lyme disease, then the estimated government cost for chronic Lyme disease for 2018 for the USA is 10.1 billion USD and in Europe 20.1 billion EUR. If governments in the USA and Europe want to minimize future costs and maximize future revenues, then they should pay for IV antibiotic treatment up to a year even if the estimated cure rate is as low as 25%. The cost for governments of having chronic Lyme patients sick in perpetuity is very large.

Keywords: *Borrelia*; Lyme disease; chronic Lyme disease; ILADS; incidence rate; cost chronic Lyme disease; CDC

1. Introduction

The objectives of this article are to investigate the incidence rate of Lyme disease in the USA and Europe, to investigate the financial cost of chronic Lyme disease and to find the most cost-efficient way for the governments to solve the current chronic Lyme disease pandemic [1]. Very few studies exist that calculate the economic impact of chronic Lyme disease [2]. According to the European Centre for Disease Prevention and Control (ECDC), Lyme disease—also known as Borreliosis—is caused by a spirochete bacteria called *Borrelia burgdorferi* [3]. An early stage *Borrelia* infection is known as acute Lyme disease and a late stage *Borrelia* infection is known as chronic Lyme disease. A Lyme disease "war" has been going for a long time [4,5] between two doctors' associations regarding the most appropriate way to diagnose and treat Lyme disease. The two doctors associations are the Infectious Diseases Society of America (IDSA) [6] and International Lyme and Associated Diseases Society (ILADS) [7]. IDSA represents infectious disease doctors that firmly believe that all Lyme disease infections, regardless of whether the infection is acute or chronic, can successfully and easily be treated with three weeks of oral antibiotic [8] despite the fact that no scientific studies currently exist that support the claim that three weeks of oral antibiotics can always cure acute or chronic Lyme disease [9] and there exist many scientific studies that have shown that the *Borrelia* bacteria can survive three weeks of oral antibiotics in vitro [10,11] and in vivo, in mice [12–15], dogs [16], horses [17], monkeys [18] and in humans [19–36]. The in vivo references have mostly been extracted from [37–39]. Alive *Borrelia* bacteria has been found in 7 out of 8 patients with chronic Lyme disease [40]. The immune system by itself can never eradicate a *Borrelia* infection [41–44] and no scientific studies exist that show that bacterial infections can simply disappear. Approximately 63% [45,46] of people today that are infected with *Borrelia*, unfortunately, develop chronic Lyme disease. Most Lyme disease patients today either do not receive any antibiotic treatment at all or they receive an insufficient amount of antibiotic treatment. The IDSA does not recognize chronic Lyme disease, nor do they recommend antibiotic treatment for chronic Lyme disease. The IDSA calls chronic Lyme disease post-treatment Lyme disease syndrome (PTLDS) [47] but it has been suggested that this term is a misnomer and should not be used [48]. Because chronic Lyme disease is classified as a syndrome instead of an infection, the IDSA therefore does not recommend antibiotic treatment for chronic Lyme disease.

In 2006, the IDSA treatment guidelines development process was subjected to an antitrust investigation by the Connecticut Attorney General [49], which found that many IDSA treatment panel members had conflicts of interest [50]. In November 2017, another antitrust lawsuit (Civil Action No 17-cv-190) [51,52] was directed at the IDSA along with several large insurance companies in the USA and several IDSA medical doctors, in a federal court in Texarkana, Texas in the USA. The allegations concern violations of the Racketeer Influenced and Corrupt Organizations (RICO) Act and the Sherman Antitrust Act. According to the Agency for Healthcare Research and Quality (AHRQ), which is part of the U.S. Department of Health and Human Services, 86% of health care costs in 2010 in the USA came from patients with one or more chronic conditions [53]. The concern is that because Intravenous (IV) antibiotic treatment for people with chronic Lyme disease costs so much money, insurance companies in the USA may gain by colluding with the IDSA to ensure chronic Lyme disease is not classified as a real disease caused by bacteria, so that IV antibiotic treatment can be denied.

The scientific process fails if it can be controlled by a group or groups with a particular agenda [54]. The IDSA's treatment guidelines for Lyme disease are problematic in the following ways: (A) They do not follow The National Academies of Sciences, Engineering and Medicine recommendations on how to develop treatment guidelines [55] because the IDSA treatment guideline panel did not consist of a diversified and balanced group of doctors nor did the panel include patient representatives; (B) More than 50% of IDSAs treatment guidelines are based only on "expert opinion" [56]; (C) The IDSA's treatment guidelines for Lyme disease do reflect the fact that, according to the CDC, Lyme disease can lead to death if not treated with antibiotics [57]. The CDC has, however, significantly underestimated the number of deaths caused by *chronic* Lyme disease. One study estimates that chronic Lyme disease and associated diseases could be the cause of over 1200 suicides per year in the USA [58].

The International Lyme and Associated Diseases Society (ILADS) represents Lyme Literate Medical Doctors (LLMDs) from around the world who recognize that chronic Lyme disease is a real and serious disease that must be treated with long-term antibiotics [59]. ILADS' treatment guidelines for Lyme disease can be found on the National Guidelines Clearinghouse (NGC) web page [60]. According to ILADS, Lyme disease is a clinical diagnosis that is based on the symptoms a patient presents. LLMDs prefer to treat chronic Lyme disease patients with IV antibiotics because IV antibiotics are more effective than oral antibiotics [61]. However, oral antibiotics are much easier to administer, and they are not as expensive as IV antibiotics. Hence, in a situation where a patient cannot afford IV antibiotics, or if a patient has difficulties finding someone to administer IV antibiotics, then oral antibiotics are always preferred over no antibiotics. LLMDs can, if necessary, treat a patient with chronic Lyme disease with oral antibiotics for the rest of the patient's life. Thus, similarities exist between chronic Lyme disease and the Human Immunodeficiency Virus (HIV) that also cannot be eradicated with oral medication.

Up until December 2017, the Centers for Disease Control and Prevention (CDC) in the USA officially endorsed the IDSA treatment guidelines for Lyme disease. What the CDC's view on treatment for chronic Lyme disease is today is unclear [62]. The CDC still uses the IDSA terminology 'post-treatment Lyme disease syndrome' (PTLDS) [63]. It is unlikely that the IDSA's lack of medical ethics when it comes to Lyme disease [64] was the reason why the CDC stopped officially endorsing IDSA treatment guidelines for Lyme disease, because in 2016 an anonymous whistleblower group of scientists from within the CDC, calling themselves CDC Scientists Preserving Integrity, Diligence and Ethics in Research (CDC SPIDER), raised concerns about the CDC's lack of independence and ethics [65], stating, "We are a group of scientists at CDC that are very concerned about the current state of ethics at our agency. It appears that our mission is being influenced and shaped by outside parties and rogue interests". The CDC therefore most likely stopped endorsing the IDSA treatment guidelines because legal and public pressure was building up. Today people are becoming more aware of chronic Lyme disease. The conflict over what the best ways are to diagnose and treat Lyme disease have gone so far that a Tick-Borne Disease Working Group was created when the 21st-century cures act became law in the USA in December 2016 [66]. The objective of the working group is to review the scientific literature, regarding for example causes, prevention, diagnosis, duration, surveillance and treatment for Lyme disease and associated diseases.

The genus *Borrelia* was named in honor of the French bacteriologist Amédée Borrel in 1907 [67]. The name Lyme comes from the name of the town in Connecticut in the USA where the disease was "first" observed in 1977 [68] this despite the fact that the German physician Alfred Buchwald published the first case of atrophy of the skin already in 1883 [69]. In 1902 Herxheimer and Hartmann named such atrophy of the skin Acrodermatitis Chronica Atrophicans (ACA) [70] which is why ACA, which is dermatological disorder mostly associated with chronic Lyme disease in Europe [71], sometimes is called Herxheimer disease. ACA presents its self as a red-bluish discoloration of the extremities [72]. The link between Lyme disease and the bacteria that cause it was first discovered by the medical entomologist Dr. Willy Burgdorfer in 1982 [73]. The bacteria, therefore, took the name after its discoverer *Borrelia* Burgdorferi. It was first in 1929 when the serendipitous discovery of penicillin was made by scientist Alexander Fleming [74] that treatment for Lyme disease became available. Penicillin was originally produced from mold. Naturally occurring antibiotics can also be produced by fermentation, an old technique that can be traced back almost 8000 years [75]. The genes that convey antibiotic resistance to bacteria have been around for at least 30,000 years [76], which means that antibiotic resistance to a large part has not been developed during the last 88 years humankind has known about antibiotics which is a fact that we rarely hear about though.

One of the first people to treat chronic Lyme, or more specifically ACA, with penicillin in 1949 was Nils Thyresson [77] who was a Swedish medical doctor and professor of Dermatology and Venereology. The first human believed to have been infected with Lyme disease was Ötzi the Iceman [78]. This 5300 years old naturally preserved mummy was discovered in 1991 in the Ötztal Alps on the border between Austria and Italy. Spirochete bacteria are believed to be much older this though. Spirochetes similar to *Borrelia* has been found in a 15 million years old tick preserved in amber in the Dominican Republic [79] which means that the spirochete bacteria that causes Lyme disease is much older than humankind. The complete *Borrelia* genome was first sequenced in 1997 [80]. The *Borrelia* bacteria has the most complex genomic architecture among known prokaryotes [81]. *Borrelia* bacteria are also very genetically diversified [82,83]. Different Borrelia strains have different antigens [84] which means that different *Borrelia* strains will produce different immune system responses in the form of antibodies in an infected host. A blood test that only test for one specific antibody cannot detect antibodies from different Borrelia strains. A person that is infected with one type of Borrelia strain will also have different symptoms compared to a person that is infected with a different Borrelia strain [85]. For example, arthritis is usually not seen in European Lyme disease patients [86] due to the different *Borrelia* strains that exist in Europe compared to the USA which means that the lack of arthritis in a patient should not be interpreted as the patient not having Lyme disease. Lyme disease diagnosis and treatment are further complicated by the fact that *Borrelia* also has many different co-infections [87] such as Babesia, Bartonella, Ehrlichia, etc. It is believed that a vector such as a tick can spread at least 237 different types of bacteria [88] and many types of viruses [89] which means that many chronic Lyme patients might be infected with many different types of microbes at the same time.

In the Lyme disease documentary Under Our Skin, Dr. Burgdorfer says: "The controversy in the Lyme disease research is a shameful affair and I say this because the whole thing is politically tainted. Money goes to the same people who have for the last thirty years produced the same thing. Nothing." [90]. The *Borrelia* bacteria has at least three different morphological forms. (1) A spirochete form [91]. (2) A round body form that is also known as cyst form [92]. (3) A biofilm form [93]. The *Borrelia* bacteria evade the immune system by for example changing morphology [94] and by changing its outer surface proteins (Osp) also known as antigens [95–98]. When the bacteria change its antigens all the time, the specific antibodies that are produced by the immune system to try to eradicate the infection becomes useless. The DNA structure that is believed to be responsible for the bacteria's antigenic variation ability is called G-quadruplex (G4) [99]. Immune system evasion by other diseases such as Amyotrophic Lateral Sclerosis (ALS) [100] and cancer [101] is also believed to be connected to G4. Exciting research is being done that is trying to find medications that block G4 for the *Borrelia* bacteria [102]. If the researchers are successful, it could mean an end to chronic Lyme disease but also to other diseases. If the immune system in combination with some drug could eradicate the *Borrelia* bacteria that would be a superior solution compared to a possible lifetime of oral antibiotics. The bacteria evade being killed by broad-spectrum antibiotics by changing morphology [103]. Note that the bacteria ability to evade broad-spectrum antibiotics should not be interpreted as antibiotic resistant. Metronidazole/Tinidazole forces the bacteria to take a spirochete form [104,105] where other broad-spectrum antibiotics such as Azithromycin can kill it off. When chronic Lyme patients are treated with a macrolide antibiotic such as Azithromycin in combination with Metronidazole/Tinidazole, then the physician can also give Plaquenil which is an anti-malaria medication. Plaquenil raises the PH level in cells so that macrolide antibiotics can work more effectively [106]. Unfortunately, Plaquenil does not work for tetracycline antibiotics [107]. It is, however, important to note that Plaquenil can cause eye problems [108] which means that not all patients can tolerate this medication.

Because different combinations of antibiotics have different effects on the different morphological forms of the *Borrelia* bacteria [109], ILADS treatment guidelines recommend combination therapy with two different types antibiotics for chronic Lyme disease [110] for example metronidazole/tinidazole in combination with azithromycin/doxycycline. The recommended treatment for chronic Lyme disease is therefore different from the recommended treatment for acute Lyme by the IDSA which is, monotherapy with one antibiotic for example doxycycline. Again, similarities exist between HIV and chronic Lyme disease because both are treated with combination therapy. The reason for combination therapy for HIV and chronic Lyme disease is however different. Combination therapy in HIV is motivated by the fact that the virus develops resistance to the medication if you only treat with one antiviral medication. For chronic Lyme disease, this is not the cases. Combination therapy for chronic Lyme disease is motivated by the fact that *the Borrelia* bacteria changes morphology which means that monotherapy is not an effective treatment for Lyme disease.

A common mistake is to describe the symptoms of Lyme disease as "flu-like". A serious Lyme disease infection should not be reduced to a simple cold. A better screening symptom for Lyme disease is paresthesia. Paresthesia manifests itself as vibrating sensation under the skin. One study estimates that 53% of patients with chronic Lyme disease develop paresthesia [111]. A second study estimates that 70% of patients with chronic Lyme disease develop paresthesia [112]. The good thing is that the paresthesia stops when antibiotics have killed off the infection [113] but also during treatment with antibiotics such as Metronidazole or Tinidazole. There are three main questions that need to be answered to justify treatment for chronic Lyme disease. (1) Do chronic Lyme disease patients without treatment suffer from a low Quality of Life (QOL) than the general population? Four National Institute of Health (NIH) studies have shown that the answer to that question is yes [114]. (2) Are the symptoms of chronic Lyme disease patients reduced because of antibiotic treatment? The answer to that question is yes [115–119]. (3) Can an untreated chronic Lyme disease lead to premature death? The answer to that question is yes according to our previous CDC reference. There exist a few studies that show that the symptoms of chronic Lyme patients do not improve with antibiotics treatment.

There exist at least two problems with these studies. (1) They usually treat chronic Lyme patients with monotherapy which again is not a recommended treatment. (2) They have used flawed statistical methods [120]. Medical doctors should be able to use their professional expertise and in consultation with their patients determine the most appropriate treatment for patients.

A European study [121] estimates the sensitivity of the Lyme disease test to 44%. Such number was found by analyzing the performance of eight different Lyme disease tests. 89 different blood samples were tested for each test manufacturer. The sample also included healthy controls. Another study [122] that conducted a meta-analysis of the American scientific literature (eight scientific articles) regarding the performance of the Lyme disease test estimates the sensitivity of the Lyme disease test to 46% and the specificity to 99%. Because the blood tests that are used today by government health agencies to detect the human body's production of antibodies against the *Borrelia* bacteria's antigens are so insensitive Lyme disease, today must be defined as a clinical diagnosis as correctly advocated by ILADS. If a patient has had a blood test that suggests a Lyme disease infection that is fine, but a positive blood test should not be a requirement for a diagnosis. A person that suspect a Lyme disease infection is today, unfortunately, better of tossing a coin and diagnosing themselves because the blood tests for Lyme disease today will miss most infections. Specific antibodies often cannot be found in patients with Lyme disease because of the bacteria ability to shift its antigens.

Testing cerebrospinal fluid instead of blood will not improve test sensitivity because the bacteria can still shift its antigens in cerebrospinal fluid which means that the probability of detecting specific antibodies in cerebrospinal fluid is not larger than in blood. Moreover, cerebrospinal fluid causes the bacteria to change its morphology from a spirochete form to a cyst from [123]. If you only diagnose Lyme disease in patients that have specific antibodies in their blood or cerebrospinal fluid, you will miss most cases. To better understand Lyme disease testing let's look at the confusion matrix [124]. All calculations can be found in the macro-enabled excel file "Lyme disease model.xlsm". We assume in Table 1 that the number of people in the disease and control groups are known and equal. In real life, however, we do not know the number of people in the disease and control group. We can only observe the total number of people that tested positive in both groups.

We can now plot the number of people that tested positive in both groups (z) and the % number of people that tested positive in both groups (zz) when the number of infected people in the disease group (x) and the number of healthy people in control groups (y) are unknown as seen in Figures 1 and 2.

Table 1. Number of people that tested positive in both groups (z) when the number of infected people in the disease group (x) and the number of healthy people in control groups (y) are known and assumed to be equal.

Assumed values			
Number of infected people in disease group (x)	100		
Number of healthy people in control group (y)	100		
Test sensitivity (se)	0.44		
Test specificity (sp)	0.99		
Formulas			
Number of infected people in the disease group that tested positive = true positive (a)	$x * se$		
Number of infected people in the disease group that tested negative = false negative (b)	$x - a = x - x * se$		
Number of healthy people in the control group that tested positive = false positive (c)	$y * (1-sp)$		
Number of healthy people in the control group that tested negative = true negative (d)	$y - c = y - y * (1-sp)$		
Confusion matrix			
Disease group		Control group	
Number of true positives (a) =	44	Number of false positives (c) =	1
Number of false negatives (b) =	56	Number of true negatives (d) =	99
Statistics			
The relationship between y and x (p)	y / x	1	
Test sensitivity (se)	$a / (a + b)$	0.44	
Test specificity (sp)	$d / (c + d)$	0.99	

Table 1. *Cont.*

Number of infected people in the disease group (x)	a + b	100
Number of healthy people in the control group (y)	c + d	100
Total number of tested people	a + b + c + d	200
Number of people that tested positive in both groups (z)	a + c = x * se + y * (1-sp)	45
% of people that tested positive in both groups (zz)	(z / (x + y)) * 100	22.5
Number of false test results in disease group	b	56
% number of false test results in disease group	(b / (a + b)) * 100	56
Number of correct test results in disease group	a	44
% number of correct test results in disease group	(a / (a + b)) * 100	44
Number of correct test results in control group	d	99
% number of correct test results in control group	(d / (c + d)) * 100	99
Number of false test results in control group	c	1
% number of false test results in control group	(c / (c + d)) * 100	1
Number of false test result in both groups	b + c	57
% number of false test results in both groups	(b + c) / (a + b +c +d)	0.285
% of people that tested positive in disease group	(a / (a +b)) * 100	44

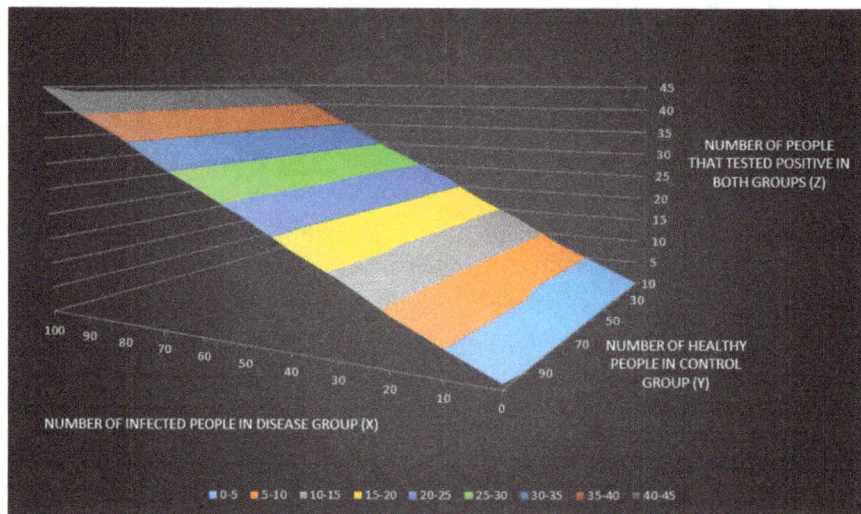

Figure 1. The number of people that tested positive in both groups (z) when the number of infected people in the disease group (x) and the number of healthy people in control groups (y) are unknown.

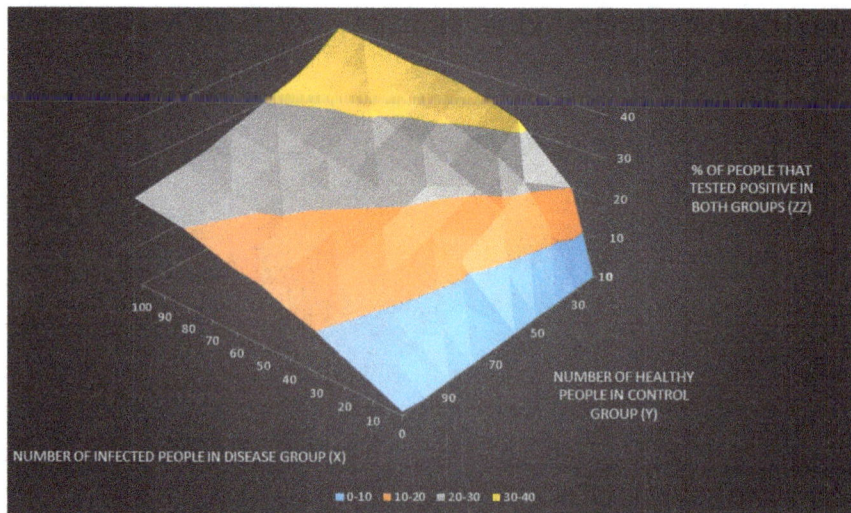

Figure 2. The % number of people that tested positive in both groups (zz) when the number of infected people in the disease group (x) and the number of healthy people in control groups (y) are unknown.

We can now assume that the number of healthy people in the control group (y) = p × the number of sick people in the disease group (x). The relationship between y, x and p can be seen in Figure 3.

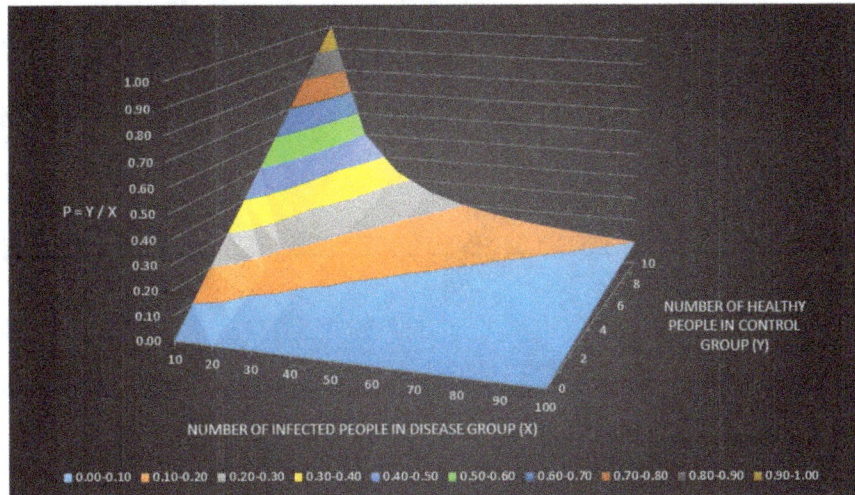

Figure 3. The relationship between y, x and p.

We now can adjust the equation for z and zz to include p as seen in Figures 4 and 5. It can be hard to see in Figure 5 (it is better to look in the excel file directly) but zz has the same value for all x values for any given value of p which means that you can never find a value for x (and a value for y thanks to y = x × p) only given values for se, sp, p and zz. I have also written a sub procedure in VBA called zzz() that also can be found in the excel file "Lyme disease model.xlsm" that can be called by simply pressing a button that calculates zz given a Lyme disease test sensitivity (se) equal to 0.44 and a Lyme disease test specificity of (sp) equal to 0.99.

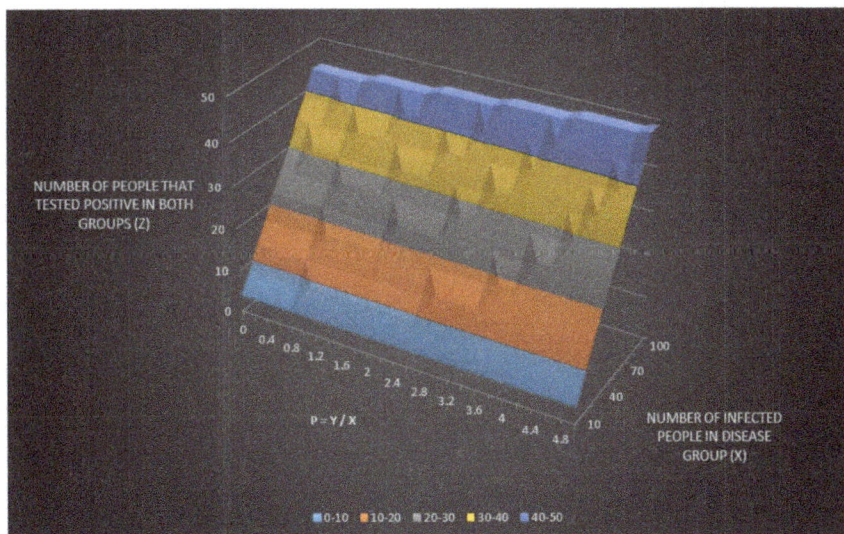

Figure 4. The number of people that tested positive in both groups (z) adjusted for the relationship between y and x (p).

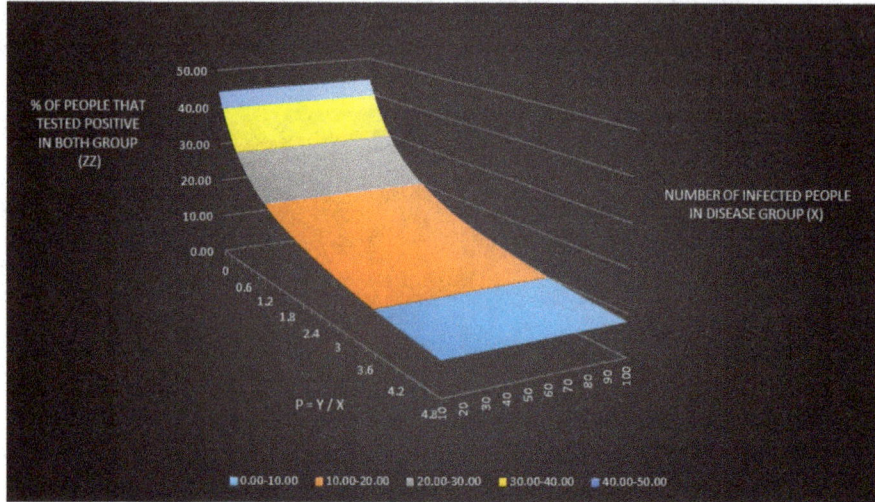

Figure 5. The % number of people that tested positive in both groups (zz) adjusted for the relationship between y and x (p).

We can now solve for the number of infected people in the disease group (x) and the number of healthy people in the control group (y) when they are unknown given a value for z with matrix algebra as seen in Table 2.

Table 2. How to find x and y with matrix algebra.

The equation we need to solve is the following:

Number of people that tested positive in both groups (z) =
the number of true positives (a) + the number of false positives (c)

where

Number of people with an infection in disease group	x
Number of people without an infection in control group	y
Total number of people in the disease and control groups	x + y
Test sensitivity (se)	0.44
Test specificity (sp)	0.99
Number of true positives (a) = x * se	x * 0.44
Number of false positives (c) = y * (1 - sp)	y * (1-0.99)
Number of people that tested positive in both groups (z)	100 000

which means:

The equation we need to solve is	z = x * se + y * (1-sp)
with constraint	z = 100 000
	se = 0.44
	sp = 0.99
	y = p*x
	p = 2.5

We can solve such equation in excel by using matrix algebra

The system of linear equations we should solve is	A * B = C	
where		
A =	0.44	0.01
	−2.5	1
B =	x	
	y	
C =	100 000	
	0	
A^-1 =	2.150538	−0.021505
	5.376344	0.946237
B = A ^ (-1) * C	x =	215 054
	y =	537 634

Table 2. *Cont.*

The relationship between y and x (p) = y / x	2.5
Number of people that test positive in the disease group = true positive (a) = x * se	94 624
Number of people that test positive in the control group = false positive (c) = y * (1-sp)	5 376
Number of people that tested positive in both groups (z) = a + c = x * se + y *(1-sp)	100 000
% of people that tested positive in both groups (zz) = (z / (x + y))*100	13.29

I have written a user defined function (udf) in VBA that does the above calculations automatically

Lyme1(se ; sp ; p ; z ; output) where output is either "x", "y" or "zz"

Lyme1(0.44;0.99;2.5;100000;"x")	x =	215 054
Lyme1(0.44;0.99;2.5;100000;"y")	y =	537 634
Lyme1(0.44;0.99;2.5;100000;"zz")	zz =	13.29

We can algebraically manipulate the previous equations further as seen in Table 3.

Table 3. Algebraic manipulation of previous equations.

We know that	We know that
z = x * se + y * (1-sp) y = p * x	z = x * se + y * (1-sp) x = y / p
which means that	which means that
z = x * se + p * x * (1 - sp)	z = (y / p) * se + y * (1 - sp)
we solve for x	we solve for y
x = z / (-sp * p + se + p)	y = p * z / (-sp * p + se + p)

For the previous example with z = 100 000 and p= 2.5 we get

x =	215 054
y =	537 634

I have again written a udf in VBA

Lyme2(se ; sp ; p ; z ; output) where output is either "x", "y" or "zz"

Lyme2(0.44;0.99;2.5;100000;"x")	x =	215 054
Lyme2(0.44;0.99;2.5;100000;"y")	y =	537 634
Lyme2(0.44;0.99;2.5;100000;"zz")	zz =	13.29

we know that	we know that
zz = (z / (x + y)) * 100 y = p * x	zz = (z / (x + y)) * 100 x = y / p
which means that	which means that
zz = (z / (x + p * x)) * 100	zz = (z / ((y / p) + y)) * 100
we solve for x	we solve for y
x = 100 * z / (p * zz + zz)	y = 100 * p * z / (p * zz + zz)

Table 3. *Cont.*

For the previous example with z=100 000, zz =13.29 and p= 2.5 we get		
x =		215 054
y =		537 634
I have again written a udf in VBA		
Lyme3(se ; sp ; p ; z ; zz ; output) where output is either "x", "y"		
Lyme3(0.44;0.99;2.5;100000;13.29;"x")	x =	215 054
Lyme3(0.44;0.99;2.5;100000;13.29;"y")	y =	537 634

We can do some further modeling and plotting as seen in Table 4, Figures 6 and 7.

Table 4. The number of infected people in the disease group (x) given total number of people (T) and the relationship between x and y = p.

Number of infected people in disease group	x
Number of healthy people in control group	y
Total number of people (T)	x + y
$T = x + y \rightarrow y = T - x$	$T = x + y \rightarrow x = T - y$
$y = p * x$	$x = y / p$
This means that	This means that
$T - x = p * x$	$T - y = y / p$
We can solve for x	We can solve for y
$x = T / (p + 1)$	$y = p * T / (p + 1)$

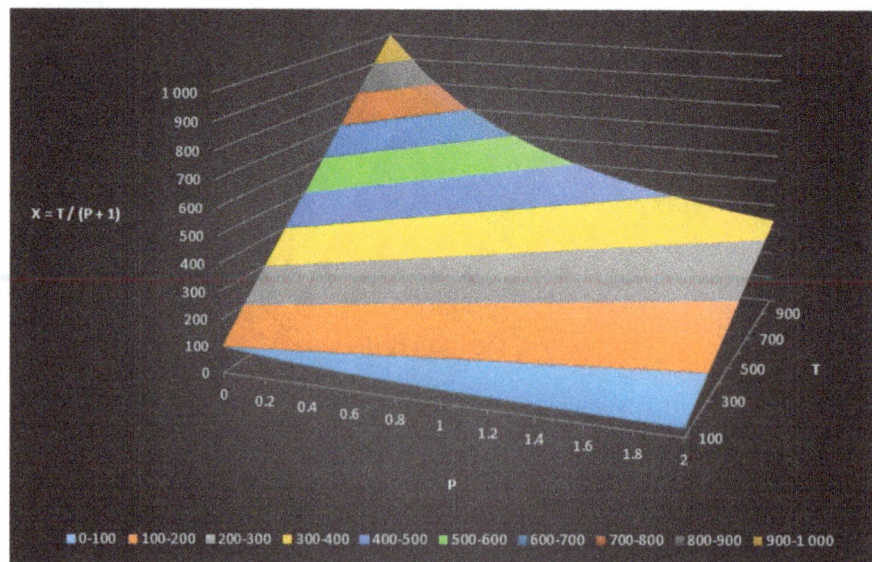

Figure 6. The number of infected people in the disease group (x) given total number of people (T) and the relationship (p) between x and y.

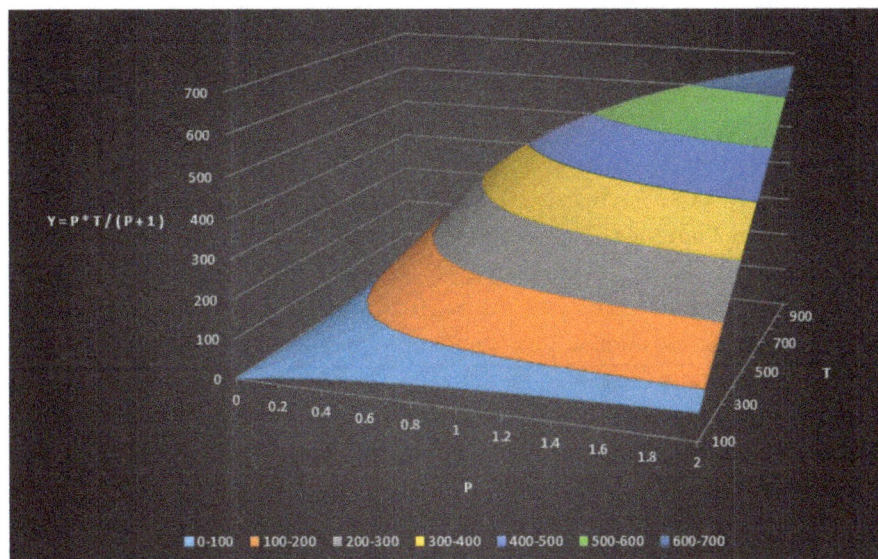

Figure 7. The number of healthy people in the control group (y) given the total number of people (T) and the relationship (p) between x and y.

2. Methods

The first limitation of this study is that we are using the incidence rate of Lyme disease from the USA on the population of Europe to get an estimate on how frequent Lyme disease is in Europe. Using the incidence rate from the USA on the population of Europe is not optimal but unfortunately, our only choice since the ECDC do not have any data on Lyme disease. Lyme disease is not spread exclusively by vectors such as ticks. One study [125] explains that Lyme disease is also a Sexually Transmitted Disease (STD). Since Lyme disease can spread sexually, the growth rate of the disease will be similar in the USA and Europe which means that it's not unrealistic to use the disease frequency from the USA on Europe's population. The second limitation of this study is that scientific literature that exists regarding Lyme disease as an STD is very limited. In a perfect world more, research should be done regarding Lyme disease as an STD but please keep in mind that Borrelia's close cousin the spirochete bacterium *Treponema pallidum* that causes syphilis is well known to spread sexually. Hence, the fact that the *Borrelia* bacteria can also or could also spread through sexual contact should not come as a surprise. Unfortunately, accurately modeling the spread of Lyme disease without sexual transmission is close to impossible because there are so many difficult questions that need to be answered regarding tick ecology [126] for example in which geographic areas are ticks most frequent?, how many different types of ticks exists?, which types of ticks spread disease?, what types of microorganisms do ticks contain?, how often do ticks reproduce?, when they reproduce how many eggs do they produce on average?, how many of these eggs survive?, what is the probability that a tick bites a human?, what is the probability that a tick bites an animal?, what is the probability of a transmission of *Borrelia* or any other microorganism after a tick bite?, what animals do ticks use for transportation deer, bird or rodent, how many of these animals that transport ticks are there in a given geographic area?, how is a tick population affected by cold temperature like a winter? As I said, the epidemiological modeling becomes close to impossible especially for an economist maybe not for a biologist.

All infectious diseases (total number of infections in a population) that are transmitted from person to person and where treatment is inadequate has by nature exponential growth over time. A pandemic initially starts with 1 infected person (total number of infections at t1 = 1) that person then goes and infect 1 more person (total number of infections at t2 = 2), these 2 infected people then go and infect 2 more people (total number of infections at t3 = 4), these 4 people then go and infect 4 more people (total number of infections at t4 = 8) etc. The % change at t2 = ((2−1)/1) × 100 = 100, the % change at t3 = ((4−2)/2) × 100 = 100, the % change at t4 = ((8−4)/4) × 100 = 100. Since the percentage change is constant over time, exponential growth models are also called constant growth rate models. For a linear growth model, the percentage change is decreasing over time. The relationship between the transmission rate of an infection that is spread through sexual contact and the annual growth rate of infection can be seen in Table 5. We can see that given that each infected person has sex with one healthy person each year then the transmission rate is equal to the annual percentage growth rate of infection for an infectious disease that is spread sexually. The third limitation of this study is that we assume that the annual growth rate for Lyme disease is 2%. To my knowledge, there does not exist any scientific literature regarding the annual growth rate of Lyme disease. The 2% number is therefore not based on empirical observation. However, we can compare such number to other infectious diseases that are also spread through sexual contact such as HIV. According to the CDC, HIV in 1977 had a transmission rate of 100% and in 2006 the transmission rate of HIV was 5% [127]. It becomes obvious that 2% is a very conservative number. The annual growth rate of Lyme disease is most likely higher than 2% because unfortunately many Lyme disease patients and especially chronic Lyme patients are struggling to find antibiotic treatment but since I lack a scientific reference for my claim and because I do not want to inflate the numbers I have chosen to report 2%. The fourth limitation of this study is that the scientific literature regarding how successful IV treatment is at curing chronic Lyme disease is very limited. However, the exact cure rate is not that important because we have known for a long time that antibiotics kill bacteria. We can simply assume that the cure rate is unknown and compare the outcome of five different assumed cure rates and scenarios: 0%, 25%, 50%, 75% and 100%.

Table 5. The transmission rate for an STD and its relationship to the annual growth rate of infection.

Total number of infections (tni1)) at year y given an annual percentage growth rateof infection (g) is given by -> $tni1(y) = tni1(y-1) * (1+g/100)$
Total number of infections (tni2) at year y given a percentage transmission rate (t) and given that each infected person has (n) number of healthy sexual partners each year is given by
-> $tni2(y) = tni2(y-1) * (1+(t/100) * n)$
We can see that given that each infected person has sex with one healthy person each year then the transmission rate is equal to the annual percentage growth rate of infection

g = 100			t = 100, n = 1			t = 100, n = 2		
Year (y)	tni1	% change	Year (y)	tni2	% change	Year (y)	tni2	% change
1	1	na	1	1	na	1	1	na
2	2	100	2	2	100	2	3	200
3	4	100	3	4	100	3	9	200
4	8	100	4	8	100	4	27	200
5	16	100	5	16	100	5	81	200
6	32	100	6	32	100	6	243	200
7	64	100	7	64	100	7	729	200

g = 2			t = 2, n = 1			t = 2, n = 2		
Year (y)	tni1	% change	Year (y)	tni2	% change	Year (y)	tni2	% change
1	1	na	1	1.0000	na	1	1.0000	na
2	1.02	2	2	1.0200	2	2	1.0400	4
3	1.04	2	3	1.0404	2	3	1.0816	4
4	1.06	2	4	1.0612	2	4	1.1249	4
5	1.08	2	5	1.0824	2	5	1.1699	4
6	1.10	2	6	1.1041	2	6	1.2167	4
7	1.13	2	7	1.1262	2	7	1.2653	4

tni2 can also be expressed as tni2(y+1) = number of old infections +number of new infections = $tni2(y) + tni2(y) * (t/100) * n$

t = 100, n = 1				t = 2, n = 1			
Year (y)	Number of old infections	Number of new infections	tni2	Year (y)	Number of old infections	Number of new infections	tni2
1	0	1	1	1	0.0000	1.0000	1.0000
2	1	1	2	2	1.0000	0.0200	1.0200
3	2	2	4	3	1.0200	0.0204	1.0404
4	4	4	8	4	1.0404	0.0208	1.0612
5	8	8	16	5	1.0612	0.0212	1.0824
6	16	16	32	6	1.0824	0.0216	1.1041
7	32	32	64	7	1.1041	0.0221	1.1262

3. Results

According to one scientific study [128], that can be found on the CDC website and published in *Clinical Infectious Diseases* which is a "scientific" journal issued by the IDSA 2.4 million individual Lyme disease blood tests were done in the USA 2008. That number comes from a survey that was sent to seven of the largest commercial laboratories in the USA. The most interesting part of such publication an equation was not included in the article itself but was present in the supplementary data [129]. The equation that the entire paper is based on is:

$$\text{Observed \% positive} = \text{\% True Infection} \times \text{Sensitivity} + (1 - \text{\% True Infection}) \times (1 - \text{Specificity})$$

If we multiply the above equation by the number of individual Lyme disease blood tests that were performed in 2008 in the USA, then we get the observed number of Lyme disease infections in the USA in 2008 by the CDC.

$$\text{Observed positive} = (\text{\% True Infection} \times \text{Sensitivity} + (1 - \text{\% True Infection}) \times (1 - \text{Specificity})) \times \text{Number of Lyme disease tests}$$

We solve the first equation for % True infection.

$$\text{\% True Infection} = (\text{Observed \% Positive} + \text{Specificity} - 1) / (\text{Specificity} + \text{Sensitivity} - 1)$$

If we multiply the above equation by the number of individual Lyme disease blood tests that were performed in 2008 in the USA, then we get CDC's predicted number of Lyme disease infections in the USA in 2008.

$$\text{True Infection} = ((\text{Observed \% Positive} + \text{Specificity} - 1) / (\text{Specificity} + \text{Sensitivity} - 1)) \times \text{Number of Lyme disease tests}$$

The CDC study estimated three different scenarios: high, low and average with an assumed test sensitivity of 66.9% and assumed specificity of 96.1%. Unfortunately, the only value for observed % positive that the CDC provides was 11.89%, which was the average scenario. The other two are not reported in the paper and need to be calculated. Why is the observed % positive variable so important for our calculations later? The observed % positive value has not been adjusted for the sensitivity and specificity of the Lyme disease blood test. Therefore, we can use our values for sensitivity and specificity. The observed % positive values do also not include any assumptions about the relationship between the number of sick people in the disease group (x) and the number of healthy people in the control group (y) that we previously defined as p. The CDC calculations can be found in Table 6.

Table 6. Comparison 1 of the CDC model and my Lyme disease model.

CDC equations	
Observed % Positive = % True Infection * Sensitivity Lyme test + (1 - % True Infection) * (1 – Specificity Lyme test)	
Observed positive = (% True Infection * Sensitivity + (1 - % True Infection) * (1 – Specificity))	
* number of performed individual Lyme disease tests	
% True Infection = (Observed % Positive + Specificity – 1) / (Specificity + Sensitivity – 1)	
True Infection = ((Observed % Positive + Specificity – 1) / (Specificity + Sensitivity – 1))	
* number of performed individual Lyme disease tests	
The performed number of individual Lyme disease test in 2008 in the USA (n)	2 400 000
Lyme disease test sensitivity assumed by the CDC (CDC se)	0.669
Lyme disease test specificity assumed by the CDC (CDC sp)	0.961

Table 6. *Cont.*

CDC scenario	Low	Average	High
% true infection also known as predicted % positive estimated by the CDC (CDC xx)	0.1	0.1189	0.185
Observed % positive in the control and disease group according to or implied by the CDC (CDC zz)	0.102	0.1189	0.15555
The number of people that tested positive in the control and disease group in the USA in 2008 according to the CDC (observed positive or CDC z)	244 800	285 360	373 320
The number of infected people in the disease group estimated by the CDC (predicted positive also known as true infection or CDC x)	240 000	285 360	444 000
CDC z = CDC x * CDC se + CDC y * (1 - CDC sp)	244 800 = 240 000 * 0.669 + y * (1-0.961)	285 360 = 285 360 * 0.669 + y * (1-0.961)	373 320 = 444 000 * 0.669 + y * (1-0.961)
The number of healthy people in the control group according the CDC (CDC y)	2 160 000	2 421 901	1 965 000
The relationship between y and x = CDC p = CDC y / CDC x	9.0000	8.4872	4.4257
Number of healthy people in the control group (y) : number of infected people in the disease group (x)	9 : 1	8.4872 : 1	4.4257 : 1
My model			
We assume p = 1, se = 0.44, sp = 0.99 and z = CDC z in Lyme2(se ; sp ; p ; z ; Output = q) where q is either "x", "y" or "zz" ?			
x =	544 000	634 133	829 600
y =	544 000	634 133	829 600
zz =	22.50	22.50	22.50
We assume p = 0.5, se = 0.44, sp = 0.99 and z = CDC z in Lyme2(se ; sp ; p ; z ; Output = q) where q is either "x", "y" or "zz" ?			
x =	550 112	641 258	838 921
y =	275 056	320 629	419 461
zz =	29.67	29.67	29.67

We can see that the CDC has unrealistically and secretly assumed without motivation or explanation that the size of the control group with healthy people is 9 (low scenario), 8.5 (average scenario) and 4.4 (high scenario) times the size of the disease group with infected people ($p = 9$, $p = 8.5$ and $p = 4.4$). These assumed p-values cannot be empirically observed because it is impossible to know the value of p by simply looking at the total number of people that test positive in the control and disease group (z). It would be more realistic to assume that the size of the control group with healthy people is the same size as the disease group with infected people ($p = 1$). Because blood testing today is so primitive (you can more or less only test for one pathogen at the time) and because the blood tests for Lyme disease are so insensitive most people today will only test to get a confirmation that they are infected. Hence, many people will only test if they are infected. It is therefore unrealistic to expect that a lot of people without an infection will demand to get tested just for "fun" because there is also a personal financial cost involved. The CDC also claims in their paper that the value of the variable observed % positive was the same as the value for the variable predicted % positive for the average scenario which is mathematically impossible as seen in Figure 8 using the same assumptions regarding Lyme disease test sensitivity and specificity as the CDC. Such claim by the CDC, therefore, does not make any sense.

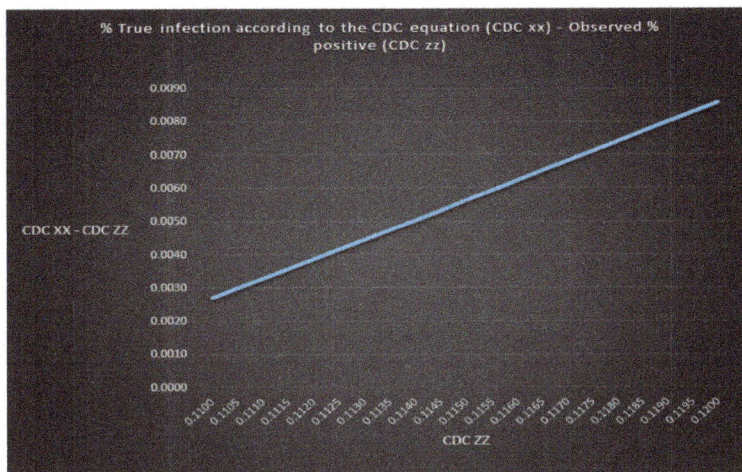

Figure 8. The value of observed % positive cannot be equal to predicted % positive for the average scenario in the CDC model.

We can now evaluate whether the CDC equation is correct and compare the CDC model with my model as seen in Table 7.

Table 7. Comparison 2 of the CDC model and my Lyme disease model.

CDC scenario	Low	Average	High
The number of infected people in the disease group estimated by the CDC (predicted positive also known as true infection or CDC x)	240 000	285 360	444 000
Assumptions	CDC z = 244 800	CDC z = 285 360	CDC z = 373 320
Lyme2(se ; sp ; p ; z ; output) = Lyme2(0.669 ; 0.961 ; 1 ; CDC z ; "x")	345 763	403 051	527 288
CDC assumptions	CDC p = 9 and CDC z = 244 800	CDC p = 8.4872 and CDC z = 285 360	CDC p = 4.4257 and CDC z = 373 320
(A) Lyme2(0.669 ; 0.961 ; CDC p ; CDC z ; "x")	240 000	285 360	443 582
CDC x - A	0	0	418
(B) Lyme2(0.44 ; 0.99 ; 1 ; CDC z ; "x")	533 333	634 133	829 600
B - A	293 333	348 773	386 018
% difference between A and B = (B - A)/B	55	55	47

Given the CDC unrealistic assumptions regarding se, sp and p, it appears that the equation is more or less correct. There is, however, an unexplained difference of +418 infections for the high scenario. We can also see that if the CDC had assumed that $p = 1$ in combination with the CDC assumptions se = 0.669, sp = 0.961, then the number of Lyme disease infections in the USA for 2008 for the high scenario would have been 527,288 instead of 444,000. We can also see that the difference between the CDC model with CDC assumptions of se = 0.669, sp = 0.961, p(low) = 9, p(average) = 8.5 and p(high) = 4.4 and my model with my assumptions of se = 0.44, sp = 0.99 and $p = 1$ is lowest for the CDC high scenario hence I will report that in 2008 in the USA the estimated number of Lyme disease infections is 829,600. The data and calculations that I will present now can be found in the excel file "Lyme disease calculations.xlsx." Given 829,600 Lyme disease infections in 2008 in the USA and an assumed annual infection growth rate of 2% then in 2018 in the USA approximately 1 million people will get infected with Lyme disease. The total number of Lyme disease infections that we can expect in the USA from 2008 to 2050 is 55.7 million. Given an annual population growth rate in the USA of 1% and given that everyone that is infected from 2008 to 2050 is still alive than 12% of the population in the USA will have been infected with Lyme disease in 2050. The plots are presented in Figures 9–12.

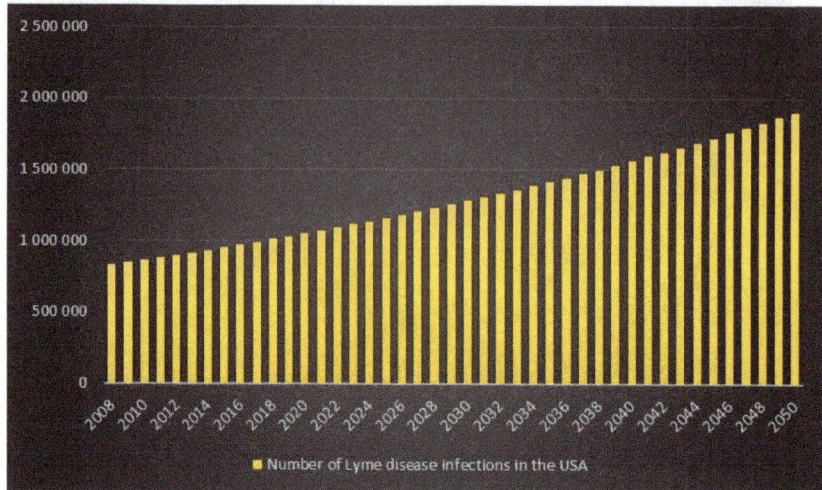

Figure 9. Number of Lyme disease infections in the USA between the years 2008 to 2050.

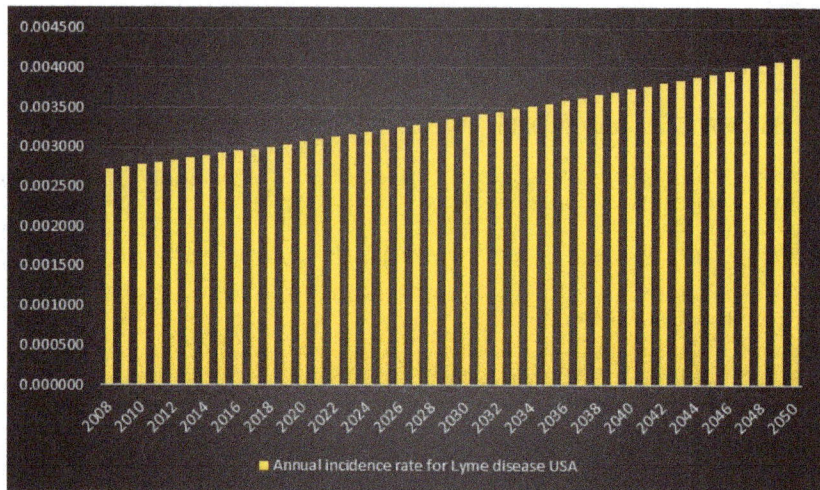

Figure 10. Annual incidence rate of Lyme disease in the USA between the years 2008 to 2050.

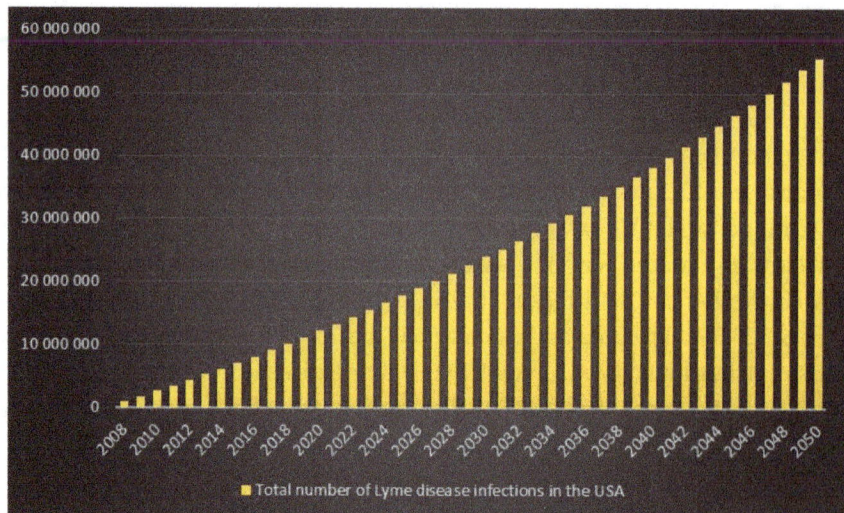

Figure 11. Total number of Lyme disease infections in the USA between the years 2008 to 2050.

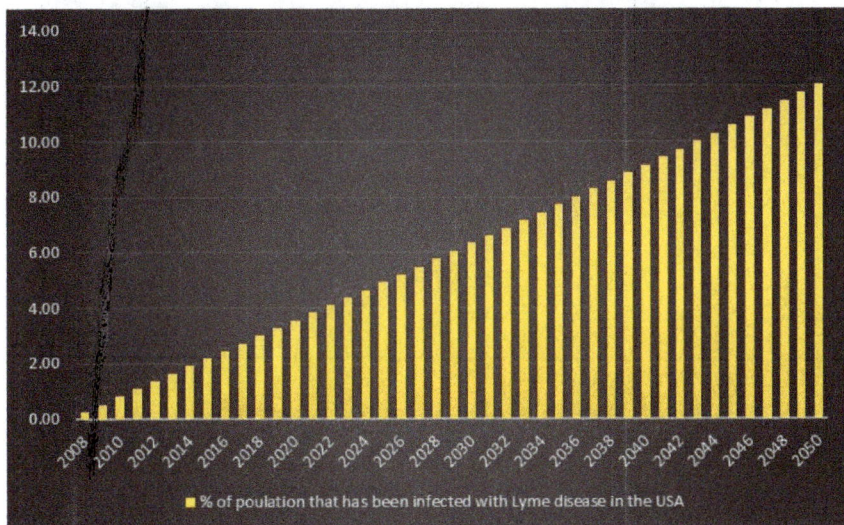

Figure 12. % of the population in the USA that have been infected with Lyme disease between the years 2008 to 2050.

Since the ECDC does not have any statistics on how frequent Lyme disease is in Europe, it is difficult to determine an exact figure for the number of Lyme disease cases in Europe in 2008. However, we can use the incidence rate (frequency) from the USA for 2008 on Europe's population for 2008 to get an estimate. The estimated number of Lyme disease infections in Europe in 2008 is 2,008,505. Given 2,008,505 Lyme disease infections in 2008 in Europe and an assumed annual infection growth rate of 2% then in 2018 in Europe approximately 2.4 million people will get infected with Lyme disease. The total number of Lyme disease infections that we can expect in Europe from 2008 to 2050 is 134.9 million. Given an annual population growth rate in Europe of 0.2% and given that everyone that is infected from 2008 to 2050 is still alive than 17% of the population of Europe will have been infected with Lyme disease in 2050. The plots are presented in Figures 13–16.

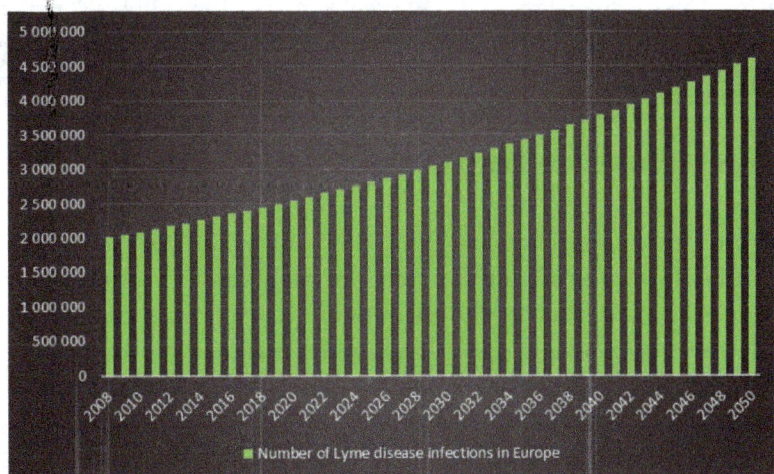

Figure 13. Number of Lyme disease infections in Europe between the years 2008 to 2050.

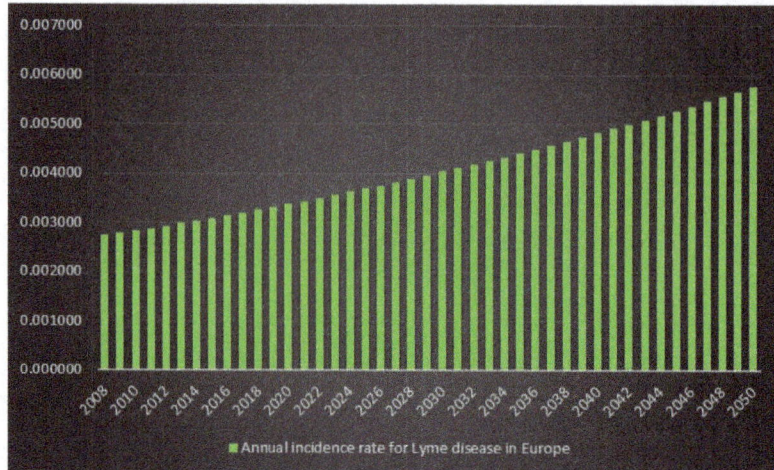

Figure 14. Annual incidence rate of Lyme disease in Europe between the years 2008 to 2050.

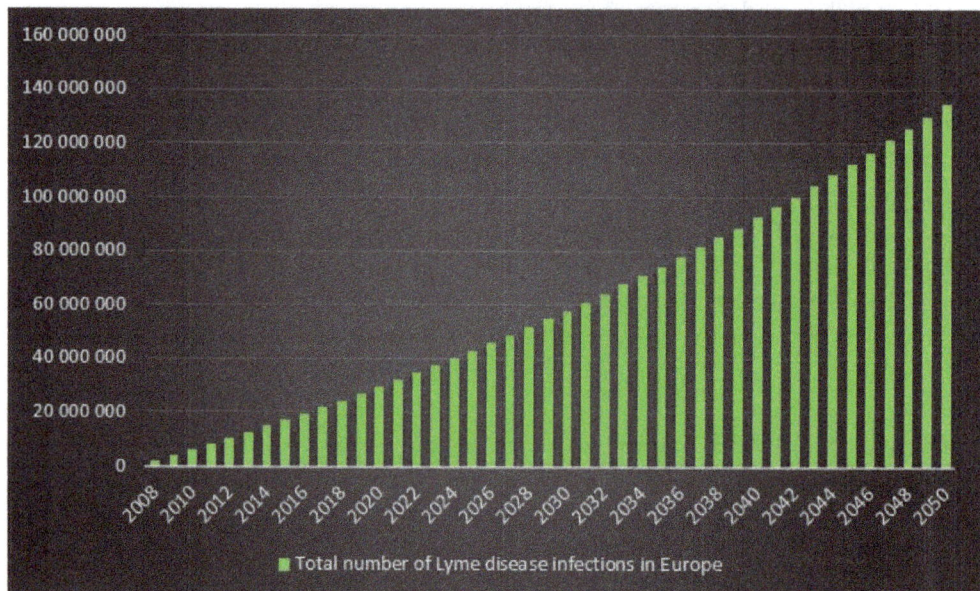

Figure 15. Total number of Lyme disease infections in Europe between the years 2008 to 2050.

According to our previous scientific reference, 63% of people that are infected with *Borrelia* develop chronic Lyme disease. The estimated number of people suffering from chronic Lyme disease in 2050 in the USA and Europe depend on the assumption we make regarding the estimated cure rate for chronic Lyme disease treatment and on the assumption that everyone that develop chronic Lyme disease from 2008 to 2050 is still alive. The last assumption is very uncertain because of how difficult it is today for chronic Lyme patients to get treatment. We can see in Table 8 and Figure 17 that the number of people that will suffer from chronic Lyme disease in 2050 in the USA with a 0% cure rate is approximately 35 million (8% of the USA population in 2050), with a 25% cure rate 26 million (6% of the USA population in 2050), with a 50% cure rate 18 million (4% of the USA population in 2050), with a 75% cure rate 9 million (2% of the USA population in 2050) and with a 100% cure rate zero (0% of the USA population in 2050).

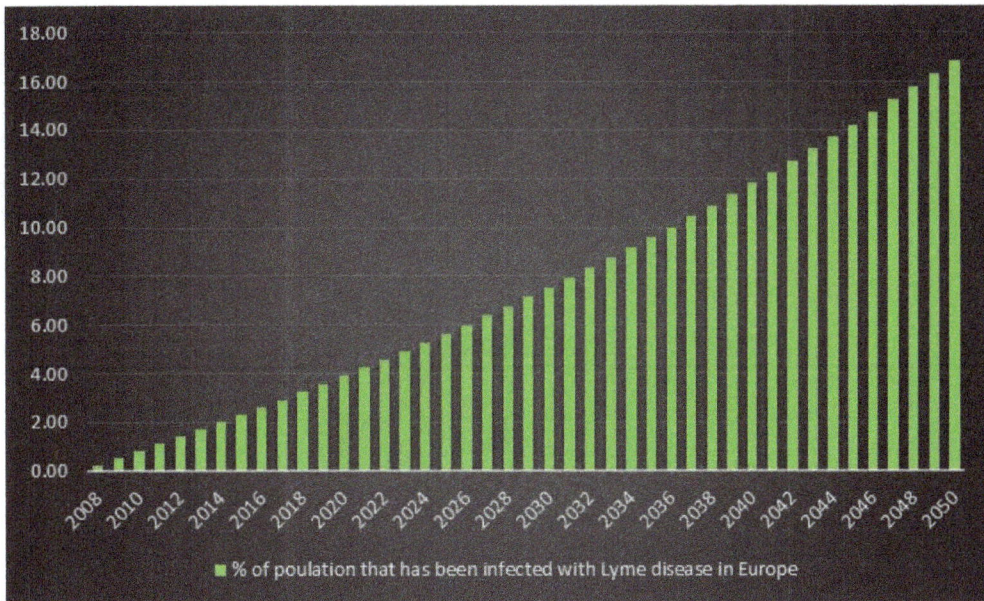

Figure 16. % of the population in Europe that have been infected with Lyme disease between the years 2008 to 2050.

Table 8. Number of people with chronic Lyme disease in 2050 in the USA.

Number of Lyme disease infections in the USA between 2008 to 2050 given an assumed 2% annual growth rate of infection	55 715 494
USA's population in 2050 given an annual population growth of 1%	461 712 128
% of the population in the USA that has been infected with Lyme disease between 2008 and 2050	12.07
People that are infected with Lyme disease that develop chronic Lyme disease	0.63
People that are infected with Lyme disease that develop an acute infection	0.37
Number of people that has had acute Lyme disease between 2008 and 2050 in the USA	20 614 733
% of population in 2050 that has had acute Lyme disease between 2008 and 2050 in the USA	4.46

Assumed cure rate	Number of people with chronic Lyme disease in 2050 in the USA	% of USA's population with chronic Lyme disease in 2050
0% cure rate	35 100 762	8
25% cure rate	26 325 571	6
50% cure rate	17 550 381	4
75% cure rate	8 775 190	2
100% cure rate	0	0

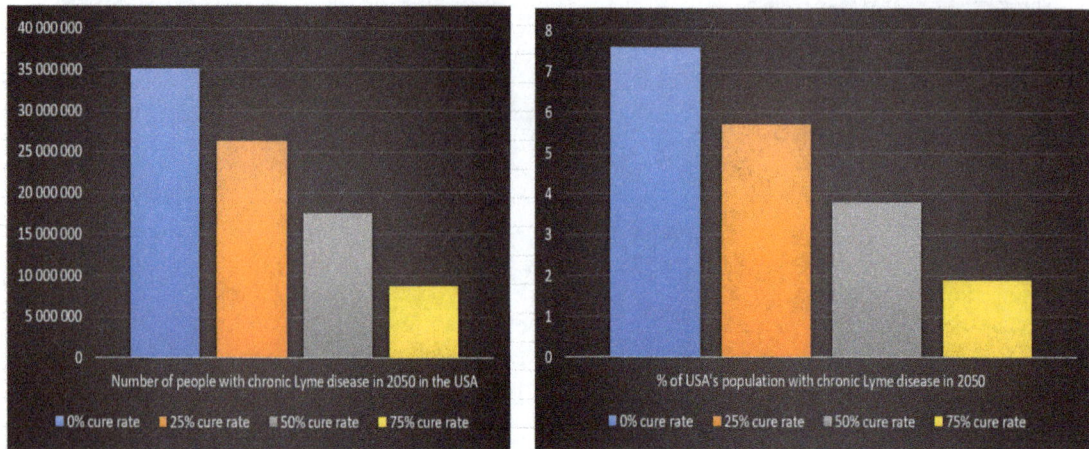

Figure 17. Number of people with chronic Lyme disease in 2050 in the USA

We can see in Table 9 and Figure 18 that the number of people that will suffer from chronic Lyme disease in 2050 in Europe with a 0% cure rate is approximately 85 million (11% of Europe's population in 2050), with a 25% cure rate 64 million (8% of Europe's population in 2050), with a 50% cure rate 42 million (5% of Europe's population in 2050), with a 75% cure rate 21 million (3% of the Europe's population in 2050) and with a 100% cure rate zero (0% of Europe's population in 2050).

Table 9. Number of people with chronic Lyme disease in 2050 in Europe

Number of Lyme disease infections in Europe between 2008 to 2050 given an assumed 2% annual growth rate of infection	134 890 144
Europe's population in 2050 given an annual population growth of 0.2%	800 427 717
% of the population in Europe that has been infected with Lyme disease between 2008 and 2050	16.85
People that are infected with Lyme disease that develop chronic Lyme disease	0.63
People that are infected with Lyme disease that develop an acute infection	0.37
Number of people that has had acute Lyme disease between 2008 and 2050 in Europe	49 909 353
% of population in 2050 that has had acute Lyme disease between 2008 and 2050 in Europe	6.24

Assumed cure rate	Number of people with chronic Lyme disease in 2050 in Europe	% of Europe's population with chronic Lyme disease in 2050
0% cure rate	84 980 791	11
25% cure rate	63 735 593	8
50% cure rate	42 490 396	5
75% cure rate	21 245 198	3
100% cure rate	0	0

If 2,008,505 people were infected with Lyme disease in Europe in 2008 and go undetected by the non-exist statistics what types of illnesses can Lyme disease patients be misdiagnosed with? It is therefore not unrealistic to assume that some Lyme disease patients are misdiagnosed with illnesses such as for example fibromyalgia, chronic fatigue syndrome (CFS), heart arrhythmia, multiple sclerosis (MS), restless legs syndrome (RLS), amyotrophic lateral sclerosis (ALS), Parkinson disease, systemic lupus erythematosus (SLE), Gulf War Syndrome (GWS) or Alzheimer's disease. The commonality between these diseases is that there is currently no known cure. Before we can start to estimate costs for Lyme disease, we need to discuss the tax on disability benefits. The tax rate on disabilities benefits is approximately 50% of the tax rate on income from work [130,131]. However, the tax on disability benefits is irrelevant to the government because assuming the government keeps the amount of disability benefit after tax fixed an increased tax rate on disability benefits will not increase the government's financial balance (government revenues + government costs) as seen in Table 10. If a government raises the tax rate on a person's disability benefit, then the increased tax revenues from such tax raise are completely offset by the larger government cost for the disability benefit.

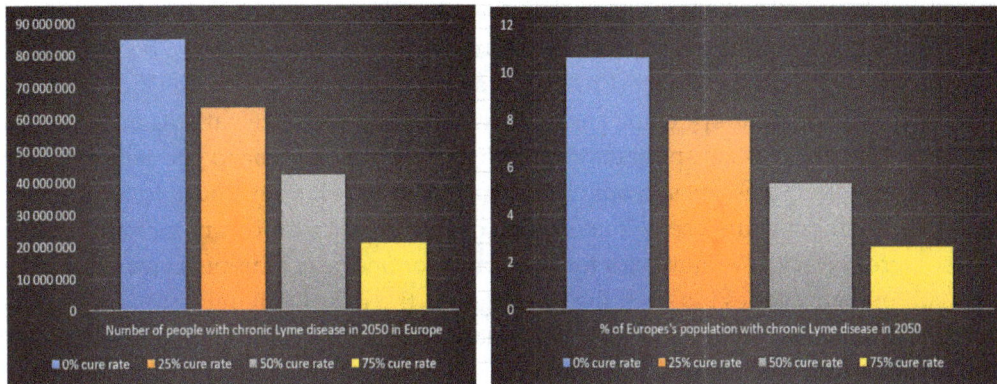

Figure 18. Number of people with chronic Lyme disease in 2050 in Europe.

Table 10. A government's financial balance (government revenues + government costs) with a disability benefit tax increase.

A government's financial balance after tax for a disabled person not working without the lost tax revenue because a chronic Lyme patient is not working			
Annual disability benefits after tax (ADAT)	13 000		
% tax rate on income from work	0.40		
Tax rate in % on disability benefits	0.20	0.40	
Annual disability benefits before tax T1 = ADAT / (1 - T1)	16 250	21 667	
			Difference
Government revenues			
Tax revenues from disability benefits (+)	3 250	8 667	5 417
Government costs for a disabled person			
Disability benefits (-)	-16 250	-21 667	-5 417
A government's financial balance = tax revenue + government cost	-13 000	-13 000	0

A government's financial balance for an enabled person working vs a disabled person not working before tax			
Annual disability benefits before tax (ADAT)	13 000		
Annual income from work before tax	35 000		
% tax rate on income from work	0.4		
	An enabled person that is working	**A disabled person that is not working**	**Difference**
Government revenues			
Tax revenues from income from work (+)	14 000	0	-14 000
Government costs for a disabled person (-)			
Disability benefits (-)	0	-13 000	-13 000
Lost tax revenues because a disabled person is not working (-)	0	-14 000	-14 000
Total costs	0	-27 000	-27 000
A government's financial balance = tax revenue + government cost	14 000	-27 000	-41 000

We can now estimate the costs for Lyme disease treatment in the USA and Europe for the year 2018. We have previously estimated that the number of infections in the USA for 2018 is approximately 1 million. In Europe, that number is approximately 2.4 million. Let's assume that in the USA for 2018 the annual cost for oral antibiotics is 1400 USD and the annual cost for IV antibiotics is 15,000 USD. In Europe, the estimated annual cost for oral antibiotics is 1200 EUR and the annual cost for IV antibiotics is 13,000 EUR. Currently, the treatment cost for IV antibiotics for chronic Lyme disease are paid by the individual and not by the government or insurance companies. Note that the cost of IV treatment for chronic Lyme disease can be different in the USA and Europe because in the USA a peripherally inserted central catheter (PICC) is preferred while in Europe an IV drip is preferred. The cost for IV treatment in Europe could easily be twice as large because patients must travel a long way and stay at a hotel close to a specialized chronic Lyme disease clinic to get daily IV treatments with a butterfly needle. Sometimes people are even forced to sell their house to afford treatment. We assume that acute Lyme disease is treated with oral antibiotics for one month and that chronic Lyme disease is treated with IV antibiotics for six months or one year. Chronic Lyme disease can also be treated with oral antibiotics but then the patient runs the risk of having to take oral antibiotics for the rest of his/her life. I have therefore not calculated the cost of treating chronic Lyme with oral antibiotics since its more realistic to assume that all chronic Lyme patients want to treat with IV antibiotics because then they will at least have a chance of getting cured of their "chronic" infection. We can see in Tables 11 and 12 that the estimated treatment cost for Lyme disease for 2018 for the USA is somewhere between 4.8 billion USD and 9.6 billion USD and for Europe somewhere between 10.1 billion EUR and 20.1 billion EUR depending on the assumptions we make regarding the length of treatment with IV antibiotics (six months vs. one year). We can also see that the cost of treating acute Lyme disease with oral antibiotics for one month only represents 0.6% of the average treatment cost for IV antibiotics. The cost of treating acute Lyme disease with oral antibiotics is so small that it barely has an impact on total treatment costs.

Table 11. The estimated total cost for the treatment of acute and chronic Lyme disease for the USA for 2018.

Treatment costs for Lyme disease for the USA for 2018	Values		
Number of infections 2018 in the USA	1 011 278		
People infected with Lyme that develop chronic Lyme	0.63	%	
People infected with Lyme that develop acute infection	0.37	%	
The assumed annual cost of oral antibiotics is	1 400	USD	
The assumed annual cost of IV antibiotics is	15 000	USD	
The cost of treating acute Lyme disease with oral antibiotics for one month for the USA for 2018 (Oral USA 2018)	43 653 490	44	million USD
The cost of treating chronic Lyme disease with IV antibiotics for 0.5 years for the USA for 2018 (IV0.5 USA 2018)	4 778 287 467	4.8	billion USD
The cost of treating chronic Lyme disease with IV antibiotics for 1 year for the USA for 2018 (IV1 USA 2018)	9 556 574 934	9.6	billion USD
Total cost of treating acute with oral antibiotics for one month and chronic with IV antibiotics 0.5 years for the USA for 2018	4 821 940 958	4.8	billion USD
Total cost of treating acute with oral antibiotics for one month and chronic with IV antibiotics 1 year for the USA for 2018	9 600 228 425	9.6	billion USD
Oral USA 2018 / ((IV0.5 USA 2018 + IV1 USA 2018)/2)	0.6	%	

Table 12. The estimated total cost for the treatment of acute and chronic Lyme disease for Europe for 2018.

Treatment costs for Lyme disease for Europe for 2018	Values		
Number of infections 2018 in Europe	2 448 357		
People infected with Lyme that develop chronic Lyme	0.63	%	
People infected with Lyme that develop an acute infection	0.37	%	
The assumed annual cost of oral antibiotics is	1 200	EUR	
The assumed annual cost of IV antibiotics is	13 000	EUR	
The cost of treating acute Lyme disease with oral antibiotics for one month for Europe in 2018 (Oral Europe 2018)	90 589 198	91	million EUR
The cost of treating chronic Lyme disease with IV antibiotics for 0.5 years for Europe for 2018 (IV0.5 Europe 2018)	10 026 020 721	10.0	billion EUR
The cost of treating chronic Lyme disease with IV antibiotics for 1 year for Europe for 2018 (IV1 Europe 2018)	20 052 041 441	20.1	billion EUR
Total cost of treating acute with oral antibiotics for one month and chronic with IV antibiotics 0.5 years for Europe in 2018	10 116 609 919	10.1	billion EUR
Total cost of treating acute with oral antibiotics for one month and chronic with IV antibiotics 1 year for Europe in 2018	20 142 630 639	20.1	billion EUR
Oral Europe 2018 / ((IV0.5 Europe 2018 + IV1 Europe 2018)/2)	0.6	%	

We have so far only looked at treatment cost. Many people are forced to leave their jobs due to the infection. So, the cost of lost personal income is also high. According to one study, approximately 42% of chronic Lyme disease patients cannot work [132]. I believe that the number is even higher but 42% is reasonable enough. The financial cost for both the individual (lost earnings from not working due to chronic Lyme disease) and for the government (lost tax revenues because chronic Lyme patients are not working and disability benefits for chronic Lyme disease patients) are therefore significant. We can now calculate the government cost for chronic Lyme disease for the USA and Europe for 2018 if governments do not finance treatment. According to the Organisation for Economic Co-Operation and Development (OECD) the average annual wage rate before tax for 2016 for the USA was 60 154 USD and for Germany 38,302 EUR [133]. The average annual wage rate in Germany represents the average annual wage rate for Europe. The global accounting firm KPMG states that the income tax rate for 2016 for the USA is 39.6% and for Germany 45% [134]. A website called disabilitysecrets.com [135] claims that the average monthly Social Security Disability Insurance (SSDI) payment after tax for the USA for 2017 is 1171 USD which means that the average annual disability benefit after tax for the USA for 2017 is 14,052 USD. This amount is on par with the lowest monthly disability payment after taxed paid in Sweden which is 11,000 Swedish kroner [136] which means that the minimum annual disability benefit after tax for Sweden is 132,000 Swedish kroner which as of October 2017 is approximately 13,778 EUR. We will use the monthly Swedish disability payment to represent the disability payment in Europe.

We can see in Tables 13 and 14 that the estimated lost personal income for chronic Lyme patients that are not working for 2018 for the USA is 16.1 billion USD and in Europe 24.8 billion EUR. If the governments in the USA and Europe do not finance IV treatment with antibiotics for chronic Lyme disease, then the estimated government costs for chronic Lyme disease (lost tax revenues because some chronic Lyme patients are not working plus disability benefits for chronic Lyme patients that not working) for 2018 for the USA is 10.1 billion USD and for Europe 20.1 billion EUR. We can also see that the government cost for chronic Lyme disease for 2018 (which does not include treatment costs) in the USA is 2.1 times larger than the cost for 6 months of IV treatment with antibiotics in the USA for 2018 and 1.1 times larger than the cost for 1 year of IV treatment with antibiotics in the USA for 2018. In Europe, the government cost for chronic Lyme disease for 2018 is two times larger than the cost for six months of IV treatment in Europe for 2018 and the government cost is on par with the cost for one year of IV treatment in Europe for 2018.

Table 13. Government cost for chronic Lyme disease for the USA for 2018 if governments do not finance IV treatment with antibiotics for chronic Lyme disease.

Government costs for chronic Lyme disease for the USA for 2018 if the government does not finance IV treatment for chronic Lyme disease			
	Values		
Number of Lyme disease infections 2018 in the USA	1 011 278		
People infected with Borrelia that develop chronic Lyme	0.63	%	
Number of chronic infections in the USA for 2018	637 105		
% of chronic Lyme patients that does not work	0.42	%	
% of chronic Lyme patients that does work	0.58		
Average annual income from work before tax for the USA for 2016	60 154	USD	
Income tax rate for the USA for 2016	0.396	%	
Average annual disability benefits after tax for the USA for 2017	14 052	USD	
Lost personal income for chronic Lyme patients not working in the USA for 2018	16 096 253 841	16.1	billion USD
Lost tax revenues because chronic Lyme patients are not working in the USA in 2018 (LTR USA 2018)	6 374 116 521	6.4	billion USD
Disability benefits for chronic Lyme patients for the USA for 2018 (DB USA 2018)	3 760 091 747	3.8	billion USD
Government cost for chronic Lyme disease for the USA in 2018 (GCL USA 2018) = LTR USA 2018 + DB USA 2018	10 134 208 268	10.1	billion USD
GCL USA 2018 / IV0.5 USA 2018	2.1		
GCL USA 2018 / IV1 USA 2018	1.1		

Table 14. Government cost for chronic Lyme disease for Europe for 2018 if governments do not finance IV treatment with antibiotics for chronic Lyme disease.

Government costs for chronic Lyme disease for Europe for 2018 if the governments do not finance IV treatment for chronic Lyme disease			
	Values		
Number of infections 2018 in Europe	2 448 357		
People infected with Borrelia that develop chronic Lyme	0.63	%	
Number of chronic infections in Europe for 2018	1 542 465	%	
People that cannot work due to chronic Lyme	0.42	%	
Average annual income from work before tax for Germany for 2016	38 302	EUR	
Income tax rate for Germany for 2016	0.45	%	
The minimum annual disability benefits after tax in Sweden for 2016 is 11 000 Swedish kroner	13 778	EUR	
Lost personal income for chronic Lyme patients not working in Europe in 2018	24 813 383 257	24.8	billion EUR
Lost tax revenues because chronic Lyme patients are not working in Europe for 2018 (LTR Europe 2018)	11 166 022 466	11.2	billion EUR
Disability benefits for chronic Lyme patients in Europe for 2018 (DB Europe 2018)	8 925 976 833	8.9	billion EUR
Government cost for chronic Lyme disease for Europe for 2018 (GCL Europe 2018) = LTR Europe 2018 + DB Europe 2018	20 091 999 298	20.1	billion EUR
GCL Europe 2018 / IV0.5 Europe 2018	2.0		
GCL Europe 2018 / IV1 Europe 2018	1.0		

Today's and future government revenues and costs for chronic Lyme disease are however much more important to look at than historical annual cost. We will again treat the cure rate for IV antibiotics for chronic Lyme disease as an unknown. We will calculate variables for five different scenarios: A cure rate of 0%, a cure rate 25%, a cure rate of 50%, a cure rate of 75% and a cure rate of 100%. The number of chronic Lyme patients that are cured with treatment/not cured with treatment and are working/not working can be seen in Table 15.

Table 15. The work/not work/cured/not cured matrix.

The number of Lyme disease infections per year	n	100 000
% of people that develops a chronic infection	%ch	63
The number of chronic infections (nn)	n * (%ch/100)	63 000
% of chronic Lyme patients that work	w	58
% of chronic Lyme patients that do not work	nw	42

% cure rate (cr)	Cured from treatment	Not cured from treatment	Sum
Number of people	C = nn * (cr/100)	NC = nn - C	C + NC
Number of people that are working	C * 1	NC * (w / 100)	C * 1 + NC * (w / 100)
Number of people that are not working	C * 0	NC * (nw / 100)	C * 0 + NC * (nw / 100)
Sum	C*1 + C*0	NC * (w / 100) + NC * (nw / 100)	C * 1 + NC * (w / 100) + C * 0 + NC * (nw / 100)

0	Cured from treatment	Not cured from treatment	Sum
Number of people	0	63 000	63 000
Number of people that are working	0	36 540	36 540
Number of people that are not working	0	26 460	26 460
Sum	0	63 000	63 000

25	Cured from treatment	Not cured from treatment	Sum
Number of people	15 750	47 250	63 000
Number of people that are working	15 750	27 405	43 155
Number of people that are not working	0	19 845	19 845
Sum	15 750	47 250	63 000

50	Cured from treatment	Not cured from treatment	Sum
Number of people	31 500	31 500	63 000
Number of people that are working	31 500	18 270	49 770
Number of people that are not working	0	13 230	13 230
Sum	31 500	31 500	63 000

75	Cured from treatment	Not cured from treatment	Sum
Number of people	47 250	15 750	63 000
Number of people that are working	47 250	9 135	56 385
Number of people that are not working	0	6 615	6 615
Sum	47 250	15 750	63 000

100	Cured from treatment	Not cured from treatment	Sum
Number of people	63 000	0	63 000
Number of people that are working	63 000	0	63 000
Number of people that are not working	0	0	0
Sum	63 000	0	63 000

Number of people that are working and not cured from treatment can also be calculated as:
nn * (w / 100) * (1 - cr / 100)
Number of people that are not working and not cured from treatment can also be calculated as:
nn * (nw / 100) * (1 - cr / 100)

Cure rate in %	Number of people that are working and not cured from treatment	Number of people that are not working and not cured from treatment
0	36 540	26 460
25	27 405	19 845
50	18 270	13 230
75	9 135	6 615
100	0	0

Now we need to answer the important question: should a government pay for IV treatment for chronic Lyme disease? From a purely economic and financial perspective which excludes any ethical aspect of not offering antibiotics treatment to patients that suffer from a bacterial infection that can lead to death a government should finance treatment with IV antibiotics for chronic Lyme disease if

Future government revenues [treatment] + future government cost [treatment] + treatment cost

> future government revenues [no treatment] + future government cost [no treatment]

where government revenues are positive values and government costs are negative values. Such governments' financial chronic Lyme disease balance sheet is presented in Table 16.

Table 16. A government's financial chronic Lyme disease balance sheet.

A government's Financial Balance	Today		Future	
	If the Government Finance IV Treatment	If the Government Does not Finance IV Treatment	If the Government Finance IV Treatment	If the Government Does not Finance IV Treatment
A government's chronic Lyme disease revenue (+)	x1 = tax revenues from chronic Lyme patients that are cured from treatment and are working	x5 = 0	x11 = future tax revenues from chronic Lyme patients that are cured from treatment and are working	x55 = 0
A government's chronic Lyme disease revenue (+)	x2 = saved disability benefits for chronic Lyme patients that are cured from treatment and are working	x6 = 0	x22 = saved future disability benefits for chronic Lyme patients that are cured from treatment and are working	x66 = 0
A government's chronic Lyme disease cost (-)	- X3 = lost tax revenues for chronic Lyme patients that are still sick after treatment and are not working	- x7 = lost tax revenues from chronic Lyme patients that are sick and have not received treatment and are not working	- x33 = lost future tax revenues for chronic Lyme patients that are still sick after treatment and are not working	- x77 = lost future tax revenues from chronic Lyme patients that are sick and have not received treatment and are not working
A government's chronic Lyme disease cost (-)	- x4 = disability payments to chronic Lyme patients that are still sick after treatment and are not working	- x8 = disability payments to chronic Lyme patients that are sick and have not received treatment and are not working	- x44 = future disability payments to chronic Lyme patients that are still sick after treatment and are not working	- x88 = future disability payments to chronic Lyme patients that are sick and have not received treatment and are not working
Treatment cost for 0.5 year of IV antibiotics (-)	- IV0.5			
Treatment cost for 1 year of IV antibiotics (-)	- IV1			
A government's revenues because of treatment	x1 + x2		x11 + x22	
A government's costs for chronic Lyme disease with IV 0.5 year	x3 + x4 + IV0.5		x33 + x44 + IV0.5	
A government's cost for chronic Lyme disease with IV 1 year	x3 + x4 + IV1		X33 + X44 + IV1	
A government's cost without treatment (-)		x7 + x8		x77 + x88
A government's financial balance based on today's revenues and costs for 0.5 year of IV treatment (GBTiv0.5)	x1 + x2 + x3 + x4 + IV0.5 - x7 - x8		A government's financial balance based on future revenues and costs for 0.5 year of IV treatment (GBFiv0.5)	x11 + x22 + x33 + x44 + IV0.5 - x77 - x88
A government's financial balance based on today's revenues and costs for 1 year of IV treatment (GBTiv1)	x1 + x2 + x3 + x4 + IV1 - x7 - x8		A government's financial balance based on future revenues and costs for 1 year of IV treatment (GBFiv1)	x11 + x22 + x33 + x44 + IV1 - x77 - x88

To justify IV treatment for 0.5 years
x11 + x22 + x33 + x44 + IV0.5 > x55 + x66 + x77 + x88
x11 + x22 + x33 + x44 + IV0.5 - (x55 + x66 + x77 + x88) > 0
GBFiv0.5 = x11 + x22 + x33 + x44 + IV0.5 - x77 - x88 > 0
To justify IV treatment for 1 year
x11 + x22 + x33 + x44 + IV1 > x55 + x66 + x77 + x88
x11 + x22 + x33 + x44 + IV1 - (x55 + x66 + x77 + x88) > 0
GBFiv1 = x11 + x22 + x33 + x44 + IV1 - x77 - x88 > 0

Note also that the previous equation become less reliable over time. The closer we get to our endpoint which is 2050 the less impact the future government revenues and future government expenditures will have on a government's financial balance. Note that tax revenues from chronic Lyme patients that are not cured with treatment and working, saved disability benefits from chronic Lyme patients that are not cured with treatment and working, tax revenues from chronic Lyme patients that are sick and have not received treatment and are working and saved disability benefits from chronic Lyme patients that are sick and have not received treatment and are working are not included in the above government financial chronic Lyme disease balance sheet because they will be the same regardless of if the government choose to treat or not. The government's purely financial treatment decision regarding chronic Lyme disease is further illustrated in Table 17.

Table 17. A government's financial IV treatment decision regarding chronic Lyme disease.

1 = If the government finance IV treatment						
2 = If the government does not finance IV treatment						
3 = is GBFT > GBFnT ?						
4 = GBFT - GBFnT						
5 = is GFBBT - GFBnT > 0 ?						
6 = Should a government finance treatment with IV antibiotics?						
	1	2	3	4	5	6
A government's future chronic Lyme disease revenues	GFR	GFRnT				
A government's future chronic Lyme disease costs	- GFC	- GFCnT				
Treatment cost today for IV antibiotics	- TCT	na				
A government's balance based on future government revenues and costs	GBFT = GFR + GFC + TCT	GBFnT = GFRnT + GFCnT				
A government's future chronic Lyme disease revenues	200	0				
A government's future chronic Lyme disease costs	-200	-100				
Treatment cost today for IV antibiotics	-500	na				
A government's balance based on future government revenues and costs	-500	-100	no	-400	no	no
A government's future chronic Lyme disease revenues	200	0				
A government's future chronic Lyme disease costs	-200	-200				
Treatment cost today for IV antibiotics	-300	na				
A government's balance based on future government revenues and costs	-300	-200	no	-100	no	no
A government's future chronic Lyme disease revenues	500	0				
A government's future chronic Lyme disease costs	-300	-200				
Treatment cost today for IV antibiotics	-200	na				
A government's balance based on future government revenues and costs	0	-200	yes	200	yes	yes
A government's future chronic Lyme disease revenues	600	0				
A government's future chronic Lyme disease costs	-400	-500				
Treatment cost today for IV antibiotics	-100	na				
A government's balance based on future government revenues and costs	100	-500	yes	600	yes	yes

We now again assume that the annual growth rate of the infection is 2% per year, the annual population growth rate in the USA is assumed to be 1% and the annual population growth rate in Europe is assumed to be 0.2%. We assume that we treat all chronic Lyme patients with IV antibiotics for either six months or one year and we again look at the value for different variables for five different cure rates 0%, 25%, 50%, 75% and 100%. All charts in this section and more can be found in the Excel file "Lyme disease calculations.xlsx" There will be only four individual group captions in this section: today's government costs and revenues in the USA over time, future government costs and revenues in the USA over time, today's government costs and revenues in Europe over time and future government costs and revenues in Europe over time. There is no point in including a caption for each chart when the same text can be found in the chart's legend. We can see in Figure 19 that the US government's financial balance based on today's cost and revenues for antibiotic IV treatment for 6 months for chronic Lyme disease GBTiv0.5 is positive for an assumed cure rate of 25% and above and for 1 year of IV treatment with antibiotics GBTiv1 is positive for an assumed cure rate of 50% and above. We can see in Figure 20 that the US government's financial balance based on future cost and revenues for antibiotic IV treatment for 6 months for chronic Lyme disease GBFiv0.5 is positive for an assumed cure rate of 25% and above and for 1 year of IV treatment GBFiv1 is also positive for an assumed cure rate of 25% and above. We can see in Figure 21 that the European governments' financial balance based on today's cost and revenues for antibiotic IV treatment for 6 months for chronic Lyme disease GBTiv0.5 is positive for an assumed cure rate of 25% and above and for 1 year of IV treatment with antibiotic GBTiv1 is positive for an assumed cure rate of 50% and above. We can see in Figure 22 that the European governments' financial balance based on future cost and revenues for IV antibiotic treatment for 6 months for chronic Lyme disease GBFiv0.5 is positive for an assumed cure rate of 25% and above and for 1 year of IV antibiotic treatment GBFiv1 is also positive for an assumed cure rate of 25% and above.

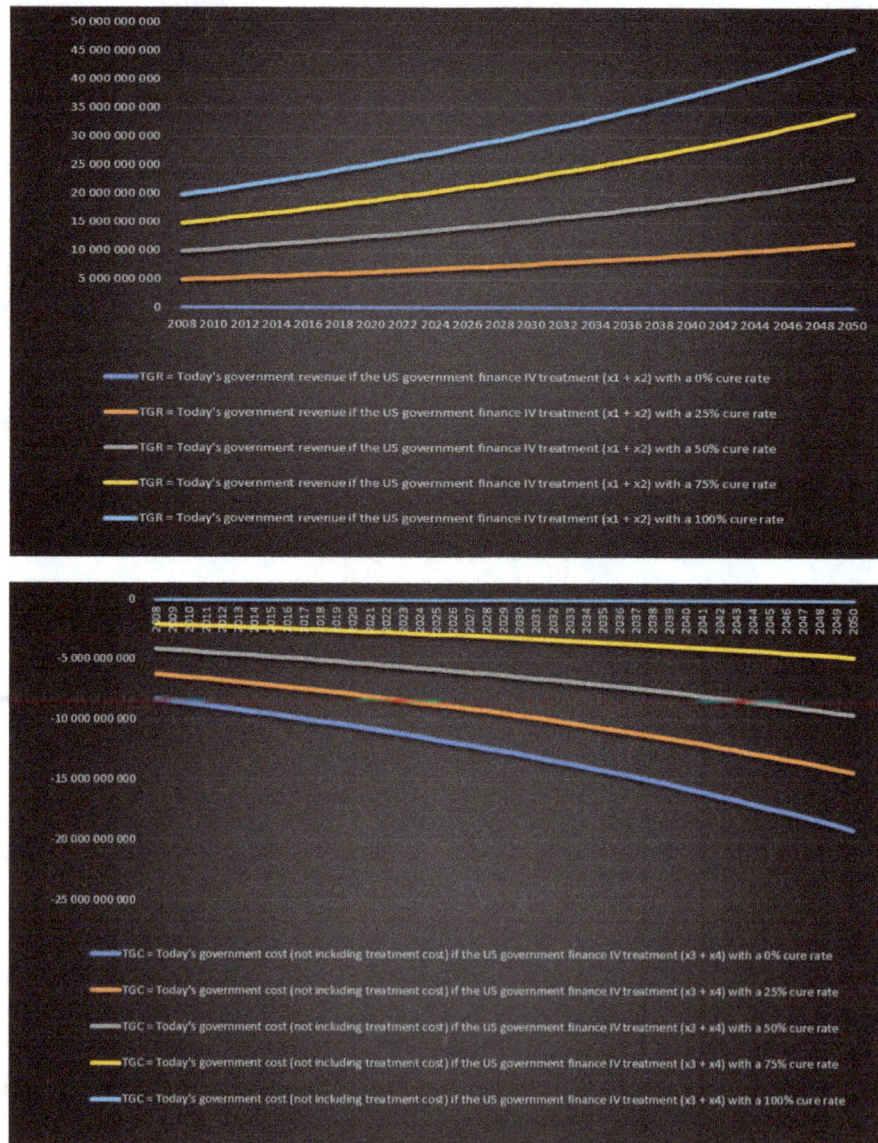

Figure 19. *Cont.*

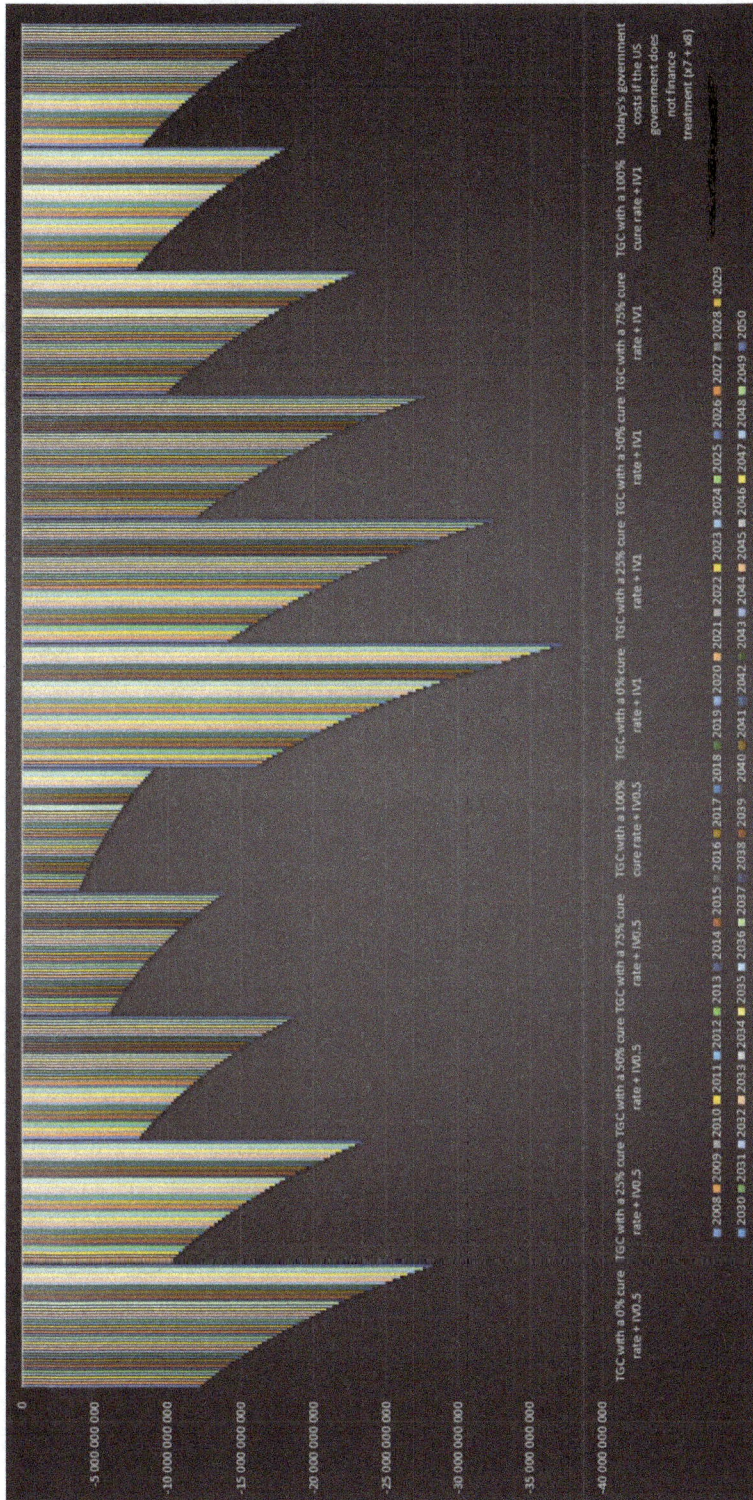

Figure 19. *Cont.*

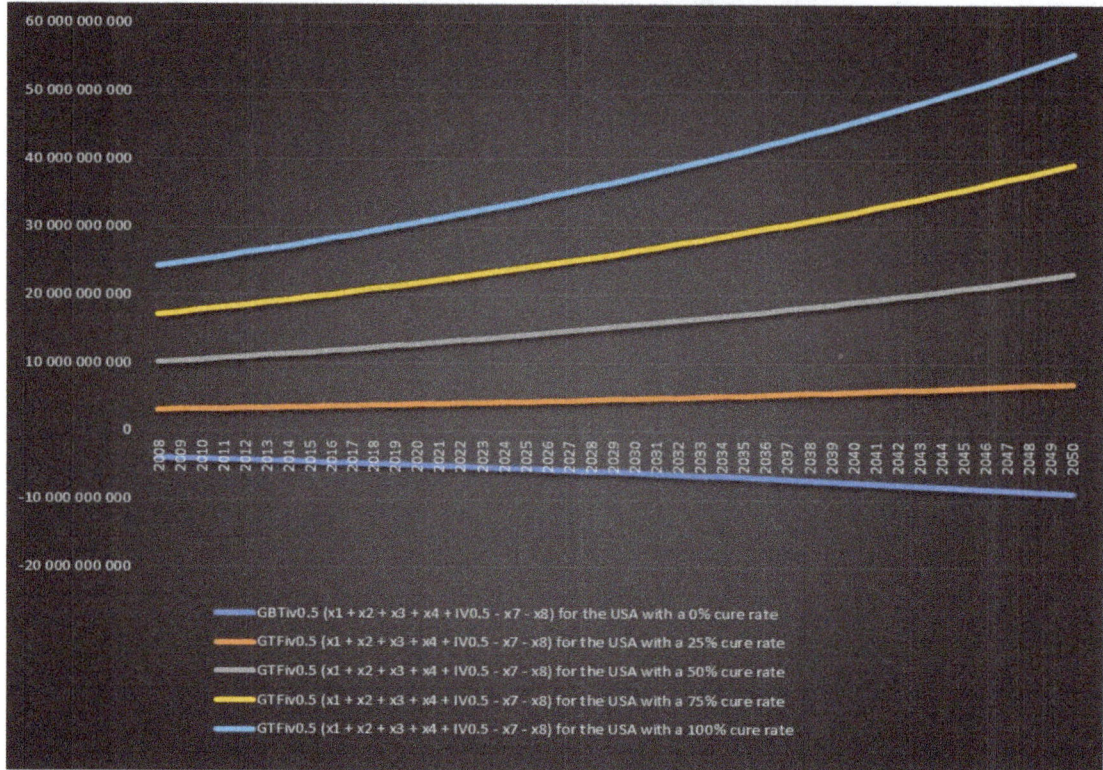

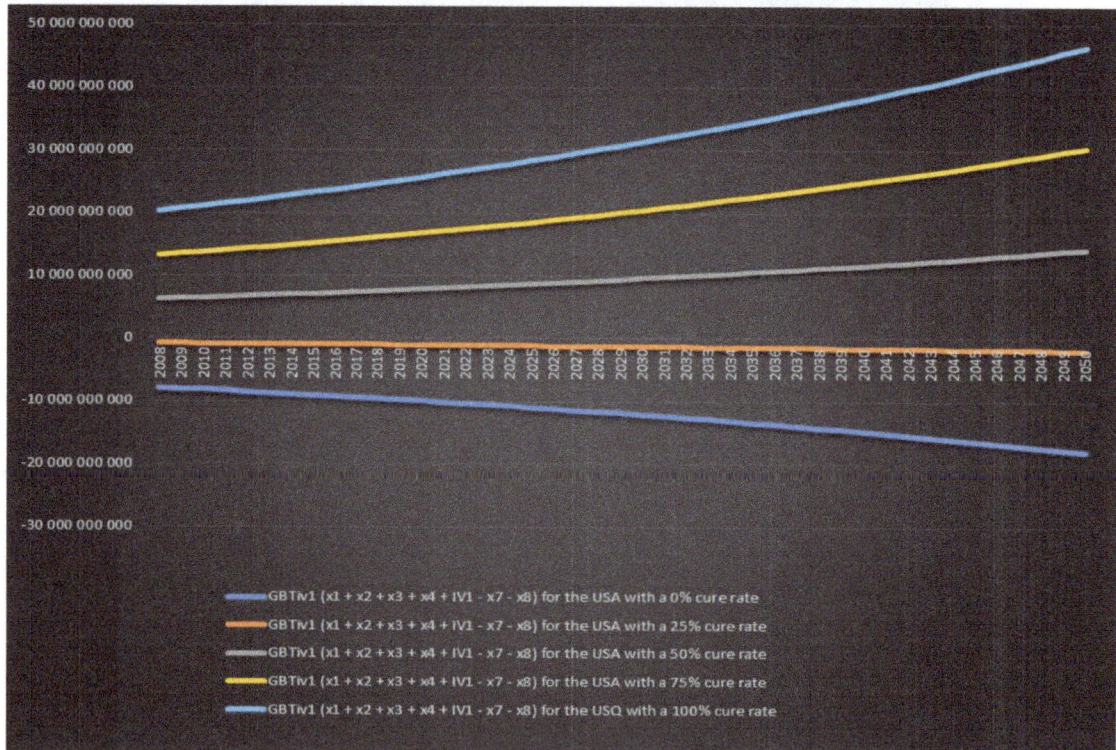

Figure 19. Today's government costs and revenues in the USA over time.

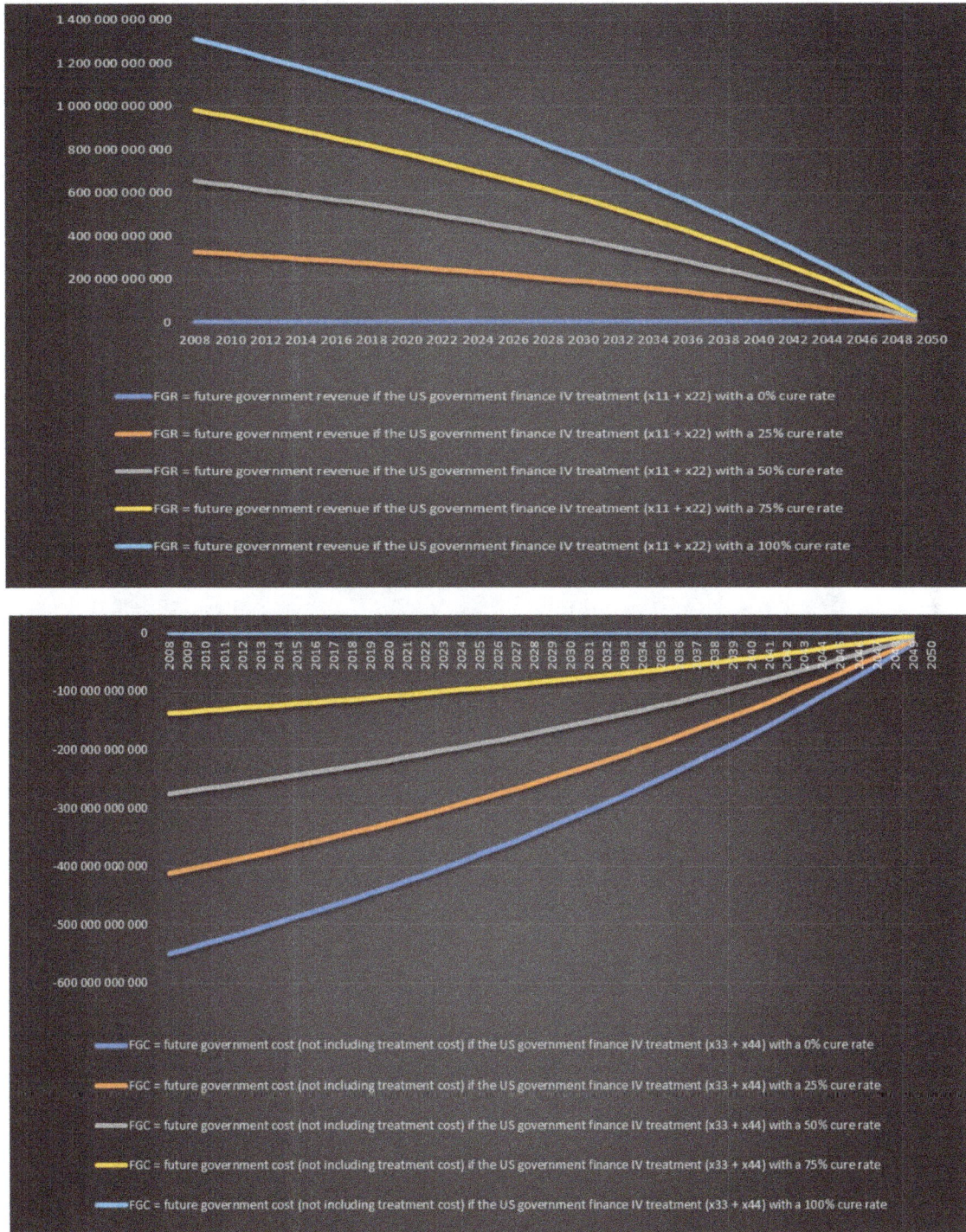

Figure 20. *Cont.*

Figure 20. *Cont.*

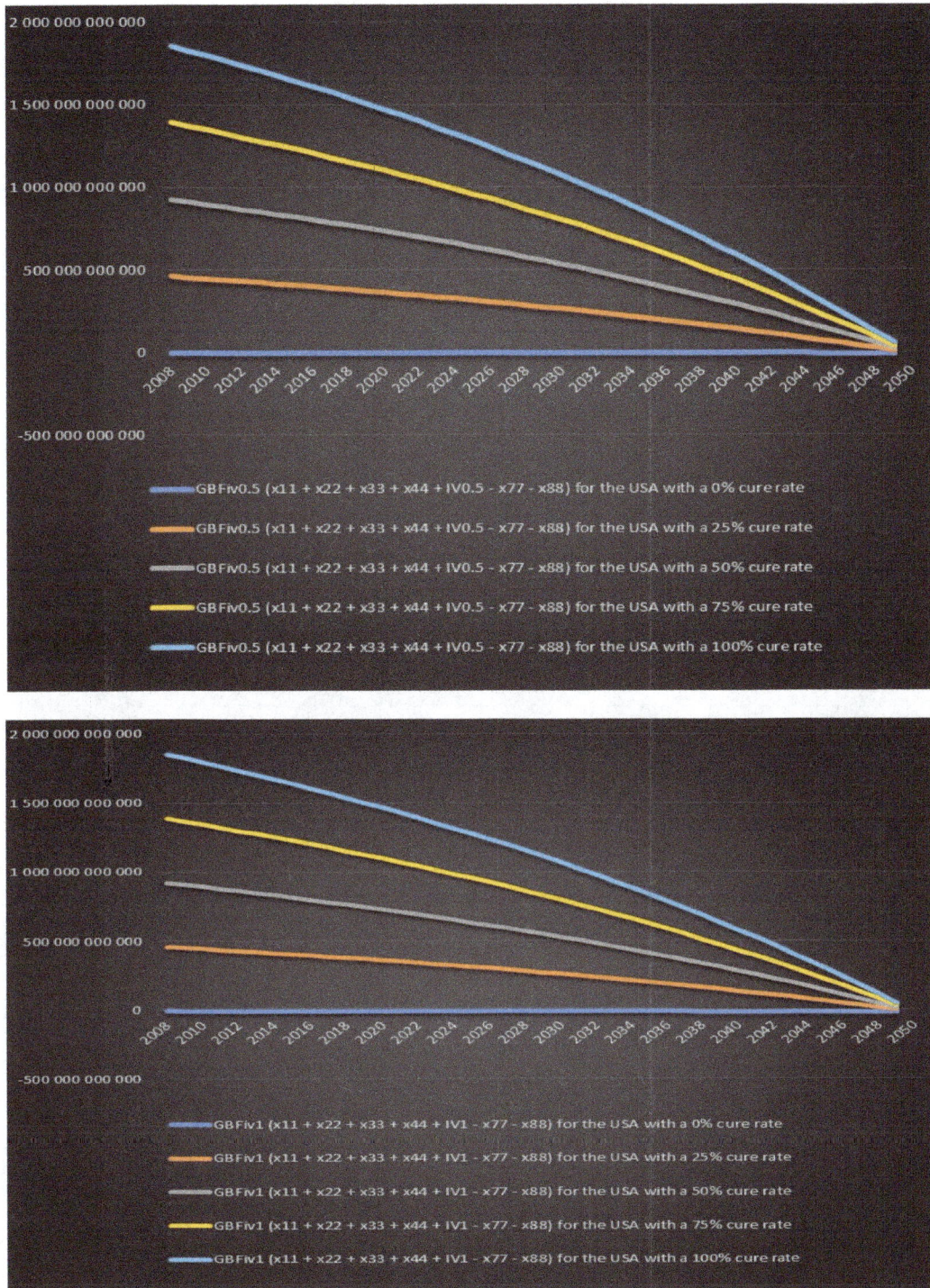

Figure 20. Future government costs and revenues in the USA over time.

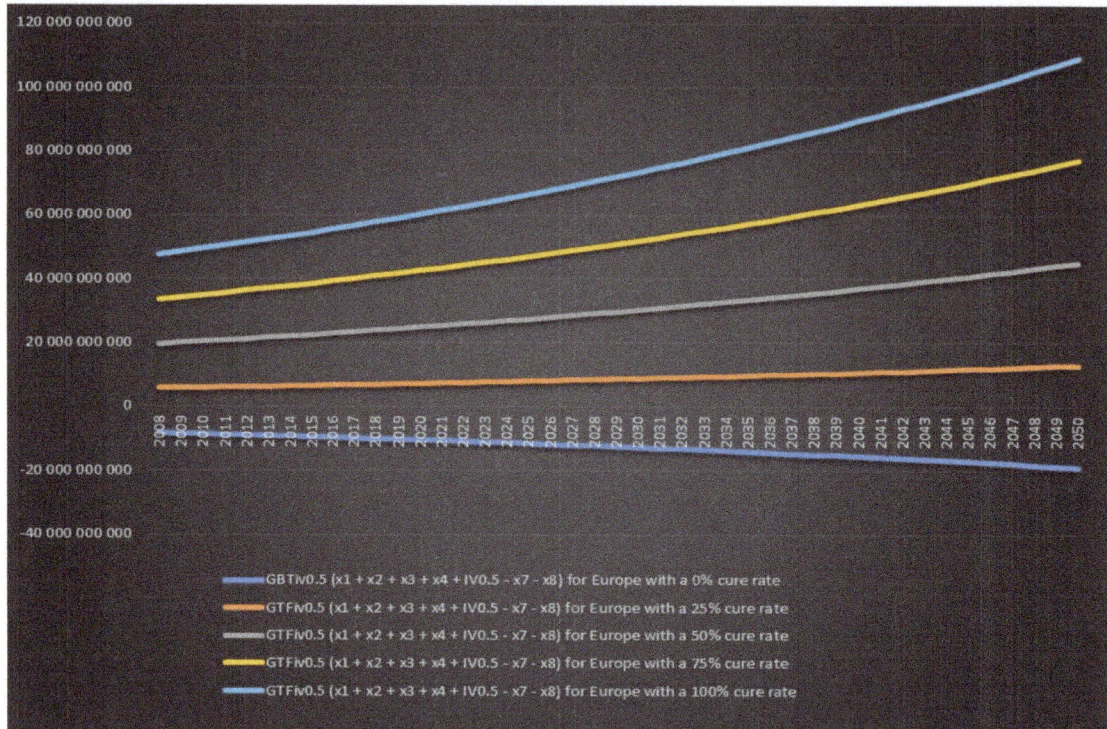

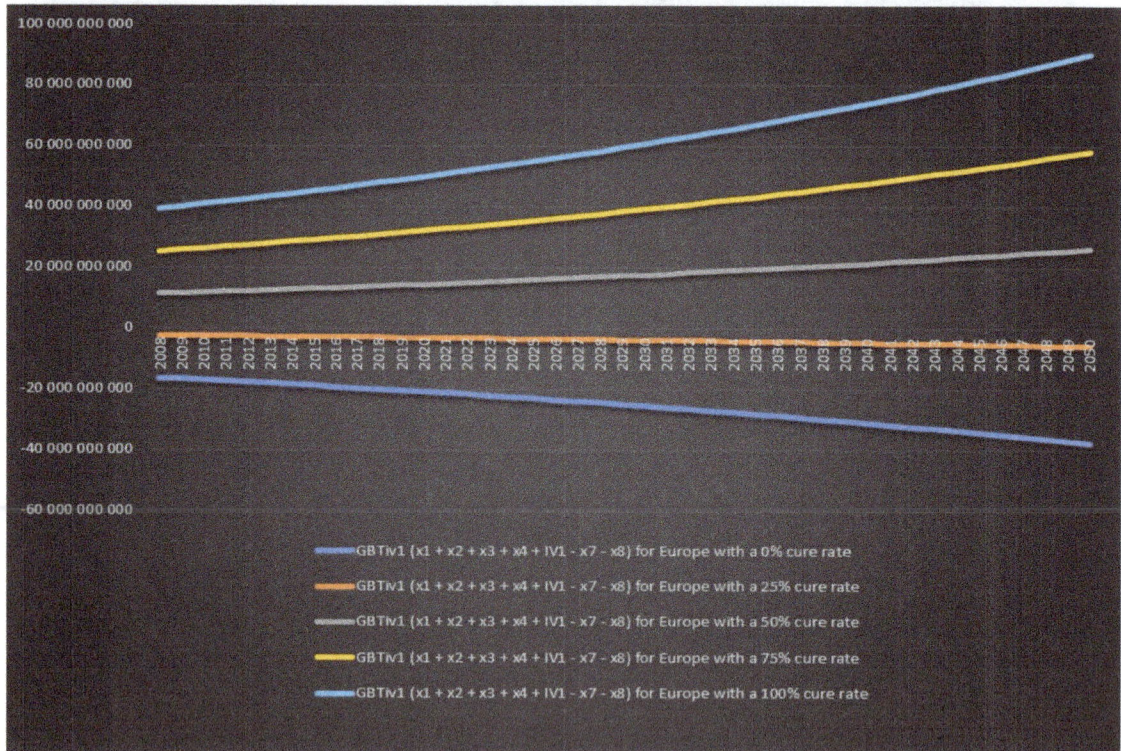

Figure 21. *Cont.*

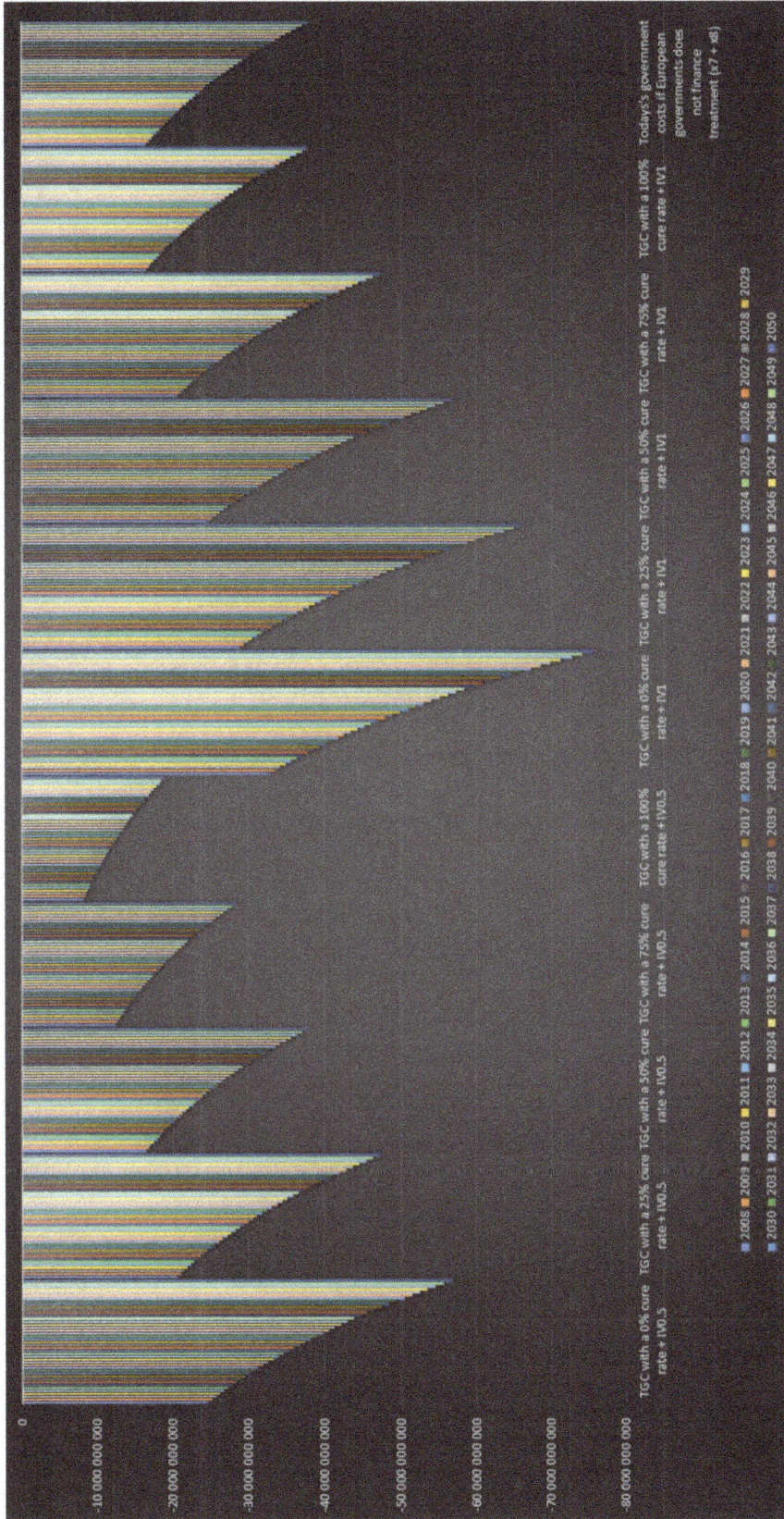

Figure 21. *Cont.*

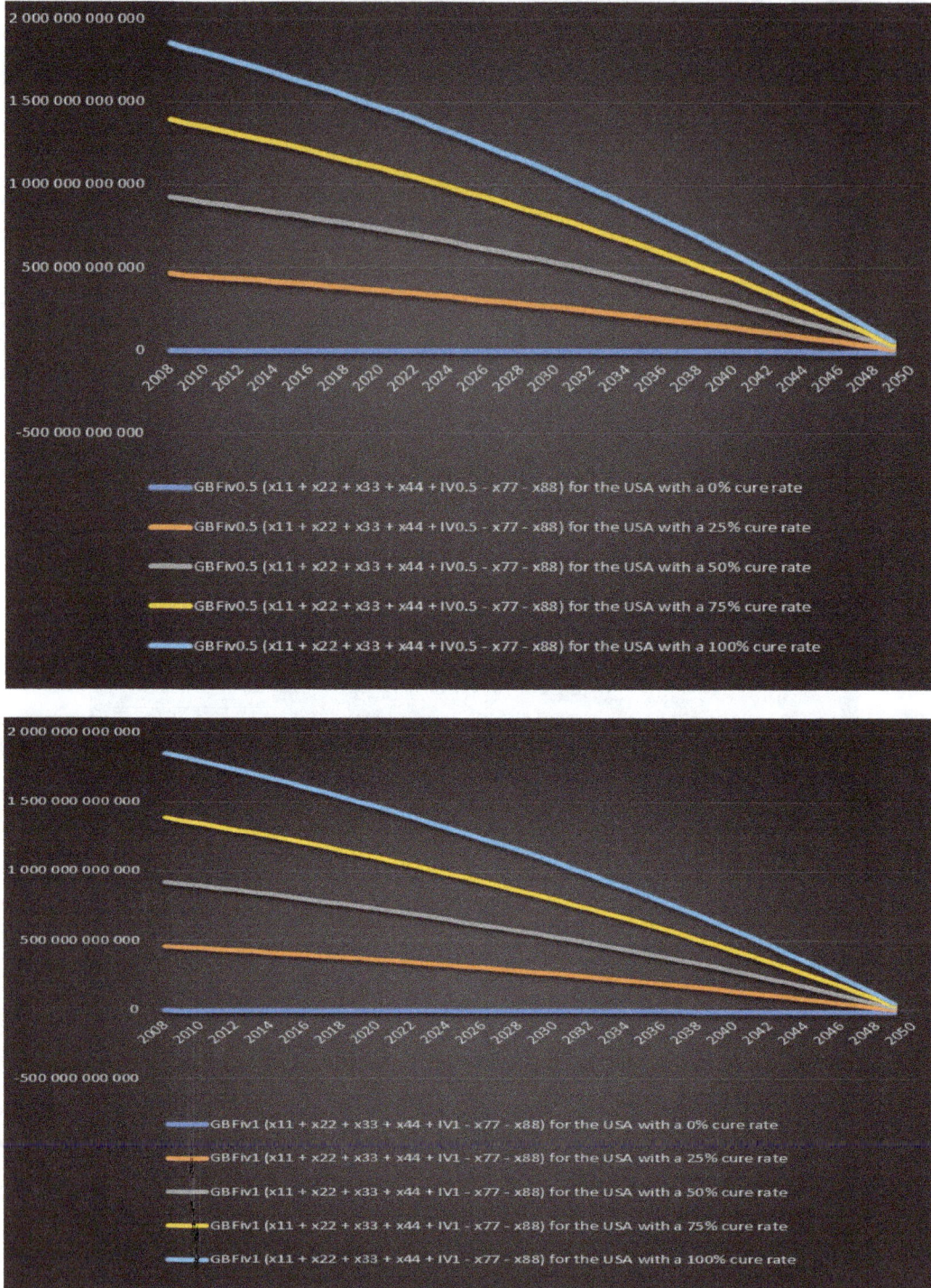

Figure 21. Today's government costs and revenues in Europe over time.

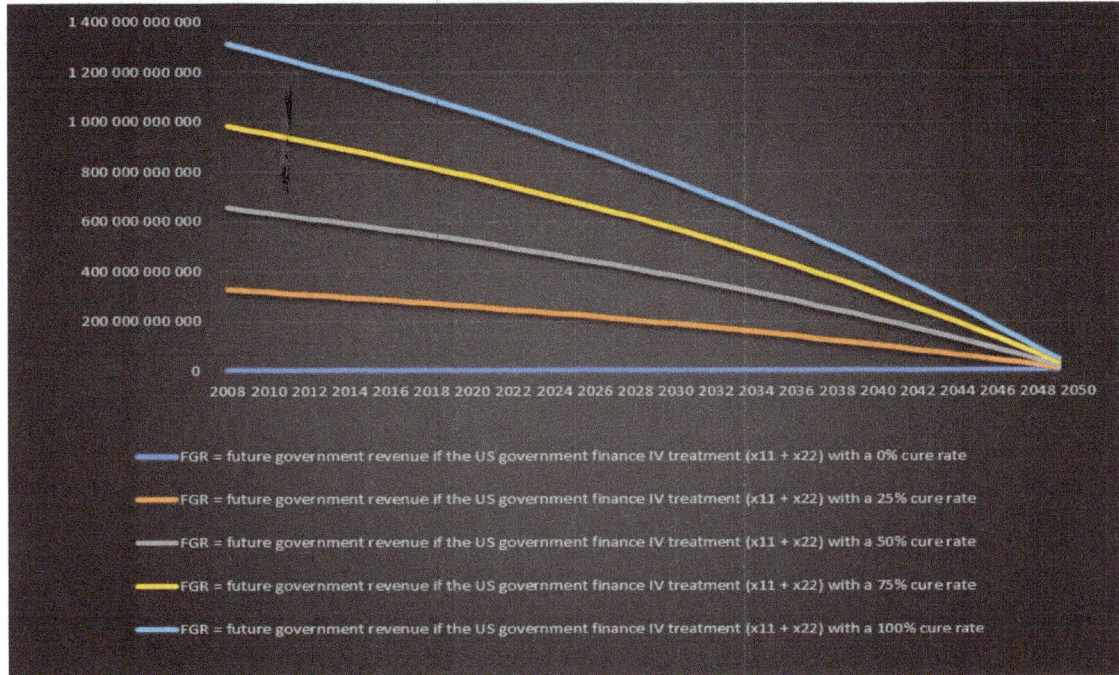

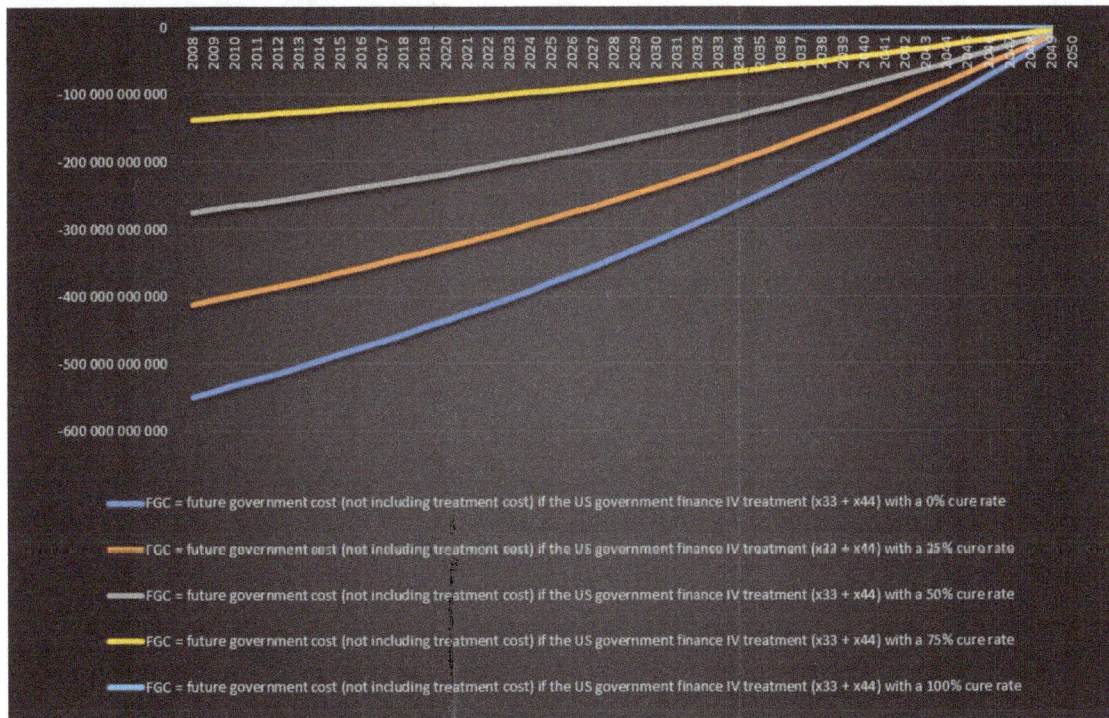

Figure 22. *Cont.*

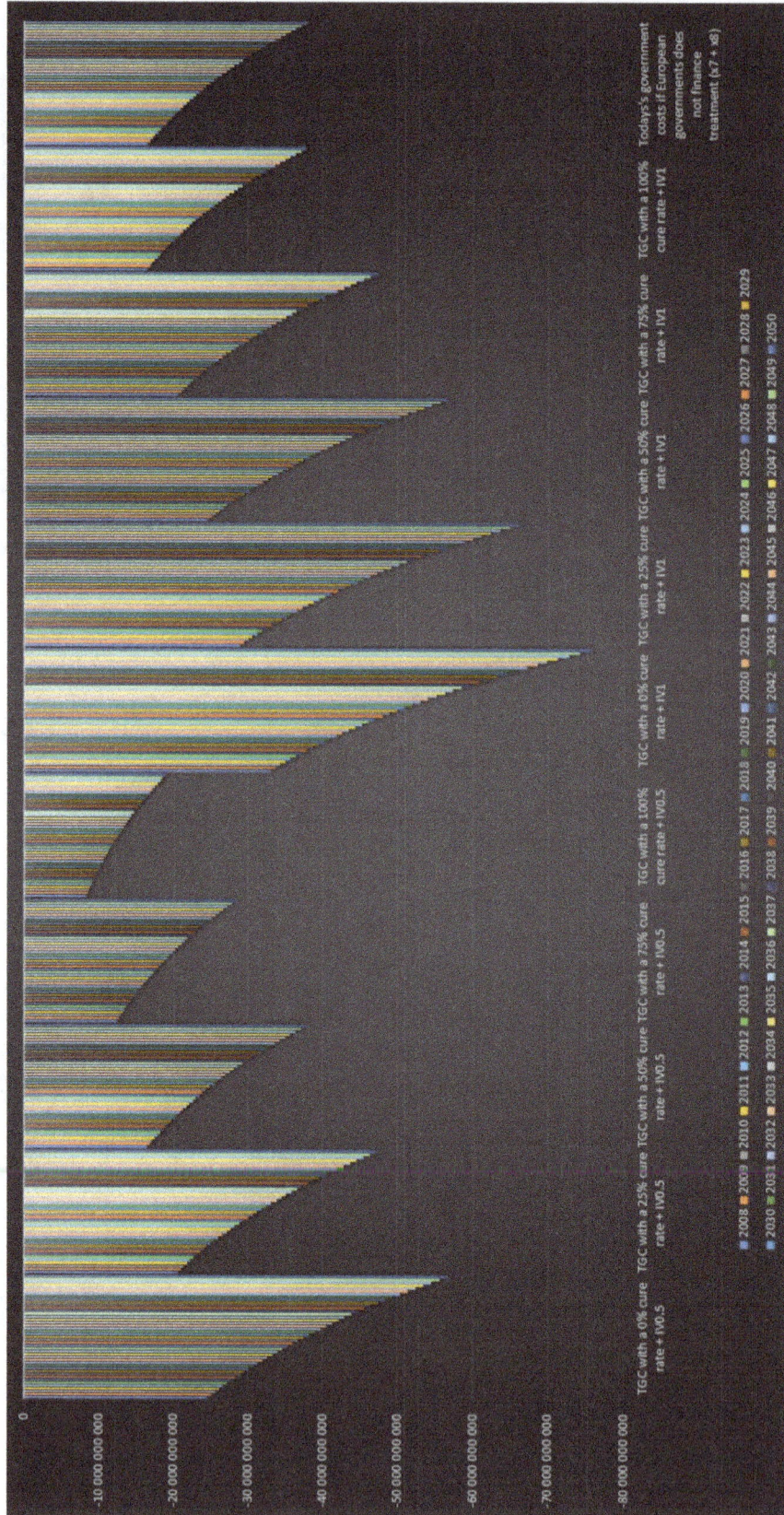

Figure 22. *Cont.*

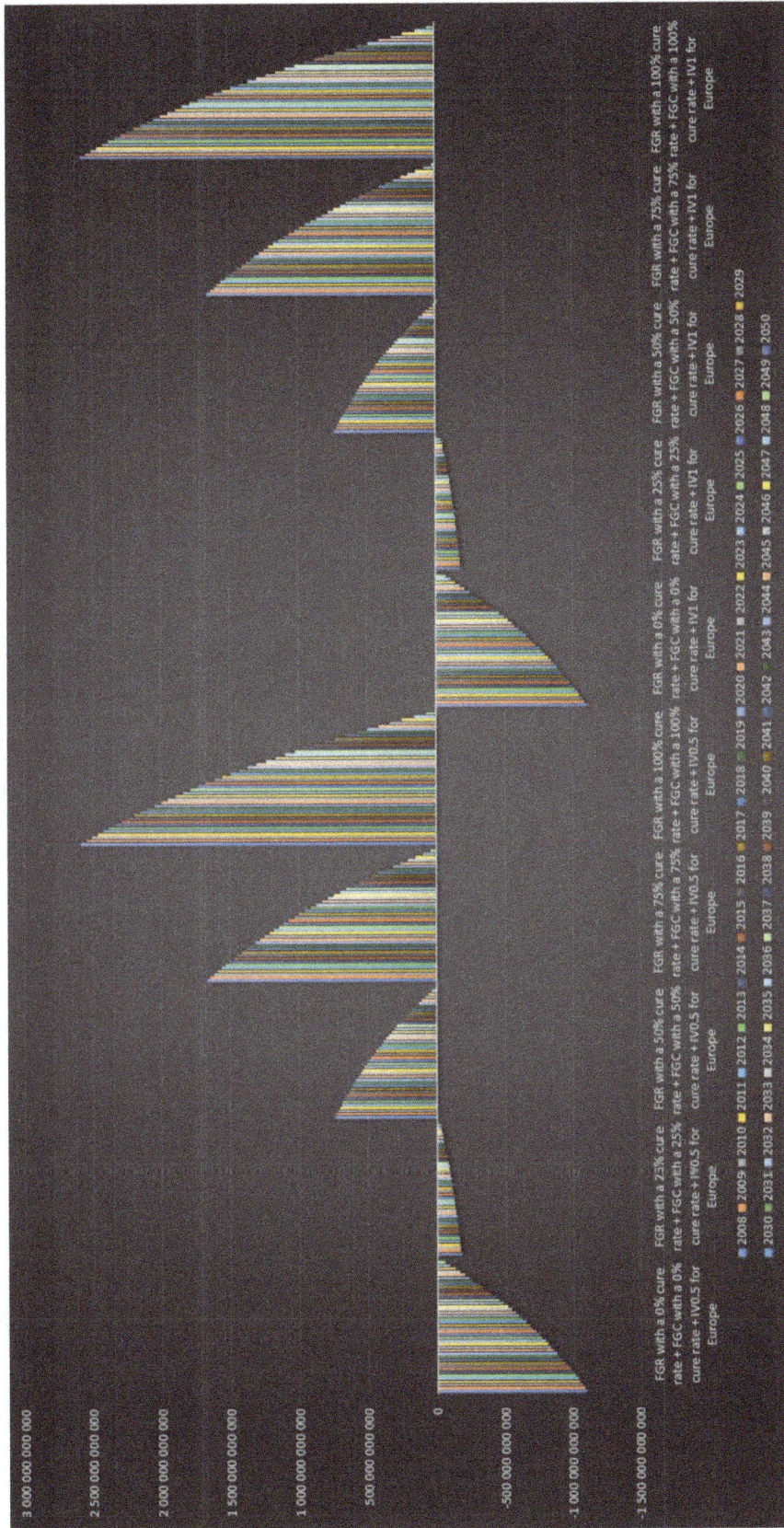

Figure 22. *Cont.*

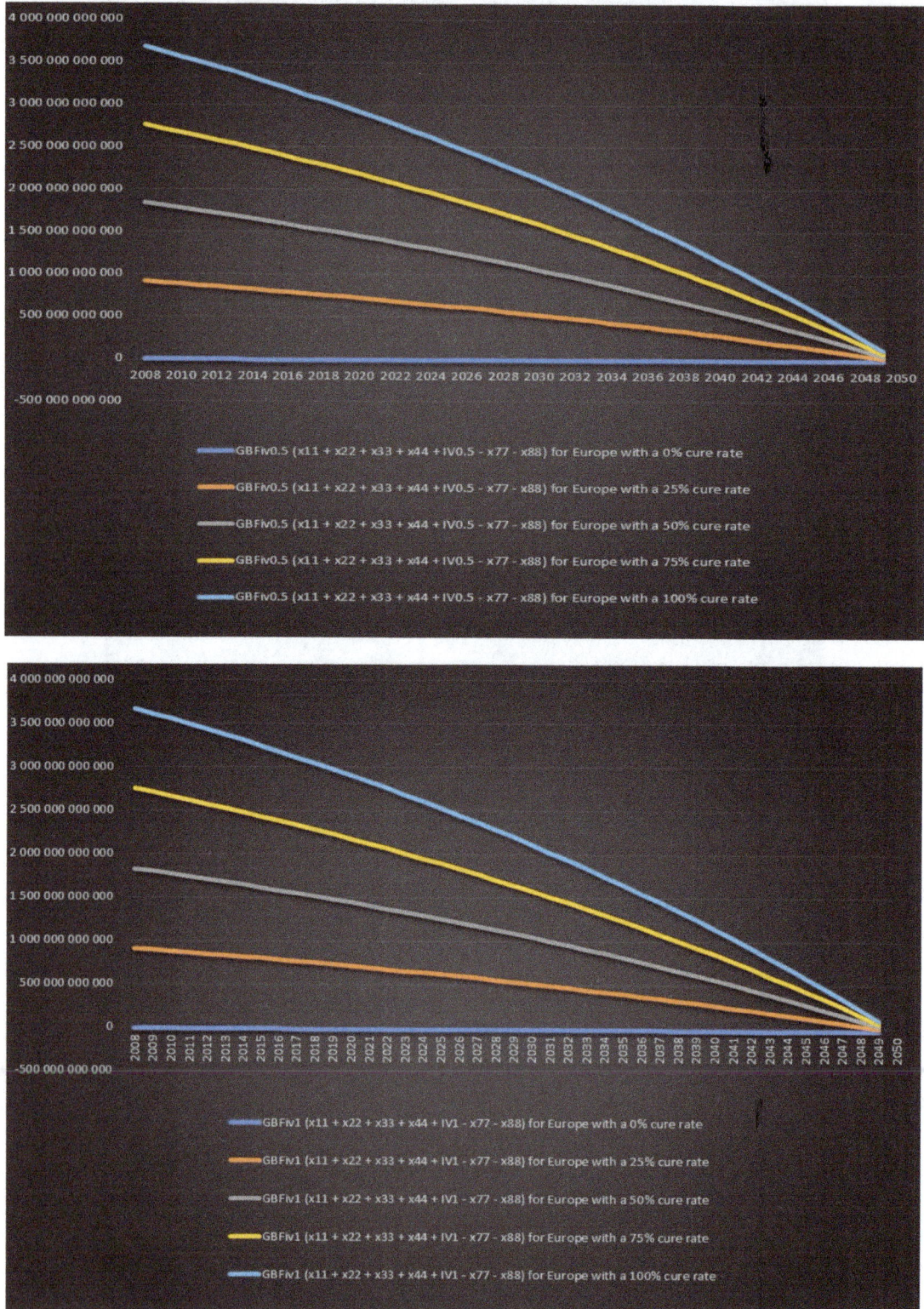

Figure 22. Future government costs and revenues in Europe over time.

4. Discussion

Independent and objective peer review is a critical component for scientific publication because of two main reasons. (1) It makes sure that only high-quality papers are published which is critical for the credibility of a scientific journal and science in general. (2) It leads to decentralization of power which is also critical for the credibility of a scientific journal and science in general. When the CDC publishes its research on Lyme disease in a private special interest group's "scientific" journal such as *Clinical Infectious Diseases* which is issued by the IDSA the probability that the paper will receive independent and objective peer review is close to zero. *The Journal of Infectious Diseases*, *Clinical Infectious Diseases and Open Forum Infectious Diseases* are all "scientific" journals published by the IDSA. Scientific publication is not democratic in a sense that everyone (including people without subject knowledge) can vote and where the majority decides which papers are published. Such undemocratic nature of science is a strength, but it can also sometimes be a weakness. Medicine is based on science, but medicine also has patients. Patients are the only ones that will be affected by a physician's decision. It is therefore not unrealistic to expect that patients can influence decision making regarding their diagnosis and treatment. Unfortunately, today medical doctors, journal editors that desk reject papers, politicians, journalists and governments are experts when it comes to centralized decision-making. It also appears that medicine and medical science today has become politicized where personal and subjective opinions govern. Government health agencies have not done an objective review of the scientific literature regarding chronic Lyme disease. There exist at least five reasons for this. (1) Governments' treatment guidelines or research on Lyme disease have not been published in high quality international scientific journals which means that such publications have not been subject to objective and independent peer review which is very unscientific. (2) Infectious disease doctors (in the USA IDSA) and government health agencies (in the USA CDC) have previously or are possibly still colluding and IDSA is colluding with insurance companies in the USA. (3) The treatment guideline panels with doctors have not been sufficiently diversified because ILADS doctors have been excluded from the decision making. (4) Chronic Lyme patients have been excluded from the treatment guideline panels for Lyme disease. (5) Governments have a fear of antibiotic resistance even though there exists no scientific evidence that the *Borrelia* bacteria have developed antibiotic resistance. Encouraging physicians to do an independent and objective evaluation of the scientific literature is more important than to force physicians to blindly follow government treatment guidelines that may or may not be ethical and up to date. Doing scientific research and reading the scientific literature are demanding work. Blindly following treatment guidelines requires little effort and does not require a degree in medicine because you don't need to be a professional chef to follow a cooking recipe. The importance of a patient voice is also something that is missing in the debate. Doctors have a responsibility to help sick patients. To deny a patient medical treatment in a situation when there exists scientific evidence to support treatment will always be controversial. Infectious disease doctors need to be more modest here. Patients have a critical role in healthcare and without them, there will be no healthcare. Some people conclude that since oral antibiotics cannot cure chronic Lyme disease patients, oral antibiotics should not be given to chronic Lyme patients. Such reasoning is a *non-sequitur* (logical fallacy). HIV is a chronic infection that cannot be eradicated with oral medication, but HIV patients still receive oral medication for life. Does there exist a general rule in medicine that states that only viral infections can become chronic? No! Is it ethical to refuse a patient treatment that reduces a patient's bacterial load, reduces a patient's symptoms and sometimes even cures them? No! Is it ethical to refuse a patient treatment for an infection that can kill them without treatment? No!

There also exist at least two problems with studies that treat chronic Lyme disease patients with IV antibiotics and conclude that such treatment did not eradicate the infection is (1) These studies usually treat chronic Lyme patients with monotherapy which is not a recommended treatment. (2) They usually do not treat for a sufficient period to make inference about how effective IV treatment is in eradicating the infection. I also want to point out that a double-blind, randomized controlled trial where neither the patient nor the treating doctor knows if the patient has received placebo or medication might, in theory, sound like a good a way to determine how effective a certain medication is. Reality is however far from theory. There also exists an ethical aspect. It is not ethical to give patients with a confirmed infection placebo in the name of science when such action could result in a lifelong infection for the patient. The estimated number of people that were infected with Lyme disease in the USA in 2008 is 829,600. If we assume that the incidence rate 2008 in the USA and Europe were the same, then approximately 2 million people were infected with Lyme disease Europe in 2008. Given an annual infection growth rate of 2% then in 2018 in the USA approximately 1 million people and in Europe 2.4 million will get infected with Lyme disease. Given an annual population growth of 1% in the USA then by 2050 in the USA 56 million people (12% of the population in the USA in 2050) will have been infected with Lyme disease. Given an annual population growth in Europe of 0.2% then by 2050 in Europe 135 million people (17% of the population Europe in 2050) will have been infected with Lyme disease. Most of these Lyme disease infections will, unfortunately, become chronic. I have also shown in this article that the financial implications of chronic Lyme disease are vast. A financial cost not only to patients but also to governments. Given that acute Lyme disease is treated with oral antibiotics for one month and chronic Lyme is treated with IV antibiotics for either 6 months or 1 year, then the estimated treatment cost for acute and chronic Lyme disease for 2018 for the USA is somewhere between 4.8 billion USD and 9.6 billion USD and for Europe somewhere between 10.1 billion EUR and 20.1 billion EUR. The estimated lost personal income for chronic Lyme patients that are not working for 2018 for the USA is 16.1 billion USD and in Europe 24.8 billion EUR. If the governments in the USA and Europe do not finance IV treatment with antibiotics for chronic Lyme disease, then the estimated government cost for chronic Lyme disease in the form of lost tax revenues because some chronic Lyme patients are not working plus disability benefits for chronic Lyme patients that not working for 2018 for the USA is 10.1 billion USD and for Europe 20.1 billion EUR. The government cost for chronic Lyme disease which does not include treatment costs for 2018 in the USA is 2.1 times larger than the cost for 6 months of IV treatment with antibiotics in the USA in 2018 and 1.1 times larger than the cost for 1 year of IV treatment with antibiotics in the USA in 2018. In Europe, the government cost for chronic Lyme disease for 2018 is two times larger than the cost for six months of IV treatment with antibiotics for Europe for 2018 and the government cost is on par with the cost, for one year of IV with antibiotics treatment for Europe for 2018. The cost for the governments of having chronic Lyme patients sick in perpetuity is very large. Future government revenues and future government costs for chronic Lyme disease are however much more important to look at than historical annual cost. Governments aggressive way to try to reduce antibiotic use unfortunately only creates more chronic infections where people can be forced to take oral antibiotics for the rest of their lives which means that the initial reduction in antibiotics use that can be observed due to the government's aggressive antibiotics reduction policy increases the use of antibiotics in the long run. No one thinks that diseases that are caused by a virus should be treated with antibiotics but when people who need antibiotics for their survival do not get access to them, then there is something wrong.

5. Conclusions

If someone acknowledges that acute Lyme disease is caused by bacteria, then they are also forced by logical reasoning to acknowledge that chronic Lyme disease is caused by bacteria because the immune system by itself can never eradicate a Borrelia infection and a bacterial infection does not magically disappear without antibiotic treatment once a person has been infected. We have known for a long time that antibiotics kill bacteria. However, sometimes oral and even IV antibiotics are unable to eradicate a Borrelia infection, but those observations are irrelevant because HIV patients receive treatment for life even though antiviral medications cannot eradicate an HIV infection and people with chronic Lyme disease die without antibiotic treatment. One single death caused by chronic Lyme disease is also enough to justify antibiotic treatment for chronic Lyme disease because a killer must "only" kill one person to become a killer. When a private special interest group such as the IDSA makes a political claim that three weeks of oral antibiotics is always enough to eradicate an acute or chronic Lyme disease infection, then the burden of proof lies with the IDSA. The IDSA must show the scientific evidence that supports their claim. I can claim that a red car is circulating the moon but unless I can show the scientific evidence that supports my claim, my claim has little meaning.

Lyme disease and chronic Lyme disease are well-hidden pandemics because: (1) the tests for Lyme disease are insensitive. Even if patients are "lucky" enough to test positive, patients will sometimes not receive antibiotic treatment because then the infectious disease physicians (in the USA IDSA) claim without scientific evidence that the antibodies are old and not a sign of an active infection. It becomes impossible for a patient to win. (2) the IDSA and CDC have previously or are possibly still colluding. (3) Because the cost of IV antibiotic treatment for chronic Lyme disease is so large insurance companies in the USA collude with IDSA to make sure IDSA deny that chronic Lyme disease is real disease that is caused by bacteria and require antibiotic treatment. This leads to that many Lyme disease patients are denied treatment and left to suffer until the infection eventually kills them. For many chronic Lyme disease patients, ILADS doctors, therefore, become heroes because these medical doctors are treating extremely sick and abandoned patients with long-term antibiotics. The CDC reported that in 2008 in the USA 444,000 people (high scenario) were infected with Lyme disease. The CDC assumption, without motivation or empirical evidence, that the number of healthy people in the control group is 4.4 times the number of infected people in the disease group for the high scenario is not realistic. If the CDC had assumed that the size of the control group with healthy people was the same size as the disease group with infected people (p = 1), then the number of Lyme disease infections in the USA for 2008 for the CDC high scenario would have been 527,288 instead of 444,000 given a Lyme disease test sensitivity of 0.669 and specificity of 0.961. If we assume a 1 to 1 relationship between the two groups and a Lyme disease test sensitivity of 0.44 and a Lyme disease test specificity of 0.99, then we get 829,600 infections in the USA in 2008. Because there exists uncertainty if the CDC is independent and objective, there also exists uncertainty about the CDC ability to protect public health. This research paper is one of the first studies that have estimated the financial cost of chronic Lyme disease both for individuals and governments. This research paper is also the first paper that can show that if the USA and European governments want to minimize future cost and maximize future revenues, then they should pay for IV treatment with antibiotics for chronic Lyme disease up to a year even if the estimated cure rate is as low as 25%. I am convinced that the history books in the future will describe controversy that exists today regarding chronic Lyme disease as one of the most shameful affairs in medicine.

Acknowledgments: The author would like to thank the two anonymous reviewers for providing valuable comments.

VBA Code

```
Public Sub zzz()

se = 0.44
sp = 0.99

np = 26
nx = 10

ThisWorkbook.Worksheets("zzz sub procedure").Range("B2:np" & np + 1).NumberFormat = "0.00"
ThisWorkbook.Worksheets("zzz sub procedure").Range("A1:np" & np + 1).HorizontalAlignment = xlCenter

Dim x As Long
Dim y As Long
Dim i As Integer
Dim j As Integer
Dim pp()
Dim xx()
Dim m()
```

```
For i = 1 To np
For j = 1 To nx

ReDim Preserve pp(i)
ReDim Preserve xx(j)
ReDim m(1 To np, 1 To nx)

pp(i) = (i - 1) / 5
xx(j) = j * 10

m(i, j) = ((xx(j) * se + pp(i) * xx(j) * (1 - sp)) / (xx(j) + pp(i) * xx(j))) * 100

ThisWorkbook.Worksheets("zzz sub procedure").Cells(1, 1).Value = "zz"
ThisWorkbook.Worksheets("zzz sub procedure").Cells(i + 1, 1).Value = pp(i)
ThisWorkbook.Worksheets("zzz sub procedure").Cells(1, j + 1).Value = xx(j)
ThisWorkbook.Worksheets("zzz sub procedure").Cells(i + 1, j + 1).Value = m(i, j)

Next j
Next i

End Sub

Public Function Lyme1(se, sp, p, z, Output As String)

Dim A(1 To 2, 1 To 2)
Dim C(1 To 2, 1 To 1) As Long

Dim x As Long
Dim y As Long

A(1, 1) = se
A(1, 2) = 1 - sp
A(2, 1) = -p
A(2, 2) = 1

C(1, 1) = z
C(2, 1) = 0

r = WorksheetFunction.MMult(WorksheetFunction.MInverse(A), C)

x = r(1, 1)
y = r(2, 1)
zz = (z / (x + y)) * 100

If Output = "x" Then Lyme1 = x
If Output = "y" Then Lyme1 = y
If Output = "zz" Then Lyme1 = zz
End Function

Public Function Lyme2(se, sp, p, z, Output As String)

Dim x As Long
```

```
Dim y As Long

x = z / (-sp * p + se + p)
y = p * z / (-sp * p + se + p)
zz = (z / (x + y)) * 100

If Output = "x" Then Lyme2 = x
If Output = "y" Then Lyme2 = y
If Output = "zz" Then Lyme2 = zz

End Function

Public Function Lyme3(se, sp, p, z, zz, Output As String)

Dim x As Long
Dim y As Long

x = 100 * z / (p * zz + zz)
y = 100 * p * z / (p * zz + zz)

If Output = "x" Then Lyme3 = x
If Output = "y" Then Lyme3 = y

End Function
```

References

1. Harvey, W.T.; Salvato, P. "Lyme disease": Ancient engine of an unrecognized borreliosis pandemic? *Med. Hypotheses* **2003**, *60*, 742–759. [CrossRef]
2. Cameron, D.J. Proof That Chronic Lyme Disease Exists. Interdiscip. Perspect. Infect. Dis. 2010. Available online: http://www.ncbi.nlm.nih.gov/pmc/articles/PMC2876246/ (accessed on 21 March 2017).
3. ECDC. Borreliosis. Borre. 2017. Available online: http://ecdc.europa.eu/en/healthtopics/emerging_and_vector-borne_diseases/tick_borne_diseases/lyme_disease/pages/index.aspx (accessed on 21 March 2017).
4. Tonks, A. Lyme wars. *BMJ* **2007**, *335*, 910–912. [CrossRef] [PubMed]
5. Stricker, R.B.; Johnson, L. Lyme Disease: Call for a "Manhattan Project" to Combat the Epidemic. *PLoS Pathog.* **2014**, *10*, e1003796. [CrossRef] [PubMed]
6. IDSA. IDSA: Infectious Diseases Society of America. Available online: http://www.idsociety.org/Index.aspx (accessed on 8 December 2017).
7. ILADS. ILADS—End Lyme disease epidemic through education, awareness & physican training. Available online: http://www.ilads.org/ (accessed on 8 December 2017).
8. Wormser, G.P.; Dattwyler, R.J.; Shapiro, E.D.; Halperin, J.J.; Steere, A.C.; Klempner, M.S.; Krause, P.J.; Bakken, J.S.; Strle, F.; Stanek, G.; et al. The Clinical Assessment, Treatment, and Prevention of Lyme Disease, Human Granulocytic Anaplasmosis, and Babesiosis: Clinical Practice Guidelines by the Infectious Diseases Society of America. *Clin. Infect. Dis.* **2006**, *43*, 1089–1134. [CrossRef] [PubMed]
9. Donta, S.T. Issues in the diagnosis and treatment of lyme disease. *Open Neurol. J.* **2012**, *6*, 140–145. [CrossRef] [PubMed]
10. Sharma, B.; Brown, A.V.; Matluck, N.E.; Hu, L.T.; Lewis, K. Borrelia burgdorferi, the Causative Agent of Lyme Disease, Forms Drug-Tolerant Persister Cells. *Antimicrob. Agents Chemother.* **2015**, *59*, 4616–4624. [CrossRef] [PubMed]
11. Caskey, J.R.; Embers, M.E. Persister Development by Borrelia burgdorferi Populations In Vitro. *Antimicrob. Agents Chemother.* **2015**, *59*, 6288–6295. [CrossRef] [PubMed]
12. Hodzic, E.; Imai, D.; Feng, S.; Barthold, S.W. Resurgence of Persisting Non-Cultivable Borrelia burgdorferi following Antibiotic Treatment in Mice. *PLoS ONE* **2014**, *9*, e86907. [CrossRef] [PubMed]

13. Hodzic, E.; Feng, S.; Holden, K.; Freet, K.J.; Barthold, S.W. Persistence of Borrelia burgdorferi following antibiotic treatment in mice. *Antimicrob. Agents Chemother.* **2008**, *52*, 1728–1736. [CrossRef] [PubMed]

14. Barthold, S.W.; Hodzic, E.; Imai, D.M.; Feng, S.; Yang, X.; Luft, B.J. Ineffectiveness of Tigecycline against Persistent Borrelia burgdorferi. *Antimicrob. Agents Chemother.* **2010**, *54*, 643–651. [CrossRef] [PubMed]

15. Yrjänäinen, H.; Hytönen, J.; Song, X.R.; Oksi, J.; Hartiala, K.; Viljanen, M.K. Anti-tumor necrosis factor-alpha treatment activates Borrelia burgdorferi spirochetes 4 weeks after ceftriaxone treatment in C3H/He mice. *J. Infect. Dis.* **2007**, *195*, 1489–1496. [CrossRef] [PubMed]

16. Straubinger, R.K.; Summers, B.A.; Chang, Y.F.; Appel, M.J. Persistence of Borrelia burgdorferi in experimentally infected dogs after antibiotic treatment. *J. Clin. Microbiol.* **1997**, *35*, 111–116. [PubMed]

17. Chang, Y.-F.; Ku, Y.-W.; Chang, C.-F.; Chang, C.-D.; McDonough, S.P.; Divers, T.; Pough, M. Antibiotic treatment of experimentally Borrelia burgdorferi-infected ponies. *Vet. Microbiol.* **2005**, *107*, 285–294. [CrossRef] [PubMed]

18. Embers, M.E.; Barthold, S.W.; Borda, J.T.; Bowers, L.; Doyle, L.; Hodzic, E.; Jacobs, M.B.; Hasenkampf, N.R.; Martin, D.S.; Narasimhan, S.; et al. Persistence of Borrelia burgdorferi in Rhesus Macaques following Antibiotic Treatment of Disseminated Infection. *PLoS ONE* **2012**, *7*, e29914. [CrossRef]

19. Rudenko, N.; Golovchenko, M.; Vancova, M.; Clark, K.; Grubhoffer, L.; Oliver, J.H. Isolation of live Borrelia burgdorferi sensu lato spirochaetes from patients with undefined disorders and symptoms not typical for Lyme borreliosis. *Clin. Microbiol. Infect.* **2016**, *22*, 267–e9. [CrossRef] [PubMed]

20. Phillips, S.E.; Mattman, L.H.; Hulínská, D.; Moayad, H. A proposal for the reliable culture of Borrelia burgdorferi from patients with chronic Lyme disease, even from those previously aggressively treated. *Infection* **1998**, *26*, 364–367. [CrossRef] [PubMed]

21. Schmidli, J.; Hunziker, T.; Moesli, P.; Schaad, U.B. Cultivation of Borrelia burgdorferi from Joint Fluid Three Months after Treatment of Facial Palsy Due to Lyme Borreliosis. *J. Infect. Dis.* **1988**, *158*, 905–906. [CrossRef] [PubMed]

22. Cimmino, M.A.; Azzolini, A.; Tobia, F.; Pesce, C.M. Spirochetes in the spleen of a patient with chronic Lyme disease. *Am. J. Clin. Pathol.* **1989**, *91*, 95–97. [CrossRef] [PubMed]

23. Treib, J.; Fernandez, A.; Haass, A.; Grauer, M.T.; Holzer, G.; Woessner, R. Clinical and serologic follow-up in patients with neuroborreliosis. *Neurology* **1998**, *51*, 1489–1491. [CrossRef] [PubMed]

24. Preac-Mursic, V.; Weber, K.; Pfister, H.W.; Wilske, B.; Gross, B.; Baumann, A.; Prokop, J. Survival of Borrelia burgdorferi in antibiotically treated patients with Lyme borreliosis. *Infection* **1989**, *17*, 355–359. [CrossRef] [PubMed]

25. Hudson, B.J.; Stewart, M.; Lennox, V.A.; Fukunaga, M.; Yabuki, M.; Macorison, H.; Kitchener-Smith, J. Culture-positive Lyme borreliosis. *Med. J. Aust.* **1998**, *168*, 500–502. [PubMed]

26. Kirsch, M.; Ruben, F.L.; Steere, A.C.; Duray, P.H.; Norden, C.W.; Winkelstein, A. Fatal Adult Respiratory Distress Syndrome in a Patient With Lyme Disease. *JAMA* **1988**, *259*, 2737–2739. [CrossRef] [PubMed]

27. Valesová, H.; Mailer, J.; Havlík, J.; Hulínská, D.; Hercogová, J. Long-term results in patients with Lyme arthritis following treatment with ceftriaxone. *Infection* **1996**, *24*, 98–102. [PubMed]

28. Asch, E.S.; Bujak, D.I.; Weiss, M.; Peterson, M.G.; Weinstein, A. Lyme disease: an infectious and postinfectious syndrome. *J. Rheumatol.* **1994**, *21*, 454–461. [PubMed]

29. Pfister, H.W.; Preac-Mursic, V.; Wilske, B.; Schielke, E.; Sörgel, F.; Einhäupl, K.M. Randomized comparison of ceftriaxone and cefotaxime in Lyme neuroborreliosis. *J. Infect. Dis.* **1991**, *163*, 311–318. [CrossRef] [PubMed]

30. Breier, F.; Khanakah, G.; Stanek, G.; Kunz, G.; Aberer, E.; Schmidt, B.; Tappeiner, G. Isolation and polymerase chain reaction typing of Borrelia afzelii from a skin lesion in a seronegative patient with generalized ulcerating bullous lichen sclerosus et atrophicus. *Br. J. Dermatol.* **2001**, *144*, 387–392. [CrossRef] [PubMed]

31. Oksi, J.; Marjamäki, M.; Nikoskelainen, J.; Viljanen, M.K. Borrelia burgdorferi detected by culture and PCR in clinical relapse of disseminated Lyme borreliosis. *Ann. Med.* **1999**, *31*, 225–232. [CrossRef] [PubMed]

32. Bayer, M.E.; Zhang, L.; Bayer, M.H. Borrelia burgdorferi DNA in the urine of treated patients with chronic Lyme disease symptoms—A PCR study of 97 cases. *Infection* **1996**, *24*, 347–353. [CrossRef] [PubMed]

33. Battafarano, D.F.; Combs, J.A.; Enzenauer, R.J.; Fitzpatrick, J.E. Chronic septic arthritis caused by Borrelia burgdorferi. *Clin. Orthop. Relat. Res.* **1993**, *297*, 238–241.

34. Häupl, T.; Hahn, G.; Rittig, M.; Krause, A.; Schoerner, C.; Schönherr, U.; Kalden, J.R.; Burmester, G.R. Persistence of Borrelia burgdorferi in ligamentous tissue from a patient with chronic Lyme borreliosis. *Arthritis Rheumatol.* **1993**, *36*, 1621–1626. [CrossRef]

35. Preac-Mursic, V.; Pfister, H.W.; Spiegel, H.; Burk, R.; Wilske, B.; Reinhardt, S.; Böhmer, R. First isolation of Borrelia burgdorferi from an iris biopsy. *J. Clin. Neuroophthalmol.* **1993**, *13*, 155–161. [PubMed]

36. Lawrence, C.; Lipton, R.B.; Lowy, F.D.; Coyle, P.K. Seronegative chronic relapsing neuroborreliosis. *Eur. Neurol.* **1995**, *35*, 113–117. [CrossRef] [PubMed]

37. Johnson, L.; Stricker, R.B. Treatment of Lyme disease: A medicolegal assessment. *Expert Rev. Anti-Infect. Ther.* **2004**, *2*, 533–557. [CrossRef] [PubMed]

38. Stricker, R.B.; Johnson, L. Persistent infection in chronic lyme disease: Does form matter? *Res. J. Infect. Dis.* **2013**, *1*, 2.

39. Stricker, R.B.; Johnson, L. Lyme disease: The next decade. *Infect. Drug Resist.* **2011**, *4*, 1–9. [CrossRef] [PubMed]

40. Melchers, W.; Meis, J.; Rosa, P.; Claas, E.; Nohlmans, L.; Koopman, R.; Horrevorts, A.; Galama, J. Amplification of Borrelia burgdorferi DNA in skin biopsies from patients with Lyme disease. *J. Clin. Microbiol.* **1991**, *29*, 2401–2406. [PubMed]

41. Pachner, A.R.; Cadavid, D.; Shu, G.; Dail, D.; Pachner, S.; Hodzic, E.; Barthold, S.W. Central and peripheral nervous system infection, immunity, and inflammation in the NHP model of Lyme borreliosis. *Ann. Neurol.* **2001**, *50*, 330–338. [CrossRef] [PubMed]

42. Goodman, J.L.; Jurkovich, P.; Kodner, C.; Johnson, R.C. Persistent cardiac and urinary tract infections with Borrelia burgdorferi in experimentally infected Syrian hamsters. *J. Clin. Microbiol.* **1991**, *29*, 894–896. [PubMed]

43. Steere, A.C.; Coburn, J.; Glickstein, L. The emergence of Lyme disease. *J. Clin. Investig.* **2004**, *113*, 1093–1101. [CrossRef] [PubMed]

44. Berndtson, K. Review of evidence for immune evasion and persistent infection in Lyme disease. *Int. J. Gen. Med.* **2013**, *6*, 291–306. [CrossRef] [PubMed]

45. Adrion, E.R.; Aucott, J.; Lemke, K.W.; Weiner, J.P. Health Care Costs, Utilization and Patterns of Care following Lyme Disease. *PLoS ONE* **2015**, *10*, e0116767. [CrossRef] [PubMed]

46. Stricker, R.B.; Johnson, L. Lyme disease: The promise of Big Data, companion diagnostics and precision medicine. *Infect. Drug Resist.* **2016**, *9*, 215–219. [CrossRef] [PubMed]

47. IDSA. IDSA: Updated Guidelines on Diagnosis, Treatment of Lyme Disease. Available online: http://www.idsociety.org/Updated_Guidelines_on_Diagnosis_Treatment_of_Lyme_Disease/ (accessed on 8 December 2017).

48. Maloney, E.L. Controversies in Persistent (Chronic) Lyme Disease. *J. Infus. Nurs.* **2016**, *39*, 369–375. [CrossRef] [PubMed]

49. Johnson, L.; Stricker, R.B. Attorney General forces Infectious Diseases Society of America to redo Lyme guidelines due to flawed development process. *J. Med. Ethics.* **2009**, *35*, 283–288. [CrossRef] [PubMed]

50. Johnson, L.; Stricker, R.B. The Infectious Diseases Society of America Lyme guidelines: A cautionary tale about the development of clinical practice guidelines. *Philos. Ethics Hum. Med.* **2010**, *5*, 9. [CrossRef] [PubMed]

51. CourtDocumentLymeDisease—11 October. 2017. Available online: https://www.courthousenews.com/wp-content/uploads/2017/11/LymeDisease.pdf (accessed on 8 December 2017).

52. Langford, C. Insurers Accused of Conspiring to Deny Lyme Disease Coverage. 2017. Available online: https://www.courthousenews.com/insurers-accused-conspiring-deny-lyme-disease-coverage/ (accessed on 8 December 2017).

53. Multiple Chronic Conditions Chartbook. 2010. Available online: https://www.ahrq.gov/sites/default/files/wysiwyg/professionals/prevention-chronic-care/decision/mcc/mccchartbook.pdf (accessed on 9 December 2017).

54. Johnson, L.; Stricker, R.B. Final Report of the Lyme Disease Review Panel of the Infectious Diseases Society of America: A Pyrrhic Victory? *Clin. Infect. Dis.* **2010**, *51*, 1108–1109. [CrossRef] [PubMed]

55. The National Academies of Sciences, Engineering, and Medicine. Standards for Developing Trustworthy Clinical Practice Guidelines: Health and Medicine Division. 2011. Available online: http://www.nationalacademies.org/hmd/Reports/2011/Clinical-Practice-Guidelines-We-Can-Trust/Standards.aspx (accessed on 17 March 2017).

56. Lee, D.H.; Vielemeyer, O. Analysis of Overall Level of Evidence behind Infectious Diseases Society of America Practice Guidelines. *Arch. Intern. Med.* **2011**, *171*, 18–22. [CrossRef] [PubMed]

57. CDC: Lyme carditis. What you need to know about Lyme carditis. 2016. Available online: https://www.cdc.gov/lyme/signs_symptoms/lymecarditis.html (accessed on 17 March 2017).

58. Bransfield, R.C. Suicide and Lyme and associated diseases. *Neuropsychiatr. Dis. Treat.* **2017**, *13*, 1575–1587. [CrossRef] [PubMed]

59. Cameron, D.J.; Johnson, L.B.; Maloney, E.L. Evidence assessments and guideline recommendations in Lyme disease: The clinical management of known tick bites, erythema migrans rashes and persistent disease. *Expert Rev. Anti-Infect. Ther.* **2014**, *12*, 1103–1135. [CrossRef] [PubMed]

60. ILADS: NGCH. Evidence assessments and guideline recommendations in Lyme disease: The clinical management of known tick bites, erythema migrans rashes and persistent disease. 2004. Available online: https://www.guideline.gov/summaries/summary/49320 (accessed on 18 March 2017).

61. Stricker, R.B.; Delong, A.K.; Green, C.L.; Savely, V.R.; Chamallas, S.N.; Johnson, L. Benefit of intravenous antibiotic therapy in patients referred for treatment of neurologic Lyme disease. *Int. J. Gen. Med.* **2011**, *4*, 639–646. [CrossRef] [PubMed]

62. CDC, C. Treatment, Lyme Disease. Available online: https://www.cdc.gov/lyme/treatment/index.html (accessed on 25 November 2017).

63. CDC PTLDS. Post-Treatment Lyme Disease Syndrome. Available online: https://www.cdc.gov/lyme/postlds/index.html (accessed on 16 June 2017).

64. Jariwala, N.; Ilyas, E.; Allen, H.B. Lyme Disease: A Bioethical Morass. *J. Clin. Res. Bioeth.* **2016**, *7*, 1–4. [CrossRef]

65. CDC Spider. CDC_SPIDER_Letter-1.pdf. 2016. Available online: https://usrtk.org/wp-content/uploads/2016/10/CDC_SPIDER_Letter-1.pdf (accessed on 17 March 2017).

66. Office of HIV/AIDS and Infectious Disease Policy O of the AS for H (OASH). 2017. Available online: https://www.hhs.gov/ash/advisory-committees/tickbornedisease/about/21-century-cures-act/index.html (accessed on 7 December 2017).

67. Wright, D.J.M. Borrel's accidental legacy. *Clin. Microbiol. Infect.* **2009**, *15*, 397–399. [CrossRef] [PubMed]

68. Steere, A.C.; Malawista, S.E.; Snydman, D.R.; Shope, R.E.; Andiman, W.A.; Ross, M.R.; Steele, F.M. Lyme arthritis: An epidemic of oligoarticular arthritis in children and adults in three connecticut communities. *Arthritis Rheumatol.* **1977**, *20*, 7–17. [CrossRef]

69. Irvine, H.G. Idiopathic atrophy of the skin with report of a case. *JAMA* **1913**, *61*, 396–401. [CrossRef]

70. Sweitzer, S.E.; Laymon, C.W. Acrodermatitis Chronica Atrophicans. *Arch. Derm. Syphilol.* **1935**, *31*, 196–212. [CrossRef]

71. Dunand, V.A.; Bretz, A.-G.; Suard, A.; Praz, G.; Dayer, E.; Péter, O. Acrodermatitis chronica atrophicans and serologic confirmation of infection due to Borrelia afzelii and/or Borrelia garinii by immunoblot. *Clin. Microbiol. Infect.* **1998**, *4*, 159–163. [CrossRef] [PubMed]

72. Biesiada, G.; Czepiel, J.; Leśniak, M.R.; Garlicki, A.; Mach, T. Lyme disease: Review. *Arch. Med. Sci.* **2012**, *8*, 978–982. [CrossRef] [PubMed]

73. Burgdorfer, W.; Barbour, A.G.; Hayes, S.F.; Benach, J.L.; Grunwaldt, E.; Davis, J.P. Lyme disease-a tick-borne spirochetosis? *Science* **1982**, *216*, 1317–1319. [CrossRef] [PubMed]

74. Fleming, A. On the Antibacterial Action of Cultures of a Penicillium, with Special Reference to their Use in the Isolation of B. influenzæ. *Br. J. Exp. Pathol.* **1929**, *10*, 226–236. [CrossRef]

75. Demain, A.L.; Sanchez, S. Microbial drug discovery: 80 years of progress. *J. Antibiot.* **2009**, *62*, 5–16. [CrossRef] [PubMed]

76. D'Costa, V.M.; King, C.E.; Kalan, L.; Morar, M.; Sung, W.W.L.; Schwarz, C.; Froese, D.; Zazula, G.; Calmels, F.; Debruyne, R.; et al. Antibiotic resistance is ancient. *Nature* **2011**, *477*, 457–461. [CrossRef] [PubMed]

77. Thyresson, N. The penicillin treatment of acrodermatitis atrophicans chronica (Herxheimer). *Acta Derm. Venereol.* **1949**, *29*, 572–621. [PubMed]

78. Keller, A.; Graefen, A.; Ball, M.; Matzas, M.; Boisguerin, V.; Maixner, F.; Leidinger, P.; Backes, C.; Khairat, R.; Forster, M.; et al. New insights into the Tyrolean Iceman's origin and phenotype as inferred by whole-genome sequencing. *Nat. Commun.* **2012**, *3*, 698. [CrossRef] [PubMed]

79. Poinar, G. Spirochete-like cells in a Dominican amber Ambylomma tick (Arachnida: Ixodidae). *Hist. Biol.* **2015**, *27*, 565–570. [CrossRef]

80. Fraser, C.M.; Casjens, S.; Huang, W.M.; Sutton, G.G.; Clayton, R.; Lathigra, R.; White, O.; Ketchum, K.A.; Dodson, R.; Hickey, E.K.; et al. Genomic sequence of a Lyme disease spirochaete, Borrelia burgdorferi. *Nature* **1997**, *390*, 580–586. [CrossRef] [PubMed]

81. Di, L.; Pagan, P.E.; Packer, D.; Martin, C.L.; Akther, S.; Ramrattan, G.; Mongodin, E.F.; Fraser, C.M.; Schutzer, S.E.; Luft, B.J.; et al. BorreliaBase: A phylogeny-centered browser of Borrelia genomes. *BMC Bioinform.* **2014**, *15*, 233. [CrossRef] [PubMed]

82. Bunikis, J.; Garpmo, U.; Tsao, J.; Berglund, J.; Fish, D.; Barbour, A.G. Sequence typing reveals extensive strain diversity of the Lyme borreliosis agents Borrelia burgdorferi in North America and Borrelia afzelii in Europe. *Microbiology* **2004**, *150*, 1741–1755. [CrossRef] [PubMed]

83. Rudenko, N.; Golovchenko, M.; Grubhoffer, L.; Oliver, J.H. Borrelia carolinensis sp. nov., a New (14th) Member of the Borrelia burgdorferi Sensu Lato Complex from the Southeastern Region of the United States. *J. Clin. Microbiol.* **2009**, *47*, 134–141. [CrossRef] [PubMed]

84. Wilske, B.; Barbour, A.G.; Bergström, S.; Burman, N.; Restrepo, B.I.; Rosa, P.A.; Schwan, T.; Soutschek, E.; Wallich, R. Antigenic variation and strain heterogeneity in Borrelia spp. *Res. Microbiol.* **1992**, *143*, 583–596. [CrossRef]

85. Baranton, G.; Seinost, G.; Theodore, G.; Postic, D.; Dykhuizen, D. Distinct levels of genetic diversity of Borrelia burgdorferi are associated with different aspects of pathogenicity. *Res. Microbiol.* **2001**, *152*, 149–156. [CrossRef]

86. Nardelli, D.T.; Callister, S.M.; Schell, R.F. Lyme Arthritis: Current Concepts and a Change in Paradigm. *Clin. Vaccine Immunol.* **2008**, *15*, 21–34. [CrossRef] [PubMed]

87. Sperling, J.; Middelveen, M.; Klein, D.; Sperling, F. Evolving Perspectives on Lyme Borreliosis in Canada. *Open Neurol. J.* **2012**, *6*, 94–103. [CrossRef] [PubMed]

88. Zhang, X.-C.; Yang, Z.-N.; Lu, B.; Ma, X.-F.; Zhang, C.-X.; Xu, H.-J. The composition and transmission of microbiome in hard tick, Ixodes persulcatus, during blood meal. *Ticks Tick Borne Dis.* **2014**, *5*, 864–870. [CrossRef] [PubMed]

89. Tokarz, R.; Williams, S.H.; Sameroff, S.; Sanchez Leon, M.; Jain, K.; Lipkin, W.I. Virome Analysis of Amblyomma americanum, Dermacentor variabilis, and Ixodes scapularis Ticks Reveals Novel Highly Divergent Vertebrate and Invertebrate Viruses. *J. Virol.* **2014**, *88*, 11480–11492. [CrossRef] [PubMed]

90. Open Eye Pictures. Excerpts from interview with Willy Burgdorfer. 2014. Available online: https://www.youtube.com/watch?v=QLIWSkQdCmU&app=desktop (accessed on 17 March 2017).

91. Brorson, O.; Brorson, S.H. Transformation of cystic forms of Borrelia burgdorferi to normal, mobile spirochetes. *Infection* **1997**, *25*, 240–246. [CrossRef] [PubMed]

92. Meriläinen, L.; Herranen, A.; Schwarzbach, A.; Gilbert, L. Morphological and biochemical features of Borrelia burgdorferi pleomorphic forms. *Microbiology* **2015**, *161*, 516–527. [CrossRef] [PubMed]

93. Sapi, E.; Bastian, S.L.; Mpoy, C.M.; Scott, S.; Rattelle, A.; Pabbati, N.; Poruri, A.; Burugu, D.; Theophilus, P.A.S.; Pham, T.V.; et al. Characterization of Biofilm Formation by Borrelia burgdorferi In Vitro. *PLoS ONE* **2012**, *7*, e48277. [CrossRef] [PubMed]

94. Smith, A.J.; Oertle, J.; Prato, D. Chronic Lyme Disease: Persistent Clinical Symptoms Related to Immune Evasion, Antibiotic Resistance and Various Defense Mechanisms of Borrelia burgdorferi. *Open J. Med. Microbiol.* **2014**, *4*, 252. [CrossRef]

95. Zhang, J.-R.; Hardham, J.M.; Barbour, A.G.; Norris, S.J. Antigenic Variation in Lyme Disease Borreliae by Promiscuous Recombination of VMP-like Sequence Cassettes. *Cell* **1997**, *89*, 275–285. [CrossRef]

96. Liang, F.T.; Yan, J.; Mbow, M.L.; Sviat, S.L.; Gilmore, R.D.; Mamula, M.; Fikrig, E. Borrelia burgdorferi Changes Its Surface Antigenic Expression in Response to Host Immune Responses. *Infect. Immun.* **2004**, *72*, 5759–5767. [CrossRef] [PubMed]

97. Coutte, L.; Botkin, D.J.; Gao, L.; Norris, S.J. Detailed Analysis of Sequence Changes Occurring during vlsE Antigenic Variation in the Mouse Model of Borrelia burgdorferi Infection. *PLoS Pathog.* **2009**, *5*, e1000293. [CrossRef] [PubMed]

98. Graves, C.J.; Ros, V.I.D.; Stevenson, B.; Sniegowski, P.D.; Brisson, D. Natural Selection Promotes Antigenic Evolvability. *PLoS Pathog.* **2013**, *9*, e1003766. [CrossRef] [PubMed]

99. Harris, L.M.; Merrick, C.J. G-Quadruplexes in Pathogens: A Common Route to Virulence Control? *PLoS Pathog.* **2015**, *11*, e1004562. [CrossRef] [PubMed]

100. Maizels, N. G4-associated human diseases. *EMBO Rep.* **2015**, *16*, 910–922. [CrossRef] [PubMed]

101. Yang, D.; Okamoto, K. Structural insights into G-quadruplexes: Towards new anticancer drugs. *Future Med. Chem.* **2010**, *2*, 619–646. [CrossRef] [PubMed]

102. Bay Area Lyme Foundation. Yuko Nakajima, PhD. Bay Area Lyme Foundation. 2017. Available online: http://www.bayarealyme.org/our-research/emerging-leader-award/yuko-nakajima-phd/ (accessed on 8 December 2017).

103. Cabello, F.C.; Godfrey, H.P.; Bugrysheva, J.; Newman, S.A. Sleeper cells: The stringent response and persistence in the Borreliella (Borrelia) burgdorferi enzootic cycle. *Environ. Microbiol.* **2017**, *19*, 3846–3862. [CrossRef] [PubMed]

104. Brorson, O.; Brorson, S.H. An in vitro study of the susceptibility of mobile and cystic forms of Borrelia burgdorferi to metronidazole. *APMIS* **1999**, *107*, 566–576. [CrossRef] [PubMed]

105. Brorson, O.; Brorson, S.-H.A. An in vitro study of the susceptibility of mobile and cystic forms of Borrelia burgdorferi to tinidazole. *Int. Microbiol.* **2004**, *7*, 139–142. [PubMed]

106. Brorson, O.; Brorson, S.H. An in vitro study of the susceptibility of mobile and cystic forms of Borrelia burgdorferi to hydroxychloroquine. *Int. Microbiol.* **2002**, *5*, 25–31. [CrossRef] [PubMed]

107. Donta, S.T. Macrolide therapy of chronic Lyme Disease. *Med. Sci. Monit.* **2003**, *9*, PI136–PI142. [PubMed]

108. Geamănu, A.; Popa-Cherecheanu, A.; Marinescu, B.; Geamănu, C.; Voinea, L. Retinal toxicity associated with chronic exposure to hydroxychloroquine and its ocular screening. *Rev. J. Med. Life* **2014**, *7*, 322–326.

109. Sapi, E.; Kaur, N.; Anyanwu, S.; Luecke, D.F.; Datar, A.; Patel, S.; Rossi, M.; Stricker, R.B. Evaluation of in-vitro antibiotic susceptibility of different morphological forms of Borrelia burgdorferi. *Infect. Drug Resist.* **2011**, *4*, 97–113. [PubMed]

110. ILADS webpage. Evidence-based guidelines for the management of Lyme disease. *Expert Rev. Anti-Infect. Ther.* **2004**, *2*, S1–S13.

111. Halperin, J.; Luft, B.J.; Volkman, D.J.; Dattwyler, R.J. Lyme neuroborreliosis. Peripheral nervous system manifestations. *Brain* **1990**, *113*, 1207–1221. [CrossRef] [PubMed]

112. Logigian, E.L.; Kaplan, R.F.; Steere, A.C. Chronic neurologic manifestations of Lyme disease. *N. Engl. J. Med.* **1990**, *323*, 1438–1444. [CrossRef] [PubMed]

113. Halperin, J.J.; Little, B.W.; Coyle, P.K.; Dattwyler, R.J. Lyme disease: Cause of a treatable peripheral neuropathy. *Neurology* **1987**, *37*, 1700–1706. [CrossRef] [PubMed]

114. Cameron, D.J. Clinical trials validate the severity of persistent Lyme disease symptoms. *Med. Hypotheses* **2009**, *2*, 153–156. [CrossRef] [PubMed]

115. Stricker, R.B. Counterpoint: Long-term antibiotic therapy improves persistent symptoms associated with lyme disease. *Clin. Infect. Dis.* **2007**, *5*, 149–157. [CrossRef] [PubMed]

116. Cameron, D. Severity of Lyme disease with persistent symptoms. Insights from a double-blind placebo-controlled clinical trial. *Minerva Med.* **2008**, *99*, 89–96.

117. Donta, S.T. Tetracycline therapy for chronic Lyme disease. *Clin. Infect. Dis.* **1997**, *25* (Suppl. S1), S52–S56. [CrossRef] [PubMed]

118. Logigian, E.L.; Steere, A.C. Clinical and electrophysiologic findings in chronic neuropathy of Lyme disease. *Neurology* **1992**, *42*, 303–311. [CrossRef] [PubMed]

119. Halperin, J.J. Abnormalities of the nervous system in Lyme disease: response to antimicrobial therapy. *Rev. Infect. Dis.* **1989**, *11* (Suppl. S6), S1499–S1504. [CrossRef] [PubMed]

120. Delong, A.K.; Blossom, B.; Maloney, E.L.; Phillips, S.E. Antibiotic retreatment of Lyme disease in patients with persistent symptoms: A biostatistical review of randomized, placebo-controlled, clinical trials. *Contemp. Clin. Trials* **2012**, *33*, 1132–1142. [CrossRef] [PubMed]

121. Ang, C.W.; Notermans, D.W.; Hommes, M.; Simoons-Smit, A.M.; Herremans, T. Large differences between test strategies for the detection of anti-Borrelia antibodies are revealed by comparing eight ELISAs and five immunoblots. *Eur. J. Clin. Microbiol. Infect. Dis.* **2011**, *30*, 1027–1032. [CrossRef] [PubMed]

122. Stricker, R.B.; Johnson, L. Lyme disease diagnosis and treatment: Lessons from the AIDS epidemic. *Minerva Med.* **2010**, *101*, 419–425. [PubMed]

123. Brorson, O.; Brorson, S.H. In vitro conversion of Borrelia burgdorferi to cystic forms in spinal fluid, and transformation to mobile spirochetes by incubation in BSK-H medium. *Infection* **1998**, *26*, 144–150. [CrossRef] [PubMed]

124. Schoonjans, F. Diagnostic test evaluation calculator. *MedCalc*. 2017. Available online: https://www.medcalc. org/calc/diagnostic_test.php (accessed on 18 March 2017).

125. Middelveen, M.J.; Burke, J.; Sapi, E.; Bandoski, C.; Filush, K.R.; Wang, Y.; Franco, A.; Timmaraju, A.; Schlinger, H.A.; Mayne, P.J.; et al. 2015. Available online: http://f1000research.com/articles/3-309/v3 (accessed on 18 March 2017).

126. Estrada-Peña, A.; de la Fuente, J. The ecology of ticks and epidemiology of tick-borne viral diseases. *Antivir. Res.* **2014**, *108*, 104–128. [CrossRef] [PubMed]

127. CDC HIV. *HIV Transmission Rates in the United States, 1977–2006. Dramatic Declines Indicate Success in HIV Prevention Nationwide—CDC_TransmissionRates_FactSheet.pdf*. 2006. Available online: https://www.cdc.gov/ nchhstp/newsroom/docs/CDC_TransmissionRates_FactSheet.pdf (accessed on 19 March 2017).

128. Hinckley, A.F.; Connally, N.P.; Meek, J.I.; Johnson, B.J.; Kemperman, M.M.; Feldman, K.A.; White, J.L.; Mead, P.S. Lyme Disease Testing by Large Commercial Laboratories in the United States. *Clin. Infect. Dis.* **2014**, *59*, 676–681. [CrossRef] [PubMed]

129. Hinckley, A.F. Supplementary data to Lyme disease testing by large commercial laboratories in the United States. 2014. Available online: https://oup.silverchair-cdn.com/oup/backfile/ Content_public/Journal/cid/59/5/10.1093_cid_ciu397/1/ciu397_Supplementary_Data.zip?Expires=1512837512& Signature=RffWKdBkXiX6hlSWu5IqE3G~VQomUI713OMhRVsa4WxGUvauJy1rq9gAAV3EYqBbojqfeBkvo~ eqvXJWk5TDNrdI0QFZ~3q5m09iW716itJ20NQgnfw~7FibPdq6OMtTE19GPgdHP~X5cbWjBvJ4VRiXB~ xYwvaJg1dnfY3NOVsNRai1i4sAgFgvtCnILZ4dWh6mt-SmjaR6nEI-Q7IfNevJjePqymCPw46IZxD7xi91E13iwH~ 1KDlct06nC0z87LPcpsfbZjklnEVUmWo5ad1RYi7TxLwfTmfdlqBPWuJTC6ZflhxqwJtlpyEO4VkdwGLvsbo1dJ5FS2GmoOqkjw_ _&Key-Pair-Id=APKAIUCZBIA4LVPAVW3Q (accessed on 10 September 2017).

130. Seemann, E. Are Social Security Disability Benefits Taxable? 2015. Available online: https://www.labovick. com/2015/02/13/social-security-disability-benefits-taxable/ (accessed on 17 October 2017).

131. Sweden's government tax agency. Skatteregler för privatpersoner SKV 330 utgåva 38. 2017. Available online: https://www.skatteverket.se/download/18.57cadbbd15a3688ff448d20/1488271841075/ skatteregler-for-privatpersoner-skv330-utgava38.pdf (accessed on 10 September 2017).

132. Johnson, L.; Wilcox, S.; Mankoff, J.; Stricker, R.B. Severity of chronic Lyme disease compared to other chronic conditions: A quality of life survey. *PeerJ* **2014**, *2*, e322. [CrossRef] [PubMed]

133. OECD Statistics. OECD. Available online: http://stats.oecd.org/index.aspx?r=659459&errocode=403& lastaction=login_submit (accessed on 17 October 2017).

134. TKPMG. Individual income tax rates table. 2016. Available online: https://home.kpmg.com/xx/en/home/ services/tax/tax-tools-and-resources/tax-rates-online/individual-income-tax-rates-table.html (accessed on 17 October 2017).

135. Disability Secrets, B. How Much in Social Security Disability Benefits Can You Get? Disability Secrets. 2016. Available online: http://www.disabilitysecrets.com/how-much-in-ssd.html (accessed on 18 March 2017).

136. Swedish government. Sjukersättning vid Sjukdom. Available online: https://www.forsakringskassan.se/ privatpers/sjuk/sjuk_minst_1_ar/sjukersattning (accessed on 17 October 2017).

## 2

Effect of Skeletal Muscle and Fat Mass on Muscle Strength in the Elderly

Koji Nonaka [1],* ⑩, Shin Murata [1], Kayoko Shiraiwa [1], Teppei Abiko [1], Hideki Nakano [1], Hiroaki Iwase [2], Koichi Naito [3] and Jun Horie [1]

[1] Faculty of Physical Therapy, Department of Health Sciences, Kyoto Tachibana University, Kyoto 607-8175, Japan; murata-s@tachibana-u.ac.jp (S.M.); shiraiwa@tachibana-u.ac.jp (K.S.); abiko@tachibana-u.ac.jp (T.A.); nakano-h@tachibana-u.ac.jp (H.N.); horie-j@tachibana-u.ac.jp (J.H.)

[2] Faculty of Physical Therapy, Department of Rehabilitation, Kobe International University, Kobe 658-0032, Japan; iwase@kobe-kiu.ac.jp

[3] Department of Physical Therapy, Hakuho College, Oji 636-0011, Japan; k.naitou@hakuho.ac.jp

*   Correspondence: nonaka-k@tachibana-u.ac.jp

Abstract: It is important for elderly people to maintain or improve muscle strength and for clinicians to know the factors that affect muscle strength. Therefore, the purpose of this study was to compare the effects of fat mass (FM) and skeletal muscle mass (SMM) on muscle strength. The participants included 192 community-dwelling elderly women. The SMM and FM, grip strength, and knee extension strength were measured. Data were evaluated using stepwise multiple linear regression analysis, which was performed with grip or knee extension strength as a dependent variable and the SMM and FM of the upper and lower limbs as the independent variables. The SMM and FM of the upper limbs were associated with grip strength, whereas the SMM but not the FM of the lower limbs was associated with knee extension strength. These findings suggest that there may be thresholds for the SMM/FM ratio to affect muscle strength.

Keywords: muscle strength; skeletal muscle mass; fat mass; grip strength; knee extension strength

---

1. Introduction

Muscle strength decreases with aging [1], and this decrease is characterized by a slow walking speed [2], which in turn is associated with mortality [3]. The risk of falling and subsequently developing a fracture is reportedly associated with a decline in walking speed [4]. Therefore, it is important for elderly people to maintain or improve muscle strength.

It is well known that skeletal muscle mass (SMM) is associated with muscle strength [5]. Additionally, fat mass (FM), which is higher in the elderly than in younger individuals [6], has been shown to affect muscle strength negatively. Intramuscular adipose tissue inhibits central activation, resulting in a reduction in muscle strength [7]. It also produces tumor necrosis factor (TNF-α) [8], which reduces muscle performance [9]. The accumulation of intramuscular adipose tissue has been shown to increase with an increase in FM, as seen in individuals with obesity [10].

We hypothesized that not only SMM but also FM affects muscle strength among the elderly. If FM negatively affects muscle strength, clinicians can target it for maintenance or improvement of muscle strength in the elderly. Therefore, the aim of this study was to test this hypothesis among community-dwelling elderly women.

2. Materials and Methods

2.1. Participants

This was a cross-sectional study that recruited 215 participants and included 192 community-dwelling elderly women according to the following inclusion criteria (Figure 1): (1) an age of more than 60 years, (2) no significant cognitive impairment, and (3) all measurements could be performed. This study was approved by the institutional ethics committee and was conducted in accordance with the Helsinki Declaration. All participants provided written informed consent to participate in the study.

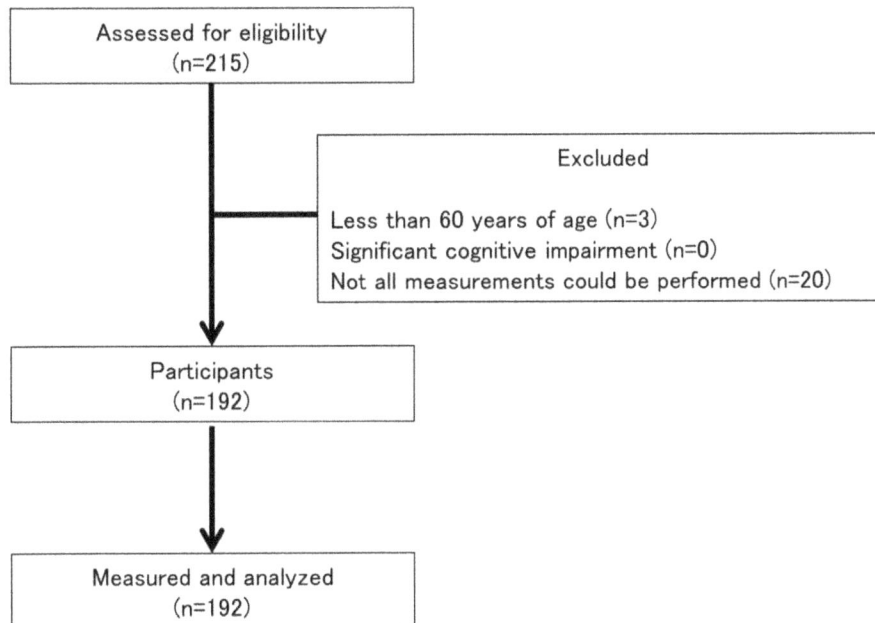

```
┌─────────────────────────┐
│  Assessed for eligibility│
│        (n=215)           │
└─────────────────────────┘
            │         ┌──────────────────────────────────────────┐
            │         │  Excluded                                │
            ├────────▶│                                          │
            │         │  Less than 60 years of age (n=3)         │
            │         │  Significant cognitive impairment (n=0)  │
            │         │  Not all measurements could be performed │
            │         │  (n=20)                                  │
            │         └──────────────────────────────────────────┘
            ▼
┌─────────────────────────┐
│     Participants         │
│        (n=192)           │
└─────────────────────────┘
            │
            ▼
┌─────────────────────────┐
│  Measured and analyzed   │
│        (n=192)           │
└─────────────────────────┘
```

Figure 1. Flowchart of participation in the present study.

2.2. Body Mass Index (BMI)

The participants were grouped into different body mass index (BMI) categories in accordance with the Japanese criteria for underweight (BMI < 18.5), normal weight ($18.5 \leq$ BMI ≤ 24.9), and obesity (BMI > 25).

2.3. Exercise Habits

In order to understand their exercise habits and physical activity, participants were asked whether they performed exercise regularly for more than 30 min/day and 3 days/week.

2.4. SMM and FM

SMM and FM were measured by the bioelectrical impedance method using Inbody 430 (Biospace Co., Ltd., Seoul, Korea) or 470 (InBody Japan Inc., Tokyo, Japan), which were used for 107 (56%) and 85 (44%) of the participants, respectively. The participants stood on two metallic electrodes and held metallic grip electrodes, and the SMM and FM of the upper and lower limbs were measured.

2.5. Grip Strength

The grip strength was measured with a hand grip dynamometer (T.K.K.58401, Takei Scientific Instruments Co., Ltd., Niigata, Japan) to assess upper limb muscle strength as described by Abe et al. [11]. The measurements were taken for both upper limbs, and the mean value was used for analysis.

2.6. Knee Extension Strength

The knee extension strength was measured to assess the muscle strength of the lower limbs as described by Bohannon [12]. The participants were instructed to sit with their knees and hips flexed at 90°. A hand-held dynamometer (μTas F-1; Anima Corp., Tokyo, Japan) was placed just proximal to the ankle on the anterior surface of the leg, and participants were instructed to perform maximal isometric muscle contraction. Knee extension strength was measured in both legs, and the mean value was used for analysis.

2.7. Statistical Analysis

Stepwise multiple linear regression analysis was performed with grip or knee extension strength as a dependent variable and the SMM and FM of the upper and lower limbs as the independent variables. Statistical analyses were performed using SPSS ver. 22.0 (IBM Japan, Ltd., Tokyo, Japan) and significance was accepted when $p < 0.05$.

3. Results

The characteristics of the participants are summarized in Table 1. The mean age, height, and weight were 73.7 ± 5.8 years, 151.5 ± 5.1 cm, and 51.0 ± 8.0 kg, respectively. In total, 66.1% of all participants regularly exercised. The percentages of underweight, normal weight, and obese were 10, 70, and 20%, respectively. The mean SMM/FM ratios of the upper and lower limbs were 1.76 ± 1.36 and 2.31 ± 1.04, respectively.

Table 1. Participant characteristics.

Variable	Mean ± SD
Age (years)	73.7 ± 5.8
Height (cm)	151.5 ± 5.1
Weight (kg)	51.0 ± 8.0
Underweight (BMI < 18.5), n (%)	19 (10%)
Normal weight (18.5 ≤ BMI < 25.0), n (%)	134 (70%)
Obese (25.0 ≤ BMI), n (%)	39 (20%)
Regular exercise, n (%)	127 (66.1%)
Upper limb SMM (kg)	3.26 ± 0.65
Upper limb FM (kg)	2.17 ± 0.85
Upper limb SMM/FM ratio	1.76 ± 1.36
Lower limb SMM (kg)	10.62 ± 1.54
Lower limb FM (kg)	5.07 ± 1.54
Lower limb SMM/FM ratio	2.31 ± 1.04
Grip strength (kg)	22.1 ± 3.7
Knee extension strength (kgf)	19.9 ± 5.0
Disease	
Hypertension, n (%)	80 (42%)
Orthopedic disease, n (%)	40 (21%)
Hyperglycemia, n (%)	30 (16%)
Cardiovascular disease, n (%)	10 (5%)
Diabetes mellitus, n (%)	6 (3%)
Pulmonary disease, n (%)	5 (3%)
Rheumatoid arthritis, n (%)	3 (2%)
Renal disease, n (%)	3 (2%)
Stroke, n (%)	2 (1%)
Cancer, n (%)	2 (1%)
Others, n (%)	34 (18%)

SMM, skeletal muscle mass; BMI, body mass index; FM, fat mass.

The results of the stepwise multiple regression analysis are shown in Table 2. The analysis showed that the SMM (standardized β = 0.691, p < 0.001) and FM (standardized β = −0.263, p < 0.001) of the upper limbs were independently associated with grip strength (R^2 = 0.358). On the other hand, knee extension strength showed an independent association only with the SMM (standardized β = 0.481, p < 0.001) but not with the FM of the lower limbs (R^2 = 0.231).

Table 2. Stepwise multiple regression analysis.

Variable	β	SE	Standardized Beta	p-Value	R^2	Adjusted R^2
Grip strength					0.358	0.351
Upper limb SMM	3.889	0.384	0.691	<0.001		
Upper limb FM	−1.137	0.294	−0.269	<0.001		
Knee extension strength					0.231	0.227
Lower limb SMM	1.563	0.207	0.481	<0.001		

SMM, skeletal muscle mass; FM, fat mass.

4. Discussion

The aim of this study was to test the hypothesis that muscle strength is affected not only by SMM but also by FM. In line with our hypothesis, grip strength was found to be affected by both SMM and FM of the upper limbs. On the other hand, knee extension strength was affected only by SMM but not FM of the lower limbs. These findings suggest that there may be thresholds for the SMM/FM ratio to affect muscle strength.

The FM of the upper limb affected the grip strength. Intramuscular adipose tissue is increased with obesity and is decreased upon weight loss [10]. Our findings suggest that intramuscular adipose tissue increases as FM increases. It has been reported to inhibit central activation [7] and produce inflammatory cytokines such as TNF-α to depress myofibrillar force via the TNF receptor [9]. TNF-α has been reported to cause a decrease in the tetanic force by reducing the reactivity of muscle myofilaments to calcium [13]. Therefore, FM of the upper limbs can negatively affect grip strength by inhibiting central activation and thereby increasing TNF-α production by adipose tissue.

On the contrary, knee extension strength was not affected by the FM of the lower limbs. This could be due to less FM in lower limbs, as suggested by the decreased SMM/FM ratio in the lower limbs compared to the upper limbs. This, therefore, suggests that the FM of the lower limbs might not be large enough to affect the muscle strength. Aerobic exercise has been reported to lower FM in the lower limbs of lean (BMI < 25.0 kg/m^2) and obese (BMI > 27.0 kg/m^2) elderly men who did not otherwise exercise regularly [14]. Resistance training has been reported to decrease the thigh intramuscular adipose tissue in older individuals [15]. These reports suggest that regular exercise can attenuate the increase in fat tissue with aging. In this study, 66.1% of the participants exercised regularly for more than 3 days/week and 30 min/day. Therefore, intramuscular adipose tissue was expected to be low in participants in this study. Yoshida et al. reported that older adults with low intramuscular adipose tissue have normal central activation [7]. Therefore, participants in this study might not have had enough lower limb FM to affect knee extension strength, because many of them performed regular exercise. In addition, there were few cases of obesity in this study, so we could not divide the participants into underweight, normal weight, and obese groups when the effect of FM on muscle strength was assessed. Individuals with obesity may have higher intramuscular adipose tissue infiltration, and their muscle strength would thus be affected by FM.

There are two limitations of this study. First, as previously mentioned, there were few participants with obesity, so we could not determine how obesity impacts the effect of FM on muscle strength. Second, we failed to investigate the effect of FM on upper limb and lower limb activity. Further studies are therefore needed to investigate the effect of FM on muscle strength in participants divided into underweight, normal weight, and obese categories; and on the activity of the upper and lower limbs.

5. Conclusions

We compared the effects of SMM and FM on muscle strength. Both the SMM and FM of the upper limbs affected grip strength. However, in the lower limbs, only SMM, but not FM, was associated with knee extension strength. These findings suggest that FM can affect muscle strength when it increases to a certain degree. Therefore, clinicians may target FM to maintain or improve muscle strength in the elderly. Future studies are needed to determine the amount of FM that can affect muscle strength.

Author Contributions: K.N. and S.M. contributed to experimental design, data collection, analysis, and manuscript preparation; K.S., T.A., H.N., H.I. and K.N. contributed to experimental design and data collection; J.H. contributed to experimental design, data collection and manuscript preparation.

Funding: This research was funded by a JSPS KAKENHI Grant (16H05602 and 17K01808).

Acknowledgments: We would like to thank Editage (www.editage.jp) for English language editing.

References

1.   Kuh, D.; Bassey, E.J.; Butterworth, S.; Hardy, R.; Wadsworth, M.E.J. Grip strength, postural control, and functional leg power in a representative cohort of British men and women: Associations with physical activity, health status, and socioeconomic conditions. *J. Gerontol. A Biol. Sci. Med. Sci.* **2005**, *60*, 224–231. [CrossRef] [PubMed]

2.   Bijlsma, A.Y.; Meskers, C.G.M.; Van Den Eshof, N.; Westendorp, R.G.; Sipilä, S.; Stenroth, L.; Sillanpää, E.; McPhee, J.S.; Jones, D.A.; Narici, M.V.; et al. Diagnostic criteria for sarcopenia and physical performance. *Age* **2014**, *36*, 275–285. [CrossRef] [PubMed]

3.   Cesari, M.; Pahor, M.; Lauretani, F.; Zamboni, V.; Bandinelli, S.; Bernabei, R.; Guralnik, J.M.; Ferrucci, L. Skeletal muscle and mortality results from the InCHIANTI study. *J. Gerontol. A Biol. Sci. Med. Sci.* **2009**, *64*, 377–384. [CrossRef] [PubMed]

4.   Studenski, S.; Perera, S.; Wallace, D.; Chandler, J.M.; Duncan, P.W.; Rooney, E.; Fox, M.; Guralnik, J.M. Physical performance measures in the clinical setting. *J. Am. Geriatr. Soc.* **2003**, *51*, 314–322. [CrossRef] [PubMed]

5.   Janssen, I.; Baumgartner, R.N.; Ross, R.; Rosenberg, I.H.; Roubenoff, R. Skeletal muscle cutpoints associated with elevated physical disability risk in older men and women. *Am. J. Epidemiol.* **2004**, *159*, 413–421. [CrossRef] [PubMed]

6.   Schutz, Y.; Kyle, U.U.; Pichard, C. Fat-free mass index and fat mass index percentiles in Caucasians aged 18–98y. *Int. J. Obes. Relat. Metab. Disord.* **2002**, *26*, 953–960. [CrossRef] [PubMed]

7.   Yoshida, Y.; Marcus, R.L.; Lastayo, P.C. Intramuscular adipose tissue and central activation in older adults. *Muscle Nerve* **2012**, *46*, 813–816. [CrossRef] [PubMed]

8.   Yudkin, J.S. Inflammation, obesity, and the metabolic syndrome. *Horm. Metab. Res.* **2007**, *39*, 707–709. [CrossRef] [PubMed]

9.   Hardin, B.J.; Campbell, K.S.; Smith, J.D.; Arbogast, S.; Smith, J.; Moylan, J.S.; Reid, M.B. TNF-α acts via TNFR1 and muscle-derived oxidants to depress myofibrillar force in murine skeletal muscle. *J. Appl. Physiol.* **2008**, *104*, 694–699. [CrossRef] [PubMed]

10.   Goodpaster, B.H.; Theriault, R.; Watkins, S.C.; Kelley, D.E. Intramuscular lipid content is increased in obesity and decreased by weight loss. *Metabolism* **2000**, *49*, 467–472. [CrossRef]

11.   Abe, T.; Yaginuma, Y.; Fujita, E.; Thiebaud, R.S.; Kawanishi, M.; Akamine, T. Associations of sit-up ability with sarcopenia classification measures in Japanese older women. *Interv. Med. Appl. Sci.* **2016**, *8*, 152–157. [CrossRef] [PubMed]

12.   Bohannon, R.W. Test-retest reliability of hand-held dynamometry during a single session of strength assessment. *Phys. Ther.* **1986**, *66*, 206–209. [CrossRef] [PubMed]

13.   Reid, M.B.; Lännergren, J.; Westerblad, H. Respiratory and limb muscle weakness induced by tumor necrosis factor-α: Involvement of muscle myofilaments. *Am. J. Respir. Crit. Care Med.* **2002**, *166*, 479–484. [CrossRef] [PubMed]

14. Lee, S.; Kuk, J.L.; Davidson, L.E.; Hudson, R.; Kilpatrick, K.; Graham, T.E.; Ross, R. Role of exercise in reducing the risk of diabetes and obesity exercise without weight loss is an effective strategy for obesity reduction in obese individuals with and without Type 2 diabetes. *J. Appl. Physiol.* **2005**, *99*, 1220–1225. [CrossRef] [PubMed]

15. Marcus, R.L.; Addison, O.; Kidde, J.P.; Dibble, L.E.; Lastayo, P.C. Skeletal muscle fat infiltration: Impact of age, inactivity, and exercise. *J. Nutr. Health Aging* **2010**, *14*, 362–366. [CrossRef] [PubMed]

## 3

Depressive Symptoms Increase the Risk of Mortality for White but Not Black Older Adults

Shervin Assari [1,2] (iD)

[1] Department of Psychiatry, University of Michigan, Ann Arbor, MI 48109, USA; assari@umich.edu

[2] Center for Research on Ethnicity, Culture and Health, School of Public Health, University of Michigan, Ann Arbor, MI 48109, USA

Abstract: *Introduction.* Long-term studies have shown that depressive symptoms predict the risk of mortality. However, it is unknown if this effect is present in shorter time intervals. In addition, recent research suggests that the salience of the negative affect on the risk of mortality is not similar across racial groups. The current study uses data from a national study of Black and White older adults to examine racial differences in the effect of baseline depressive symptoms on mortality risk over three years in the United States. *Methods.* This study used a longitudinal prospective design and followed 1493 older adults who were either White ($n = 759$) or Black ($n = 734$) for three years from 2001 to 2004. Depressive symptoms measured at baseline was the independent variable. Demographic factors, socio-economic characteristics (education, income, marital status), health behaviors (smoking and drinking), and health (self-rated health) measured at baseline in 2001 were covariates. The dependent variable was all-cause mortality between 2001 and 2004. Race was the moderator. Logistic regressions were used for data analysis. *Results.* In the pooled sample, high depressive symptoms at baseline were not associated with the three-year risk of mortality. In the pooled sample, we found a significant interaction between race and depressive symptoms on mortality, suggesting a stronger effect for Whites in comparison to Blacks. In race stratified models, depressive symptoms at baseline were predictive of mortality risk for Whites, but not Blacks. *Conclusions.* In the United States, Black-White differences exist in the effects of depressive symptoms on mortality risk in older adults. White older adults may be more vulnerable to the effects of depressive symptoms on mortality risk.

Keywords: race; ethnic groups; African Americans; mortality; depression; depressive symptoms

1. Introduction

Psychosocial resources (e.g., education, income, employment, and marital status) and psychological assets (e.g., affect and coping) are essential for maintaining health and well-being [1,2]. Individuals with high levels of psychosocial risk factors are at a higher risk of poor health [3,4], physical functioning [5], chronic disease [6], and mortality [7]. Negative affect and depressive symptoms also increase the risk of mortality [8,9].

In a number of studies, race, ethnicity, and class have been found to alter the effects of psychosocial resources and assets on chronic disease [10] and health [11]. Race, ethnicity, and class also mitigate the effects of depression on physical health [12–19]. Racial and ethnic groups differ in separate [20] and combined [21] effects of depression and anxiety on obesity, [20–22] cardiovascular diseases (CVDs) [11,22–24], and well-being [12]. All this literature suggests that race and ethnicity operate as moderators for the effects of psychosocial factors on physical health outcomes [15–19,24–27].

Although Cooper et al. [28], Lewis et al. [11,23], Assari et al. [22,24,29], and Capistrant et al. [30] have all documented Black-White differences in the effect of depression on coronary artery disease

(CAD) and CAD risk factors, the results of these studies are inconsistent. Cooper et al. showed that among individuals with depression, comorbid Posttraumatic Stress Disorder (PTSD) was linked to a lower and higher risk of CAD for Whites and Blacks, respectively [28]. In a longitudinal study by Lewis et al., high depressive symptoms predicted CVD and stroke mortality for Blacks but not Whites [11]. In another prospective study by Capistrant et al., race did not modify the effect of depression on CVD mortality [30].

Racial differences are not specific to the effects of depressive symptoms [8,9,31–33] as similar patterns are shown for a wide range of other psychosocial factors such as mastery [33,34], sleep [35], and perceived health [36]. The effects of education [37], income [38], employment [39], neighborhood quality [40], and social network [41] are shown to be stronger for Whites than Blacks. It is, however, not only race, but also SES, that buffers the effects of these resources and assets on mortality [7]. As race and social class have a strong overlap [42], it is still unknown whether it is race or SES that moderates the effects of these risk and protective factors.

To replicate and extend the results of the previous studies, we conducted this study to compared Black and White older adults in the United States (USA) for the effects of depressive symptoms on the short-term risk of mortality over a three year period.

2. Methods

2.1. Design and Setting

Religion, Aging, and Health Survey, 2001–2004, was a longitudinal panel study of older adults in the United States with three years of follow-up. We used data from Wave 1 and Wave 2 of the panel study [43].

2.2. Ethics

The Religion, Aging, and Health Survey protocol was approved by the University of Michigan Institutional Review Board (IRB). All participants provided informed consent.

2.3. Participants

The current study only included Black or White older adults. The sample was limited to non-institutionalized, English-speaking individuals, 65 years old or older at the time of enrollment. The study sampling was restricted to the coterminous (not Contiguous) United States (i.e., not including Alaska and Hawaii). The study sample was limited to Christians or those who were never associated with any faith. The study oversampled Blacks, so almost half of the sample is Black [43].

2.4. Sampling Frame

The study used random sampling to recruit a national sample. The sampling frame consisted of all eligible individuals in the Medicare Beneficiary list that were maintained by the Centers for Medicare and Medicaid Services (CMS) at the time of survey in 2001 [44]. The study used a five-step sampling process to draw individuals from the CMS file.

2.5. Data Collection

Data were collected by Louis Harris and Associates (now Harris Interactive, New York, NY, USA). Wave 1 interviews were performed between March and August of 2001 [43].

2.6. Measures

Race, demographic factors (age and gender), SES (education, income, and marital status), depressive symptoms, health risk behaviors (smoking and drinking), and health (self-rated health) were measured at baseline in 2001.

Sociodemographic Factors. Demographic factors were age (continuous measure) and gender (1 female 0 male). Socioeconomic characteristics included educational level (high school diploma 1 lower education 0), marital status (married 1 versus others 0), and income of the respondent (10 level categorical variable). Higher scores were indicative of higher SES.

Health Behaviors. Data were collected on self-reported history of smoking and drinking. We used dichotomous variables for smoking (current smoker = 1, never or ex-smoker = 0) and drinking (1 = current drinker and 0 = non-drinker). Single-item measures were previously used to measure smoking and drinking [45].

Self-rated health (poor). Individuals were asked a single question: "How would you rate your overall health at the present time?" Response items included: (1) Excellent, (2) Good, (3) Fair, and (4) Poor. We dichotomized the responses to excellent to fair (0) or poor (1). This single-item measure has shown high reliability and validity for the prediction of all-cause mortality of adults.

Depressive Symptoms. An eight-item version of the Center for Epidemiological Studies-Depression scale (CES-D) [46] was used to measure depressive symptoms. Respondents were asked about their negative emotions such as (1) blues, (2) felt depressed, (3) crying spells, (4) feeling sad, (5) not feel like eating (poor appetite), (6) feeling that everything is an effort, (7) restless sleep, and (8) could not get going. These items measure the negative affect and somatic symptoms. The eight-item CES-D measure has shown acceptable reliability and validity [47] as compared to the original 20-item CES-D measure [48–50]. Response items ranged from "rarely or none" (score 1) to "most or all of the time" (score 4). A mean score was calculated with a potential range from 1 to 4. This measure was operationalized as a continuous measure, with a higher score indicating more depressive symptoms (Cronbach Alpha = 0.87 for all, 0.85 for Whites, 0.89 for Blacks).

Mortality. Mortality data were obtained through various sources including the national death index, the death certificate, and the informants. Mortality was operationalized as a dichotomous variable (1 deceased, 0 alive). Mortality during the three year follow-up period was considered regardless of its time and cause. From all 1493 participants, 208 individuals were deceased during the follow up period.

2.7. Statistical Analysis

We used SPSS 22.0 for data analysis. Mean (SD) and frequency tables were used to describe the sample overall, and by race. We used logistic regressions in the pooled sample, and specific to race, for our multivariable models. In all models, depressive symptoms were the independent variable. All-cause mortality over the three year follow up period was the dependent variable. Demographic factors, socio-economic characteristics, health risk behaviors, and health at baseline were the covariates. Race was the focal moderator. We reported odds ratios (OR), associated 95% confidence intervals (CIs), and p values. p values less than 0.05 were considered as statistically significant.

3. Results

3.1. Sample

The study followed 1493 individuals for three years. All participants were older adults (age 65 or older). This sample was either Black (n = 734) or White (n = 759). From the 1493 participants, 208 individuals were deceased during follow up. From all the individuals who were deceased over the follow up period, 112 (54%) were Black and 96 (46%) were White.

3.2. Descriptive Statistics

Table 1 summarizes the descriptive statistics at baseline for the overall sample, as well as based on race. While age was similar between Black and White individuals, Blacks and Whites differed in gender, as the Black sample had a higher composition of females than Whites. Black participants also had a lower education, lower income, and were less frequently married. Blacks were smokers more frequently than Whites. However, they were less likely to be a drinkers, compared to Whites. Compared to Whites, Blacks had poorer self-rated health. Depressive symptoms were also higher among Black than White participants.

Table 1. Descriptive statistics in the pooled sample and by race.

Characteristics	All (n = 1439)		Whites (n = 1439)		Blacks (n = 734)	
	Mean	SD	Mean	SD	Mean	SD
Age	75.14	6.67	75.37	6.82	74.91	6.49
Income *	4.59	2.49	5.63	2.49	3.49	1.96
Depressive Symptoms *	1.56	0.62	1.54	0.59	1.59	.65
	n	%	n	%	n	%
Gender *						
Male	573	38.20	314	41.37	256	34.88
Female	927	61.80	445	58.63	478	65.12
Education *						
Low	609	40.98	200	26.60	407	55.98
High	877	59.02	552	73.40	320	44.02
Married *						
No	778	52.28	306	40.53	467	64.33
Yes	710	47.72	449	59.47	259	35.67
Smoking *						
No	1342	89.59	698	92.08	638	87.04
Yes	156	10.41	60	7.92	95	12.96
Drinking *						
No	1030	68.76	451	59.50	574	78.31
Yes	468	31.24	307	40.50	159	21.69
SRH Poor *						
No	1322	88.37	694	91.80	622	84.86
Yes	174	11.63	62	8.20	111	15.14

Source: Religion, Aging, and Health Survey, 2001–2004. * $p < 0.05$.

3.3. Models in the Pooled Sample

Table 2 shows the results of two logistic regressions in the pooled sample. While depressive symptoms were not a predictor of mortality in the pooled sample (*Model 1*), we found a significant interaction between race and depressive symptoms on mortality, suggesting a larger effect of depressive symptoms on mortality for Whites, compared to Blacks (*Model 2*).

Table 2. Association between baseline depressive symptoms (2001) and all-cause mortality (2001–2004) using logistic regression in the pooled sample (n = 1439).

Characteristics	All (n = 1439) Model 2		All (n = 1439) Model 1	
	OR	95% CI	OR	95% CI
Race (Black)	0.96	0.63–1.47	2.37	0.83–6.73
Age	1.07 ***	1.05–1.10	1.07 ***	1.05–1.10
Gender (Female)	0.61 *	0.40–0.94	0.62 *	0.40–0.96
Education	1.46 #	0.94–2.27	1.47 #	0.95–2.28
Marital Status (Married)	0.83	0.52–1.31	0.84	0.53–1.32
Income	0.92	0.83–1.03	0.93	0.83–1.03
Smoking	0.80	0.43–1.49	0.83	0.45–1.56
Drinking	0.81	0.51–1.29	0.84	0.53–1.34
Self-Rated Health (SRH)	3.96 ***	2.40–6.52	4.12 ***	2.50–6.80
Depressive Symptoms	1.18	0.87–1.58	1.58 *	1.03–2.42
Depressive Symptoms × race (Black)	-	-	0.59 *	0.34–1.00
Intercept	0.00 ***		0.00 ***	

Source: Religion, Aging, and Health Survey, 2001–2004. # $p < 0.1$, * $p < 0.05$, ** $p < 0.01$, *** $p < 0.001$.

3.4. Models by Race

Table 3 summarizes the results of two race-specific models to estimate the association between depressive symptoms and the subsequent risk of mortality among Blacks and Whites. *Model 3* showed that, in Whites, depressive symptoms at baseline were associated with an increased risk of mortality. *Model 4*, however, showed that this association could not be found for Blacks.

Table 3. Association between baseline depressive symptoms (2001) and all-cause mortality (2001–2004) using logistic regression among Whites (*n* = 759) and Blacks (*n* = 734).

Characteristics	Whites (*n* = 759) Model 3		Blacks (*n* = 734) Model 4	
	OR	95% CI	OR	95% CI
Age	1.08 **	1.04–1.12	1.08 **	1.03–1.12
Gender (Female)	0.70	0.38–1.30	0.56 #	0.30–1.03
Education	1.11	0.58–2.10	1.89 *	1.04–3.41
Marital Status (Married)	0.91	0.48–1.72	0.79	0.41–1.52
Income	0.93	0.81–1.07	0.95	0.80–1.12
Smoking	1.60	0.67–3.86	0.49	0.19–1.25
Drinking	0.95	0.51–1.77	0.73	0.35–1.51
Self-Rated Health (SRH)	2.54 *	1.17–5.53	5.98 **	3.05–11.72
Depressive Symptoms	1.74 *	1.12–2.68	0.87	0.57–1.34
Intercept	0.00 **		0.00 **	

Source: Religion, Aging, and Health Survey, 2001–2004. # $p < 0.1$, * $p < 0.05$, ** $p < 0.001$.

4. Discussion

The current study had two findings. Based on the first finding, baseline depressive symptoms did not predict the three-year mortality risk for older adults in the overall sample. Based on our second finding, however, race altered this association. High depressive symptoms at baseline increased the short-term risk of mortality for White but not Black older adults. The second finding replicates some recent findings on other cohorts, age groups, and follow up durations [8,9,51].

In a 25-year follow up study of Black and White adults, [8] high depressive symptoms at baseline were predictive of mortality risk for Whites but not Blacks [8]. The same pattern is shown for the effects of depressive symptoms and anger on mortality due to heart disease [9] and renal disease [51]. This is not because our tools do not correctly measure depressive symptoms in Blacks [52,53]. It is possible because Blacks who are depressed maintain high levels of positive emotions that can potentially undo the harmful physiological effects of negative affect [54,55].

Depressive symptoms [56] and neuroticism [57] predict long-term risk of MDD for Whites, but not Blacks. Black-White differences in the predictive role of negative affect on future risk of MDD suggests that a single measurement of negative affect is not sufficient to evaluate the future risk of MDD for Black individuals. Depressive symptoms and neuroticism, however, reflect the future risk of depression for Whites very well [56,57].

Racial and ethnic differential effects are not limited to the effects of depression. In line with findings on negative affect [8,9,31–33], health effects of mastery [33,34], sleep [35], and perceived health [36] are all larger for Whites, compared to Blacks. The same pattern also holds for the health effects of education [37], income [38], employment [39], neighborhood quality [40], and social network [41], which are all larger for Whites than Blacks. These findings collectively suggest that the health effects of psychosocial factors are not universal across all racial groups, and may be race-specific.

The above differential effects align with the Minorities' Diminished Return Theory [58,59], defined as smaller health effects of economic resources and psychological assets for the minority compared to the majority population. Given that existing racism adds societal barriers to the lives of minority individuals, the very same resources and assets (and lack thereof) show smaller effects on the lives of Blacks than Whites. Blacks experience a decline in health regardless of their baseline mental health [60], Blacks develop MDD regardless of their previous depressive symptoms [56,57], and Blacks develop poor health outcomes regardless of their economic status [38,61–63]. These should be seen as a systemic inequality in health gain from resources and assets [58,59]. Unless these differential gains are addressed, the existing racial gap between the health of Blacks and Whites may widen.

Limitations

Our study had a few limitations. First, the database was old, dating from 2001–2004. However, the results are in line with other studies that have used more recent data [8,9,51]. Demographic and socio-political changes are extremely important, and impact findings related to race and minority status. Second, the validity of depressive symptoms and negative affect may depend upon race. In addition, the current study failed to control for some important confounders such as baseline medical conditions, stress, and access to and use of health care. Finally, the study only included Blacks and Whites. Future research should include other racial groups. A major strength of this study was the enrollment of a national sample.

5. Conclusions

In summary, depressive symptoms increase the risk of mortality over a three-year period in White but not Black older adults. This finding is in line with other psychosocial constructs showing health effects that are not universal but specific to race. This finding also has implications for healthcare and public health.

Acknowledgments: Shervin Assari is supported by the Heinz C. Prechter Bipolar Research Fund and the Richard Tam Foundation at the University of Michigan Depression Center. The Religion, Aging, and Health Survey was supported by the National Institute on Aging (PI: Neal Krause; R01 AG014749), and per the NIH Public Access Policy requires that peer-reviewed research publications generated with NIH support are made available to the public through PubMed Central. Data were accessed through the Interuniversity Consortium for Political and Social Research (ICPSR), Institute of Social Research, University of Michigan.

References

1. Ross, C.; Sastry, J. The sense of personal control: Social-structural causes and emotional consequences. In *Handbook of the Sociology of Mental Health*; Aneshensel, C.S., Phelan, J.C., Eds.; Kluwer Academic/Plenum: New York, NY, USA, 1999; pp. 369–394.
2. Lachman, M.E.; Neupert, S.D.; Agrigoroaei, S. The relevance of control beliefs for health and aging. In *Handbook of the Psychology of Aging*; Schaie, K.W., Willis, S.L., Eds.; Elsevier: New York, NY, USA, 2011; pp. 175–190.
3. Mirowsky, J.; Ross, C.E. Well-being across the life course. In *A Handbook for the Study of Mental Health: Social Contexts, Theories, and Systems*; Horwitz, A.V., Scheid, T.L., Eds.; Cambridge University Press: New York, NY, USA, 1999; pp. 328–347.
4. Keeton, C.P.; Perry-Jenkins, M.; Sayer, A.G. Sense of control predicts depressive and anxious symptoms across the transition to parenthood. *J. Fam. Psychol.* **2008**, *22*, 212–221. [CrossRef] [PubMed]
5. Infurna, F.J.; Gerstorf, D.; Zarit, S.H. Examining dynamic links between perceived control and health: Longitudinal evidence for differential effects in midlife and old age. *Dev. Psychol.* **2011**, *47*, 9–18. [CrossRef] [PubMed]
6. Surtees, P.G.; Wainwright, W.J.; Luben, R.; Wareham, N.J.; Bingham, S.; Khaw, K.T. Mastery is associated with cardiovascular disease mortality in men and women at apparently low risk. *Health Psychol.* **2010**, *29*, 412–420. [CrossRef] [PubMed]
7. Turiano, N.A.; Chapman, B.P.; Agrigoroaei, S.; Infurna, F.J.; Lachman, M. Perceived control reduces mortality risk at low, not high, education levels. *Health Psychol.* **2014**, *33*, 883–890. [CrossRef] [PubMed]
8. Assari, S.; Moazen-Zadeh, E.; Lankarani, M.M.; Micol-Foster, V. Race, Depressive Symptoms, and All-Cause Mortality in the United States. *Front. Public Health* **2016**, *4*, 40. [CrossRef] [PubMed]

9. Assari, S. Hostility, Anger, and Cardiovascular Mortality among Blacks and Whites. *Res. Cardiovasc. Med.* **2017**, *6*. [CrossRef]

10. Assari, S. Race and Ethnic Differences in Additive and Multiplicative Effects of Depression and Anxiety on Cardiovascular Risk. *Int. J. Prev. Med.* **2016**, *7*, 22. [CrossRef] [PubMed]

11. Lewis, T.T.; Guo, H.; Lunos, S.; Mendes de Leon, C.F.; Skarupski, K.A.; Evans, D.A.; Everson-Rose, S.A. Depressive symptoms and cardiovascular mortality in older black and white adults: Evidence for a differential association by race. *Circ. Cardiovasc. Qual. Outcomes* **2011**, *4*, 293–299. [CrossRef] [PubMed]

12. Assari, S. Separate and combined effects of anxiety, depression and problem drinking on subjective health among black, Hispanic and non-Hispanic white men. *Int. J. Prev. Med.* **2014**, *5*, 269–279. [PubMed]

13. Assari, S.; Lankarani, M.M.; Lankarani, R.M. Ethnicity modifies the additive effects of anxiety and drug use disorders on suicidal ideation among black adults in the United States. *Int. J. Prev. Med.* **2013**, *4*, 1251–1257. [PubMed]

14. Assari, S. Synergistic effects of lifetime psychiatric disorders on suicidal ideation among blacks in the USA. *J. Racial Ethn. Health Disparities* **2014**, *1*, 275–282. [CrossRef]

15. Assari, S. The link between mental health and obesity: Role of individual and contextual factors. *Int. J. Prev. Med.* **2014**, *5*, 247–249. [PubMed]

16. Assari, S. Chronic medical conditions and major depressive disorder: Differential role of positive religious coping among African Americans, Caribbean blacks and non-Hispanic whites. *Int. J. Prev. Med.* **2014**, *5*, 405–413. [PubMed]

17. Assari, S. Race and ethnicity, religion involvement, church-based social support and subjective health in United States: A case of moderated mediation. *Int. J. Prev. Med.* **2013**, *4*, 208–217. [PubMed]

18. Krok-Schoen, J.L.; Baker, T.A. Race differences in personality and affect between older white and black patients: An exploratory study. *J. Racial Ethn. Health Disparities* **2014**, *1*, 283–290. [CrossRef]

19. Bruce, M.A.; Beech, B.M.; Hamilton, G.E.; Collins, S.M. Knowledge and perceptions about clinical trial participation among African American and Caucasian College Students. *J. Racial Ethn. Health Disparities* **2014**, *1*, 337–342. [CrossRef]

20. Assari, S. Association between obesity and depression among American blacks: Role of ethnicity and gender. *J. Racial Ethn. Health Disparities* **2014**, *1*, 36–44. [CrossRef]

21. Assari, S. Additive effects of anxiety and depression on body mass index among blacks: Role of ethnicity and gender. *Int. Cardiovasc. Res. J.* **2014**, *8*, 44–51. [PubMed]

22. Assari, S.; Caldwell, C.H. Gender and ethnic differences in the association between obesity and depression among black adolescents. *J. Racial Ethn. Health Disparities* **2015**, *2*, 481–493. [CrossRef] [PubMed]

23. Lewis, T.T.; Everson-Rose, S.A.; Colvin, A.; Matthews, K.; Bromberger, J.T.; Sutton-Tyrrell, K. Interactive effects of race and depressive symptoms on calcification in African American and white women. *Psychosom. Med.* **2009**, *71*, 163–170. [CrossRef] [PubMed]

24. Assari, S. Race and ethnic differences in associations between cardiovascular diseases, anxiety, and depression in the United States. *Int. J. Travel Med. Glob. Health* **2014**, *2*, 103–109.

25. Wysocki, J.; Newby, C.; Balart, L.; Shores, N. HCV triple therapy is equally effective in African-Americans and Non-African-Americans. *J. Racial Ethn. Health Disparities* **2014**, *1*, 319–325. [CrossRef]

26. Insaf, T.Z.; Shaw, B.A.; Yucel, R.M.; Chasan-Taber, L.; Strogatz, D.S. Lifecourse Socioeconomic Position and Racial Disparities in BMI Trajectories among Black and White Women: Exploring Cohort Effects in the Americans Changing Lives' Study. *J. Racial Ethn. Health Disparities* **2014**, *1*, 309–318. [CrossRef] [PubMed]

27. Hicken, M.T.; Lee, H.; Mezuk, B.; Kershaw, K.N.; Rafferty, J.; Jackson, J.S. Racial and ethnic differences in the association between obesity and depression in women. *J. Women's Health* **2013**, *22*, 445–452. [CrossRef] [PubMed]

28. Cooper, D.C.; Trivedi, R.B.; Nelson, K.M.; Reiber, G.E.; Beaver, K.A.; Eugenio, E.C.; Fan, V.S. Post-traumatic Stress Disorder, Race/Ethnicity, and Coronary Artery Disease among Older Patients with Depression. *J. Racial Ethn. Health Disparities* **2014**, *1*, 163–170. [CrossRef]

29. Assari, S.; Sonnega, A. Racial Differences in the Predictive Role of High. Depressive Symptoms on Incident Heart Disease over 18 Years: Results from the Health and Retirement Study. *Res. Cardiovasc. Med.* **2017**, *6*. [CrossRef]

30. Capistrant, B.D.; Gilsanz, P.; Moon, J.R.; Kosheleva, A.; Patton, K.K.; Glymour, M.M. Does the association between depressive symptoms and cardiovascular mortality risk vary by race? Evidence from the Health and Retirement Study. *Ethn. Dis.* **2013**, *23*, 155–160. [PubMed]

31. Assari, S.; Lankarani, M.M.; Burgard, S.A. Black White Difference in Long Term Predictive Power of Self-Rated Health on All-Cause Mortality in United States. *Ann. Epidemiol.* **2016**, *26*, 106–114. [CrossRef] [PubMed]

32. Assari, S.; Burgard, S.A.; Zivin, K. Long Term Reciprocal Associations between Depression and Chronic Medical Conditions; Longitudinal Support for Black-White Health Paradox. *J. Racial Ethn. Health Disparities* **2015**, *2*, 589–597. [CrossRef] [PubMed]

33. Assari, S.; Lankarani, M.M. Chronic Medical Conditions and Negative Affect; Racial Variation in Reciprocal Associations over Time. *Front. Psychiatry* **2016**, *24*, 140. [CrossRef] [PubMed]

34. Assari, S. Race, sense of control over life, and short-term risk of mortality among older adults in the United States. *Arch. Med. Sci.* **2017**, *13*, 1233–1240. [CrossRef] [PubMed]

35. Assari, S.; Sonnega, A.; Leggett, A.; Pepin, R.L. Residual Effects of Restless Sleep over Depressive Symptoms on Chronic Medical Conditions: Race by Gender Differences. *J. Racial Ethn. Health Disparities* **2017**, *4*, 59–69. [CrossRef] [PubMed]

36. Assari, S. General Self-Efficacy and Mortality in the USA; Racial Differences. *J. Racial Ethn. Health Disparities* **2017**, *4*, 746–757. [CrossRef] [PubMed]

37. Assari, S.; Lankarani, M.M. Race and Urbanity Alter the Protective Effect of Education but not Income on Mortality. *Front. Public Health* **2016**, *4*, 100. [CrossRef] [PubMed]

38. Assari, S. The Benefits of Higher Income in Protecting against Chronic Medical Conditions Are Smaller for African Americans than Whites. *Healthcare* **2018**, *6*, 2. [CrossRef] [PubMed]

39. Assari, S.; Assari, S. Life Expectancy Gain Due to Employment Status Depends on Race, Gender, Education, and Their Intersections. *J. Racial Ethn. Health Disparities* **2018**, *5*, 375–386. [CrossRef] [PubMed]

40. Assari, S. Perceived Neighborhood Safety Better Predicts 25-year Mortality Risk among Whites than Blacks. *J. Racial Ethn. Health Disparities* **2016**. [CrossRef]

41. Assari, S. Whites but Not Blacks Gain Life Expectancy from Social Contacts. *Behav. Sci.* **2017**, *74*, 68. [CrossRef] [PubMed]

42. Drake, K.A.; Galanter, J.M.; Burchard, E.G. Race, ethnicity and social class and the complex etiologies of asthma. *Pharmacogenomics* **2008**, *9*, 453–462. [CrossRef] [PubMed]

43. Krause, N. *Religion, Aging, and Health Survey, 2001, 2004 [United States] ICPSR03255-v2*; Inter-university Consortium for Political and Social Research: Ann Arbor, MI, USA, 2006; Available online: http://doi.org/10.3886/ICPSR03255.v2 (accessed on 20 February 2018).

44. Centers for Medicare & Medicaid Services. Medicare Beneficiary Characteristics. Available online: https://www.cms.gov/Research-Statistics-Data-and-Systems/Statistics-Trends-and-Reports/Chronic-Conditions/Medicare_Beneficiary_Characteristics.html (accessed on 20 February 2018).

45. Harvey, I.S.; Alexander, K. Perceived social support and preventive health behavioral outcomes among older women. *J. Cross Cult. Gerontol.* **2012**, *27*, 275–290. [CrossRef] [PubMed]

46. Radloff, L.S. The CES-D scale: A self-report depression scale for research in the general population. *Appl. Psychol. Meas.* **1977**, *1*, 385–401. [CrossRef]

47. Van de Velde, S.; Levecque, K.; Bracke, P. Measurement equivalence of the CES-D 8 in the general population in Belgium: A gender perspective. *Arch. Public Health* **2009**, *67*, 15. [CrossRef]

48. Amtmann, D.; Kim, J.; Chung, H.; Bamer, A.M.; Askew, R.L.; Wu, S.; Cook, K.F.; Johnson, K.L. Comparing CESD-10, PHQ-9, and PROMIS depression instruments in individuals with multiple sclerosis. *Rehabil. Psychol.* **2014**, *59*, 220–229. [CrossRef] [PubMed]

49. Andresen, E.M.; Malmgren, J.A.; Carter, W.B.; Patrick, D.L. Screening for depression in well older adults: Evaluation of a short form of the CES-D (center for epidemiologic studies depression scale). *Am. J. Prev. Med.* **1994**, *10*, 77–84. [CrossRef]

50. Zhang, W.; O'Brien, N.; Forrest, J.I.; Salters, K.A.; Patterson, T.L.; Montaner, J.S.; Hogg, R.S.; Lima, V.D. Validating a shortened depression scale (10 item CES-D) among HIV-positive people in British Columbia, Canada. *PLoS ONE* **2012**, *7*, e40793. [CrossRef] [PubMed]

51.   Assari, S.; Burgard, S.A. Black-White differences in the effect of baseline depressive symptoms on deaths due to renal diseases: 25 year follow up of a nationally representative community sample. *J. Renal Inj. Prev.* **2015**, *4*, 127–134. [PubMed]

52.   Assari, S.; Moazen-Zadeh, E. Confirmatory Factor Analysis of the 12-Item Center for Epidemiologic Studies Depression Scale among Blacks and Whites. *Front. Psychiatry* **2016**, *7*, 178. [CrossRef] [PubMed]

53.   Assari, S.; Moazen-Zadeh, E. Ethnic Variation in the Cross-sectional Association between Domains of Depressive Symptoms and Clinical Depression. *Front. Psychiatry* **2016**, *7*, 53. [CrossRef] [PubMed]

54.   Lankarani, M.M.; Assari, S. Positive and Negative Affect More Concurrent among Blacks than Whites. *Behav. Sci.* **2017**, *7*, 48. [CrossRef] [PubMed]

55.   Assari, S.; Lankarani, M.M. Depressive Symptoms Are Associated with More Hopelessness among White than Black Older Adults. *Front. Public Health* **2016**, *4*, 82. [CrossRef] [PubMed]

56.   Moazen-Zadeh, E.; Assari, S. Depressive Symptoms Predict Major Depressive Disorder after 15 Years among Whites but Not Blacks. *Front. Public Health* **2016**, *4*, 13. [CrossRef] [PubMed]

57.   Assari, S. Neuroticism Predicts Subsequent Risk of Major Depression for Whites but Not Blacks. *Behav. Sci.* **2017**, *7*, 64. [CrossRef] [PubMed]

58.   Assari, S. Unequal Gain of Equal Resources across Racial Groups. *Int. J. Health Policy Manag.* **2017**, *7*, 1–9. [CrossRef] [PubMed]

59.   Assari, S. Health disparities due to diminished return among black Americans: Public policy solutions. *Soc. Issues Policy Rev.* **2018**, *12*, 112–145. [CrossRef]

60.   Assari, S.; Burgard, S.; Zivin, K. Long-Term Reciprocal Associations between Depressive Symptoms and Number of Chronic Medical Conditions: Longitudinal Support for Black-White Health Paradox. *J. Racial Ethn. Health Disparities* **2015**, *2*, 589–597. [CrossRef] [PubMed]

61.   Assari, S. Combined Racial and Gender Differences in the Long-Term Predictive Role of Education on Depressive Symptoms and Chronic Medical Conditions. *J. Racial Ethn. Health Disparities* **2017**, *4*, 385–396. [CrossRef] [PubMed]

62.   Assari, S. Social Determinants of Depression: The Intersections of Race, Gender, and Socioeconomic Status. *Brain Sci.* **2017**, *7*, 156. [CrossRef] [PubMed]

63.   Assari, S.; Nikahd, A.; Malekahmadi, M.R.; Lankarani, M.M.; Zamanian, H. Race by Gender Group Differences in the Protective Effects of Socioeconomic Factors against Sustained Health Problems across Five Domains. *J. Racial Ethn. Health Disparities* **2017**, *4*, 884–894. [CrossRef] [PubMed]

## 4

Striking a Balance: A Qualitative Study of Next of Kin Participation in the Care of Older Persons in Nursing Homes in Sweden

Birgitta Wallerstedt [1], Lina Behm [2], Åsa Alftberg [3], Anna Sandgren [1] (iD), Eva Benzein [1],
Per Nilsen [4] and Gerd Ahlström [2,*] (iD)

[1] Center for Collaborative Palliative Care, Department of Health and Caring Sciences,
Faculty of Health and Life Sciences, Linnaeus University, SE-351 95 Växjö, Sweden;
birgitta.wallerstedt@lnu.se (B.W.); anna.sandgren@lnu.se (A.S.); eva.benzein@lnu.se (E.B.)

[2] Department of Health Sciences, Faculty of Medicine, Lund University, SE-221 00 Lund, Sweden;
lina.behm@med.lu.se

[3] Department of Social Work, Faculty of Health and Society, Malmö University, SE-205 06 Malmö, Sweden;
asa.alftberg@mah.se

[4] Department of Medical and Health Sciences, Linköping University, SE-581 83 Linköping, Sweden;
per.nilsen@liu.se

* Correspondence: gerd.ahlstrom@med.lu.se

Abstract: Most of the care in nursing homes is palliative in nature, as it is the oldest and the frailest people who live in nursing homes. The aim of this study was to explore next of kin's experiences of participating in the care of older persons at nursing homes. A qualitative design was used, based on semi-structured interviews with 40 next of kin, and analyzed using qualitative content analysis. An overarching theme emerged, a balancing act consisting of three categories: (1) visiting the nursing home; (2) building and maintaining relationships; and (3) gathering and conveying information. The next of kin have to balance their own responsibility for the older person's wellbeing by taking part in their care and their need to leave the responsibility to the staff due to critical health conditions. The next of kin wanted to participate in care meetings and conversations, not only in practical issues. The findings indicate the need to improve the next of kin's participation in the care as an equal partner. Increased knowledge about palliative care and decision-making of limiting life-prolonging treatment may lead to a higher quality of care.

Keywords: end-of-life care; family member; involvement; life-limiting disease; next of kin; palliative care; participation; sheltered housing; significant others; relatives

1. Introduction

Assisting an older person in moving into a nursing home is a challenge for the next of kin [1–3]. It often involves mixed feelings of guilt, relief, and remorse [4,5]. In the nursing home setting, the relationships between the elderly and their next of kin may alter to a great extent [6]. Not only the move in itself, but also the continually declining health of the older person contributes to this change [7].

The current policy in the Swedish welfare system for caring for older people is "Aging in place", which means that older people remain living in their own homes for as long as possible, even when they are in need of health care due to illness and multi-morbidity. The view behind this policy is that older people prefer this care model as it enables them to maintain their independence, autonomy, and connection with their family and friends [8,9]. It is also favored by policymakers since this policy avoids the costly option of institutional care [10]. According to "aging in place", the Swedish policy is applied even in nursing homes where old people live in a small apartment with their own leasing contract. The right to an apartment in a nursing home is based on the older person's need for everyday care around the clock. This typically happens when the resident is too ill and frail to continue living in their own home or when there are no next of kin available to be a care provider [2,11]. Forty-nine percent of all people over 64 years of age who died in Sweden during 2016 were living in a nursing or group home [12]. This means that nursing homes are a workplace for assistant nurses and nurses involved in the care of the dying.

The literature shows that most of the care in nursing homes is palliative in nature. Research on palliative care in nursing homes is often descriptive and there is great interest in applying palliative care principles. However, there are relatively few published studies on palliative care interventions in a nursing home setting [13]. It is also important to focus on next of kin satisfaction with the care offered in nursing homes as they fill an important role for older persons since they participate in or are sometimes needed to take over the decision-making process when the older person's health deteriorates. After the person has died, they will live on with the memories. Next of kin participation in their care can make it easier for the physician to know if the wish of the next of kin is not to pursue a pointless extension of life or if the opposite is the case, i.e., the older person wishes to live as long as possible [14]. Studies show that resuscitation and hospitalization for older relatives are the issues most discussed, often shortly after admission to a nursing home. This generally results in a do-not-resuscitate and a do-not-hospitalize agreement [13,14].

The implementation of palliative care in nursing homes to a higher degree can be difficult because few next of kin are familiar with the term palliative care, which can be seen in a descriptive study about the use of an Advanced Care Plan (ACP) with 20 next of kin to people with dementia [14]. ACP is a process of discussion between the older person, the next of kin, the physician, the registered nurse, and assistant nurse in order to ensure the families' wishes and preferences are taken into account. However, ACP is rarely used in nursing homes, and decision-making in palliative care may therefore lead to conflict between the staff and next of kin [15]. Another barrier causing delayed decisions regarding treatment and care are the different views within the family or between the family and the physician and other staff [14].

A considerable barrier is the lack of education provided for professionals regarding knowledge and training in the principals of palliative care [16]. Recognition of this barrier provided the impetus for the present research project, which involved the provision of educational intervention concerning knowledge-based palliative care for nursing home staff and managers. The intervention consisted of five seminars over six months for staff and managers at 20 nursing homes in two counties in Sweden [11]. The intervention was evaluated using a non-randomized experimental design with intervention and control groups as well as pre- and post-assessments [11,17]. This study provided a baseline investigation before the implementation of the principles of palliative care in nursing homes by means of the educational intervention, with the intention of achieving the best possible palliative care while at the same time involving the older persons and their next of kin in the care process. Thus, this study explored the next of kin's experiences participating in the care of older persons residing in nursing homes.

2. Materials and Methods

2.1. Study Design

The study consisted of an explorative qualitative design based on semi-structured interviews with the next of kin, which were analyzed using qualitative content analysis [18,19].

2.2. Sample

The next of kin were selected from two counties in the south of Sweden that are involved in the Implementation of Knowledge-Based Palliative Care for Frail Older Persons in Nursing Homes project (acronym: KUPA project from Swedish: KUnskapsbaserad PAlliativ vård [11]). The nursing homes consisted of both larger (≥100 older persons) and smaller (<25 older persons) nursing homes situated in both urban and rural areas in both counties. The participants of this study were recruited from 20 nursing homes in each of the two counties. The distribution of participants per nursing home was related to the size of the accommodation, from four participants in a large nursing home to one participant in a small one. The inclusion criteria were to be a next of kin to an older person living in a nursing home who often visited that person, and to be able to speak and understand Swedish. Forty next of kin were invited to participate in the study and all chose to participate in the interview. The contact person primarily asked those next of kin who frequently visited the nursing home and had a close relation with the older person.

2.3. The Procedure of the Data Collection

The next of kin were selected by a contact person (a nurse assistant, a manager, or an administrator) at each of the nursing homes according to the inclusion criteria stated above. The contact person informed the next of kin about the study and then asked if they were interested in participating. If positive, the contact person passed on the name and telephone number of the participant to the researchers, who contacted them by telephone informing them once again about the study and asking them to confirm their interest in participating. Following this, a time and place for an interview were determined according to the next of kin's wishes. Before the interview began, oral and written information about the study was offered once again and written consent was provided. The interviews were performed at a place chosen by the next of kin (e.g., a conference room at the nursing home or in the next of kin's private home).

2.4. Interviews with the Next of Kin

The interviews were performed in a similar manner by four researchers, all of whom were registered nurses with a long experience of working with older persons as well as conducting research interviews. The interviews were based on a semi-structured interview guide about the ways the next of kin participated in the care, how they would like to participate, if they experienced any obstacles for participation, and what information they had received about palliative care (only asked if there was relevance for this question). These questions were related to the focus in the KUPA project described earlier.

After the opening question, "In what ways do you participate in the care of your relative at the nursing home?", follow-up questions were asked. The number and formulation of the follow-up questions depended on the richness of the participant's initial answers, and were expressed as: "Could you tell me more about your experiences?", "What did you think in that situation?", and "What did you do in that situation?" The interviews were conducted from April 2015 to May 2016 and ranged between 8 and 77 min (median 41 and mean 42 min). All interviews were audio recorded and transcribed verbatim.

2.5. Data Analysis

The data were analyzed using qualitative content analysis, which is a method used to identify categories and themes through a systematic process of coding data based on an interpretation of the content of a text [19]. A stepwise methodological approach described by Graneheim and Lundman [18] was applied, using NVIVO 11 [20] to code the data. The analysis was conducted by the first and second authors (Birgitta Wallerstedt, Lina Behm) The first step was to read the transcribed interviews several times in order to obtain an overall impression of its content regarding participation. In the second step, meaning units were identified; in the third step, they were condensed into shorter units in NVIVO (QSR International Pty Ltd, Doncaster, Victoria, Australia). In the fourth step, a preliminary interpretation of the underlying meaning was expressed in terms of codes. These steps were conducted separately by the first (Birgitta Wallerstedt) and second authors (Lina Behm). with 20 interviews each. In the fifth step, the two authors discussed together and sorted all of the codes into tentative sub-categories and categories related to the aim. In the sixth step, all authors discussed the tentative theme and categories until consensus was reached and the theme, categories, and sub-categories were established (Table 1). Selected quotations were used to illustrate the findings. The COREQ (COnsolidated criteria for REporting Qualitative research) 32-item checklist [21] was used as a guide for the reporting of the study.

Table 1. Characteristics of the participating next of kin (n = 40).

Characteristics	No.	%
Age, years		
40–49	1	2.5
50–59	11	27.5
60–69	18	45
70–79	8	20
80–89	2	5
Gender		
Men	10	25
Women	30	75
Marital status		
Married/living together	32	80
Unmarried/divorced	6	15
Widower/widow	2	5
Relation to the old person		
Husband/wife	7	17.5
Daughter/son	31	77.5
Sibling	1	2.5
Other	1	2.5
Educational level *		
Elementary school	9	25
High school	8	22
Trade school	4	11
University/college	15	42
Work status		
Full time	13	32.5
Part time	9	22.5
Not working	18	45
The frequency of visits to the old person		
Every day	6	15
Weekly	31	77.5
Monthly	2	5
Yearly	1	2.5

* Four people were missing this information.

2.6. Ethical Considerations

This study is part of the KUPA project approved by the Regional Ethics Review Board in Lund, Sweden (No. 2015/69), and with trial registration: NCT02708498. The research project is guided by the ethical principles for medical research (the Declaration of Helsinki). The participants' confidentiality was taken into account when reporting the findings that had been done at a group level. Information related to the next of kin having the right to withdraw from the study at any time without suffering any consequences was given before each interview and written informed consent was received from each participant.

3. Results

The participation by the next of kin in the care of the old person in a nursing home was presented as one theme, three categories, and nine sub-categories. An overarching theme emerged from the analysis: a balancing act. This theme describes how the next of kin tried to balance their own sense of responsibility for the old person's wellbeing by taking part in the care with their need to also leave the responsibility to the staff. The three categories comprising the theme are: visiting at the nursing home, building and maintaining relationships, and gathering and conveying information (Table 2).

Many of the next of kin described their participation in care as a routine, often having been involved in different ways for many years when the person was still living at home. Even as a routine, they had to balance their engagement in relation to their other duties and tasks in daily life. Some expressed that they wanted to participate in the care processes because of their close relation to the older person; others indicated that they did not participate at all. However, the majority were involved in the care of the old person in some way.

Table 2. The result presented in theme, categories, and sub-categories.

Theme	Category	Sub-Category
The balancing act (between having and leaving responsibility)	Visiting the nursing home	Helping with practicalities Helping with private matters Enabling activity Controlling and supervising the care
	Building and maintaining relationships	The care relationship The private relationship Adapting to new roles
	Gathering and conveying information	Having dialogue with the staff Calling and writing letters

3.1. Visiting the Nursing Home

One practical effort was to visit the nursing home. The visits were expressed as more or less frequent, alone, or together with the other parent, siblings, children, or grandchildren. Full-time work or a long distance to travel to the nursing home as well as eventual personal disability were factors that affected the possibility of visiting the old person. Other participants noted that it was all about how to prioritize.

The visits had both positive and negative aspects. It was satisfying to talk to and socialize with the old person and make sure that they felt satisfied, but there was also concern over the old person's condition and the feelings in relation to the situation, e.g., their own sadness over a deteriorating state.

And she remembers us and is very pleased when we visit which in some ways helps one to cope and helps provides the energy required to make the effort to visit her. Sometimes one can feel quite exhausted when it is time to leave (Daughter, 57 years).

3.1.1. Helping with Practicalities

An important reason for participating in the care was to make sure that everything worked well for the old person in the nursing home. One participant compared it to having two jobs at the same time. If it was impossible for the next of kin to visit, some engaged others to replace them. During a visit, the next of kin could help with, for example, pushing the older person's wheel-chair to the dining room, feeding, or to take the old person outside for some fresh air. Another practicality was being able to transport the old person to different appointments such as a visit to the doctor or dentist. Several next of kin used their own car to provide more comfort. Often older people feel more secure when being accompanied to outside appointments.

In the last few years I have been following my mother to every doctor's visit. She sees and hears badly and I have supported her and have been acting as her "memory" too. Then I have to drive her by car to and from visits when she has been able to walk with walker (Daughter, 68 years).

3.1.2. Helping with Private Matters

The next of kin also participated in matters of hygiene such as helping the old person to the toilet or to take a shower. Other ways of participation were doing the older person's laundry and buying clothes for them, and further handling other private things where necessary, sometimes together with the old person. Some next of kin took responsibility for the older person's paperwork, finances, and contacts with authorities. Visits to the bank could be accomplished with the help of a next of kin, for errands such as preparing their will. Cleaning the room was sometimes seen as a responsibility for the participants who also made the effort to make the room as home-like as possible.

They have a lot of photographs and pictures on the walls and shelves. And I . . . I had said to the staff at an early stage that we have no requirement towards them that they should dust or clean these items; we will do that ourselves (Daughter, 68 years).

3.1.3. Enabling Activity

Some next of kin participated in social gatherings together with the old person on a regular basis but also suggested and arranged their own activities at the nursing home. To take the older person to their home or that of one of their children is an excellent way to reduce the risk that the old person should be institutionalized. For example, being able to visit a church could be very important for some residents. Another way to participate was to take responsibility for the more frequent training of the old person's remaining abilities, for example, walking, when this was not organized by the staff. One next of kin brought an exercise bike to a nursing home where no rehab training was offered.

When father came here, he came directly from rehab after he had been fitted with his first prosthesis. They had trained him enough so that he could walk quite well. He should train continually to keep him going. However, no training was available here so he lost his ability (Daughter, 68 years).

3.1.4. Controlling and Supervising the Care

Knowing that help, support, and nutritious food were offered at the nursing home around the clock and that acute situations were handled without delay created a sense of security for everyone. It required the staff's sensitivity, understanding, and knowledge about the person. However, many next of kin found it necessary to participate in the care in a controlling function when they questioned whether the old persons' needs were being met. Earlier troubles and irritation surrounding caregiving increased the engagement by the next of kin and the need for control, which was sometimes due to inexperienced or ignorant staff. The large number of staff involved in the care and the low trust and confidence in the staff by the next of kin (because of missed care visits) increased their desire to take control.

This was the reason why I was there those days. I was suspicious that the staff were not able feeding her properly (Daughter, 67 years).

The next of kin's need to control resulted in their making more frequent visits to the nursing home, and sometimes they had to advocate care initiatives and be the one that made things happen.

But if I had not seen what was happening to her she would have died, of that I am sure. The staff had not noticed and the nurses are never there so I had to ask the night staff to be kind enough to take her temperature etc. during the coming night. They would not have done it otherwise. That demonstrates not following up situations that arise (Son, 64 years).

Phone calls to a next of kin during the night from a confused and frightened family member living at the nursing home also illuminated the need for control, since this situation arose when staff did not respond to the alarm. The next of kin had to support and calm down the old person until the staff finally arrived. A more responsible care of the old person was instigated following pressure from frustrated and disappointed next of kin.

Inexperienced staff who lacked knowledge about caring for older persons and unengaged physicians were perceived as a concern. The staff's lack of action regarding the implementation of necessary changes in care, disrespect for persons' wishes, and missing personal belongings at the nursing home, coupled to the cleaning, were also noted by next of kin. The need for improvements in the older person's accommodation increased the next of kin's desire for better control, and enabled some next of kin to argue their point and question the staff's methods. Such situations created a need to intervene and to speak up and act on behalf of the older people to ensure their wellbeing, as they were not always able to complain themselves. At the same time, even though it may be difficult to question the staff's behavior without sufficient background knowledge, it is important to have the courage to do so. In some difficult cases, the next of kin wanted to remove the person from the nursing home to a hospital in order to get the best care.

3.2. Building and Maintaining Relationships

When participating in the old person's care, the next of kin became part of both a care and a private relationship. Several visits to the nursing home per week gave the next of kin time to talk to the older person about other things than, for example, symptoms or wellbeing. It could be important to tell about what was happening outside the nursing home or just to socialize without needing to do so much, just be with each other. This was explained as being very satisfying for both parts. The visit often gave the parties the opportunity to look and talk about photos on a tablet computer or in a photo album, or simply to read books or newspapers together.

3.2.1. The Care Relationship

The next of kin wanted the best care for the old person, with the opportunity to be as autonomous as possible. Being part of a care relationship was one way for the next of kin to also be involved in the care. It was important to have quality in the care relationship in terms of of how they as next of kin were treated, what possibilities there were for cooperation, and that their participation was regulated by their own wishes. Many next of kin experienced that their visits to the nursing home were appreciated by the staff and that the staff also cared about them. Being asked by the staff about their own wellbeing was especially important during the end of life phase, and being validated increased their energy and desire to participate in the care. However, in disrespectful care situations where the old person might lose their dignity, the next of kin complained and spoke to the staff on their behalf.

There were hints from the staff that she was faking or that she did it on purpose to be a bit difficult, then I felt the need to shout out and said, "She is not being difficult it is just that she is unable to do it" (Daughter, 67 years).

According to the participating next of kin, being a resource to the care team for the old person, for example, by helping with their hygiene and feeding them—was appreciated by the staff. Their involvement in the care was described as almost being a member of the staff group. It also meant that others could participate in the way they wanted to, even if they did not manage all of the practical things.

In practice I did not need to take care of her as the staff did that. Rather I was simply present.

It was good to have the staff otherwise I would need to be more involved in the practical. Yes, the purpose of my participation was to be there, to be close to her (Daughter, 67 years).

Responsibilities could also be shared between the staff and the next of kin, e.g., for washing clothes. Sometimes the next of kin needed to act as intermediaries between the old persons and the staff in order to obtain the required help or to organize a meeting concerning the old person's wellbeing. In other cases, no cooperation from the staff was offered at all; instead, the next of kin were obliged to carry out the staff's duties as the staff were elsewhere doing other things.

I don't really think I am participating in anything more than being involved in her as a person. Definitely nothing in her care. I don't feel that kind of cooperation exists at all down there (Daughter, 62 years).

3.2.2. The Private Relationship

The private relationship between the next of kin and the old person as well as with other next of kin meant closeness, support, joy, natural togetherness, reciprocity, and being a lifeline, which are the conditions for a care relationship. It was seen as as a point of security that the old person now lived in a nursing home. However, illness and deterioration partly changed the relationship and limited private dialogue, implying a risk of loneliness and exposure on the part of the older person according to the next of kin. A conversation could concern everyday events, but also more difficult topics such as the matter of the eventual disposal of the older person's property. The old person's difficulty in speaking up about their own wishes and needs to the staff could be another matter for discussion.

The staff are not mind readers so one must speak up. They cannot know what she wants if she doesn't tell them and it doesn't help to tell me as I am only here once a week. (Daughter, 68 years).

Sometimes the old person's present life situation was experienced by the next of kin as being sad and not a real life. This promoted worry with feelings of disappointment and anger. Furthermore, feelings of guilt arose for not being with the old person as much as they ought to or because they felt fit while the old person deteriorated. The old person's wishes at the end of their life was also a hard topic to talk about and almost none of the next of kin had succeeded in doing that. Neither the next of kin nor the old person really wanted to talk about that, even though the old person was deteriorating.

I don't know! I almost said that I don't wish to imagine it. We have talked so much about it so I know that my father has chosen a place at the cemetery where he would like to be interred. It also came up a while back (Daughter, 68 years).

One reason for the difficulty of talking about this topic was that it could be interpreted as wishing away someone's life. It seemed to be more manageable to talk with the old person about their wishes concerning their funeral than dying and death.

According to the next of kin, participation in the care of the older person at this stage in life was important to consider and a shared responsibility for the care was crucial for their participation. They felt it important to have symptom relief available and that the older person did not have to die alone.

3.2.3. Adopting to New Roles

In their participation in the person's care, the next of kin talked about taking responsibility and the need to prioritize. Relinquishing responsibilities was not easy and some next of kin struggled with changing priorities. Some next of kin thought they still had the overarching responsibility for the old person. They continued to be engaged even if they did not need to because they were used to taking the old person into account. However, since this person was now living in a nursing home the situation was more relaxed. Other next of kin accepted that the staff had taken over the responsibility for caring and their task was to make sure that the old person was doing well and to offer a silver lining to their life. However, some next of kin could not leave the responsibility to the staff but felt it necessary to be available in case something untoward should happen to the old person.

Some next of kin who took their vacations still visited regularly, others thought they did not need to. There were also opinions that the nursing home care was safe; therefore, there was no need to worry to check or take special responsibility. Still, the old person was always on their mind. Others argued that they as next of kin should have a life of their own without so much responsibility. It was also noted that the responsibility for the old person was often divided among the family, for example, among siblings, which created an imbalance as often one took more responsibility than the others.

> *I have two brothers and a sister and I kind of felt that it is mostly I who had to take the responsibility. Yes, it did seem that way and she lived a little closer to me than the others. Yes, it was tough but then she moved to the nursing home so now everything functions very well (Daughter, 62 years).*

The reason for such an imbalance was that the next of kin all had different personalities, qualifications, depths of engagement, and time available, although all tried to do their best. It was also said that the level of responsibility varied between men and women and that age was an important factor for the level of engagement. Sickness on the part of a next of kin could prevent their participation in the care. However, in some way or another, the responsibility for visits and tasks was divided up among them and thereby they complemented each other. Overall, it was noted that if the next of kin had not participated to the degree they did, a contact person or a legally appointed guardian would be obliged to take on the responsibility for the older person. Leaving the responsibility for the old person's care to the nursing home staff made it possible for the next of kin to run their daily lives in another way. Some next of kin had learnt through experiences in life and training that it was not possible to be engaged in all matters, and that you had to leave some. To have a choice was described as a relief, but a prerequisite was the trust that the older person received adequate help and was cared for with dignity.

3.3. Gathering and Conveying Information

Contact with the staff and the quality of information that the next of kin received had an impact on both the care and private relationships with the old person as well as the next of kin's participation in care. Basic information was usually given at the time the older person moved to the nursing home.

3.3.1. Having a Dialogue with the Staff

Prerequisites for developing a continuous dialogue concerning the care of the elderly included the staff's interest and openness to take the time to learn the older person's background history, their needs, and wishes, in addition to those of the next of kin. A key person to keep the dialogue alive was the contact person. Furthermore, a notebook placed in the room was also important for making notes and sharing information related to the older person.

> *He and I and his carer talk all the time. So we sort of have a dialog on what's going on all the time which I find important. I can't really just come here and say "Hi", talk for a bit, then go home. I want to be a part of things (Son, 51 years).*

Sometimes communication just happened, perhaps over a cup of coffee or via a text message. It was highly important for the next of kin to be invited to care meetings at the nursing home.

Additionally important was the ability to receive information about what had taken place since their last visit to the older person. The possibility to ask questions about the current situation and communicate information about and together with the old person was valuable. The management of delusions or deterioration could increase the need for dialogue and closer contact with the staff via more frequent visits and communication.

For example, information about deterioration could be difficult to receive, but it was important to understand that in such a situation it was necessary for a next of kin to visit the old person without delay. Also, it was essential to communicate correct information to other next of kin about the actual situation. In some cases, discussions about resuscitation or other active management to prolong life took place. Routines concerning dying and death at the nursing home was sometimes conveyed to the next of kin, but almost none of them had received any background information concerning palliative care and its meaning.

> There was a deterioration and I thought she had perhaps sustained a small blood clot or something like that. Then they rang and talked, first they talked here and then they rang and talked to me. So I feel that I was involved. That is to say, as much as was possible (Daughter, 57 years)

Sometimes the dialogue about the old person's wellbeing was scant. The next of kin did not talk much to the staff, and the staff did not ask the next of kin any questions or request their opinions. Lacking communication within the organization and between the care levels concerning the care of the older person was highlighted. Some of the next of kin had requested a visit from a physician for the old person, but had received no answer about when that would happen, so they gave up attempting to get in touch with a physician. In some cases, the next of kin had not been invited to meetings involving follow-up of the care, and decisions were made without either the older person or the next of kin being involved.

3.3.2. Calling and Writing Letters

Using telephone calls to ask for information as an alternative to visiting the nursing home would give the next of kin the possibility to be involved in the old person's life and care.

> If I do not have the opportunity to come here, I always ask how she is. It is very rare that someone has said "X is not so good" rather they reply that she is well. Then, as a rule, I take the opportunity to also talk to her (Daughter, 57 years).

If the ability to communicate in this way with the old person was lost, it became difficult for the next of kin to know and understand the old person's actual situation, which raised the question whether there was an urgent need to visit the old person. Sometimes letters were used to communicate, for example, when it was hard to visit the old person due to distance, own disability, or relationship problems.

4. Discussion

This study sought to explore how the next of kin experienced their participation in the care of older persons (family members) at nursing homes. An overarching theme emerged, that of a balancing act, which concerns the balancing of, on the one hand, wanting to maintain and, on the other, wanting to let go of their responsibility for the old person's care. This balancing act was managed by means of visiting the nursing home, building and maintaining relationships, and gathering and conveying information.

The overarching theme of the balancing act reflects the next of kin's ambivalence towards the responsibility for the care and wellbeing of the older person. Other studies have described this in terms of mixed feelings. For example, Eika et al. [3] noted that the next of kin of an older family member who had moved to a nursing home in Norway were relieved, but also felt apprehensive about the quality of care the older person received. Similar to our findings, they observed that many next of kin continued feeling responsible for the older person, although they recognized that they were in a critical condition and there was need for nursing home care. In an ethnographic study of a nursing home ward in Sweden, Whitaker [7] concluded that the motives for involvement in the older person's life consisted of, on the one hand, love, responsibility, obligation, and repayment, and on the other hand, guilt and a bad conscience.

The balancing act by the next of kin may be understood in terms of attitudinal ambivalence, a concept introduced by Scott [22], which has been defined by Gardner as a psychological state in which "a person holds mixed feelings (positive and negative) towards some psychological object" [23]. Hence, attitudes are said to be ambivalent when something such as the responsibility for the older person's care is evaluated both positively and negatively at the same time [24]. Research has shown that higher levels of attitudinal ambivalence create discomfort, which leads people to seek out consensus information in order to solve the conflict and reduce dissonance [25]. People are also more open to persuasion when they experience high attitudinal ambivalence toward the target object [26]. This points to the importance of nursing home staff reassuring the next of kin of the quality of the care and allowing the next of kin to become involved to the extent they wish. Eika et al. [3] emphasized the importance of the next of kin and the older person feeling appreciated in the nursing home environment and of the feeling of being at home in the nursing home [27].

We found that the visits concerned both more practical day-to-day care (i.e., instrumental care) and care that served more social and emotional purposes (i.e., non-instrumental care) as expressed in the category of "Visiting the nursing home" and the four sub-categories of "Helping with practicalities", "Helping with private matters", "Enabling activity", and "Controlling and supervising the care". In a study of family involvement in nursing home care in Australia, Irving [28] showed that the next of kin who participated in assisting with instrumental care, including activities of daily living, were less satisfied with the nursing home care and that the next of kin usually wanted to limit their level of involvement in instrumental care. Greater value was placed on the possibility of providing non-instrumental support such as advocacy, advice on the older person's preferences, and care oversight [28]. Our study showed that the visits by the next of kin to the nursing home involved different types of activities. In addition, our findings revealed that the next of kin who were dissatisfied with the quality of care felt the need to control and supervise the care at the nursing home. Some of the next of kin in our study expressed frustration with the care provided by the staff, resulting in a lack of trust and confidence in the nursing home. Whitaker [7] observed that during visits to the nursing home, the next of kin often looked for signs of neglect or lack of proper care of the older person. This represents a form of control of the staff in order to preserve the older person's dignity. Whitaker calls this "the impossible" role of the next of kin; they cannot always be present and constantly guard the older person's integrity or make sure that she or he is well cared for and respected [7].

While research on family involvement in nursing home care has tended to focus on the instrumental caring role of the next of kin, Whitaker [7] argued that describing next of kin involvement according to the extent to which the next of kin carried out certain instrumental tasks was misleading and did not do justice to all of the caring activities characterized by the concern and interest in the old person's care and wellbeing.

Viewed from a broader perspective of the next of kin's visits in our study that concerned both instrumental and non-instrumental care, Whitaker [7] believed that the next of kin's visits to nursing homes had both a symbolic and ritual meaning besides their practical nature. The visits reinforced the feeling that the old person was not alone, but part of a larger community beyond the nursing home. Thus, the visits may be seen to represent a promise of the continuance of life despite the nearness of death.

Our findings showed that the next of kin were anxious to maintain the relationship with the old person, i.e., the sub-category "The private relationship". Transfer to a nursing home involves a change for both the next of kin and the older person that disrupts their previous routines, but new habits develop in the nursing home [29]. While the frequency and duration of visits by next of kin tend to vary considerably [6], our study underscored that the next of kin wanted to remain involved in the life of the older person. Whitaker [7] argued that visits to the nursing home "represent" the relationship, regardless of whether it was a parent-child relationship, friendship, or marital relationship. Although the relationship depends on the physical and mental condition of the older person, other studies have confirmed the importance of the relational links outside the nursing home [30,31].

The relationship between the next of kin and the nursing home staff was also important, as seen in our sub-category "The care relationship". We found that the next of kin, in general, felt appreciated by the staff, but other studies have suggested that this relationship could be somewhat difficult.

For example, Eika et al. [3] noted that many of the next of kin had little communication with the nursing home staff and some felt that they disturbed the nursing home's routines. The next of kin who perceived that they had limited support from the nursing home staff were unsure about what to expect from the staff.

It is important that the nursing home staff are aware of and are able to support the next of kin's process of adapting to new roles after the older person's move to a nursing home, which represents a profound life transition for both the older person and their next of kin. They continue to be involved and struggle to adjust their relationship with the older person and establish new roles [3,30]. Many of the next of kin in our study appeared to have trouble letting go of their responsibility for the older person's care, but others argued that the responsibility had now been taken over by the nursing home. The importance of the roles that emerge when an older person moves to a nursing home has been increasingly emphasized in the research [7]. The literature describes a wide range of roles played by the next of kin [32,33].

The next of kin's need for participation in the older persons care was additionally illustrated in our findings under the category "Gathering and conveying information". Phone calls and email were used when the next of kin had no possibility of visiting the older person due to other duties or when they could no longer talk with the older person due to dementia. This became a way to follow the health condition of the older person every day, but the most valuable support perceived by the next of kin was when they were invited to participate in care meetings and had the possibility to ask questions about things such as illness deterioration. The next of kin expected staff to recognize their need for information and guidance in their involvement; however, they often felt that this guidance was lacking [34]. Furthermore, many of the next of kin argued that they were not invited to be equal partners in decisions about the care [35]. Furthermore, the next of kin were sometimes afraid of being perceived as troublemakers and therefore many of them did not ask too much or complain too much about the staff [36].

The interviews with the next of kin in this study were made before the implementation of knowledge-based palliative care through an educational intervention for the staff [11]. With staff that have only a limited knowledge about palliative care, it is not surprising that communication with the next of kin about palliative care was unusual. However, it would have been expected that they were invited more frequently by the staff to take part in the care of the older person. Insufficient participation by the next of kin was also found in an interview study from Norway with the next of kin that took place 2–12 months after the death of a patient, concerning their involvement and experiences of decision-making processes related to the issues of limiting life-prolonging treatment [37]. Their results showed distinct shortcomings regarding the next of kin's participation in decisions on life-prolonging treatment in nursing homes. The staff only first contacted the next of kin for a discussion when the patient's condition had deteriorated and their life was approaching its end. If conversations did take place early in the process, this was a result of the next of kin having asked for a dialogue [37]. Most relatives wanted to be involved in the decision-making process, as well as to receive information about the patient's health condition. The next of kin wanted the staff to initiate the conversation about these issues since they felt they were emotionally challenging [38]. Research has described communication about the end of life as a challenge for nursing home staff [39] and revealed the need for education and training for this task [40,41]. However, the crucial point was that the benefits for the next of kin of using a palliative approach of care [42] in nursing homes for old persons must be fully understood [43,44].

Choosing participants with a diversity of experiences enhanced the credibility of this study [18,45]. Interviews with 40 next of kin in two counties in Sweden and from 20 nursing homes, large as well as small, situated in both urban and rural areas, were the procedures undertaken to attain credibility and transferability of the results. Therefore, the next of kin in this study represented nursing homes providing varying qualities of care and had different cultures, norms, and organization sizes. This indicates that our findings may have better transferability to other nursing homes compared to a study in which the interviewees were few and selected from only one nursing home. However, the limitations were that none of the next of kin were younger than 40 years and that we did not know the level of palliative care or end-of-life care that their older relative received when the interviews were made.

The use of four different researchers to conduct the interviews may have had a negative effect on the credibility of the findings. On the other hand, they were all nurses with a long experience of aged care. The fact that two of the researchers who conducted the interviews also analyzed the text independent of each other and had several meetings together concerning the interpretation of the texts, i.e., investigator triangulation, may have conferred a positive effect. In addition, the analyses were scrutinized by all of those in the research group to manage the bias embedded in close engagement. For the sake of credibility, the analytical process has been carefully described so the reader may follow the researchers' interpretations. The interviews served as a point of reference throughout the analytical process when a deeper understanding was required of the meaning units, codes, and categories. Hence, to make the results more credible, the quotations represent different next of kin and different relationships with older persons.

5. Conclusions

Being a next of kin of an older person in a nursing home involves an act of balance between keeping the overall responsibility for the older persons' care themselves, or trusting the nursing home staff and leaving the responsibility for the care to them. The findings confirmed previous research that the next of kin were anxious to be engaged in how the care at the nursing homes was performed. They wanted to participate in care meetings, and not only in practical tasks; however, they considered their practical participation in the daily care as an important dimension for the wellbeing of their loved ones under care. The attitudes and culture of the staff in welcoming the next of kin as equal partners needs to be supported by education as well as increased knowledge about palliative care and decision-making related to limiting life-prolonging treatment.

Author Contributions: B.W. drafted the article, performed interviews with the next of kin, conducted the analysis, and wrote the results. L.B. drafted parts of the article, performed interviews with the next of kin, and conducted the analysis. Å.A. performed a critical revision of the results and drafted parts of the article. P.N. drafted parts of the article and performed a critical revision of the manuscript. E.B. contributed to the design of the project and drafted parts of the article. A.S. contributed to the design of the project, drafted parts of the article, and performed a critical revision of the manuscript. The project leader G.A. was the recipient (PI) of national research grants, applied for ethical permission, contributed to the design of the study, drafted parts of the article, and performed a critical revision of the method and results. All of the authors contributed to the content of the manuscript and approved the final manuscript.

Funding: This study is part of the KUPA project and is funded by The Swedish Research Council, grant number 2014-2759; The Vårdal Foundation, grant number 2014-0071; Medical Faculty, Lund University; The Faculty of Health and Life Sciences, Linnaeus University; The City of Lund; The Institute for Palliative Care, Region Skane and Lund University; Greta and Johan Kocks Foundation; and the Ribbingska Memorial Fund.

Acknowledgments: We are extremely grateful to the next of kin who took part in this research and we would like to thank the contact person at each nursing home who helped with recruitment. We also thank Anne Molina Tall, RN, Helene Åvik Persson, who conducted interviews with the next of kin and research administrator Magnus Persson for support with practical tasks.

References

1. Ryan, A.A.; Scullion, H.F. Nursing home placement: An exploration of the experiences of family carers. *J. Adv. Nurs.* **2000**, *32*, 1187–1195. [CrossRef] [PubMed]
2. Sandberg, J.; Lundh, U.; Nolan, M. Moving into a care home: The role of adult children in the placement process. *Int. J. Nurs. Stud.* **2002**, *39*, 353–362. [CrossRef]

3. Eika, M.; Espnes, G.A.; Soderhamn, O.; Hvalvik, S. Experiences faced by next of kin during their older family members' transition into long-term care in a norwegian nursing home. *J. Clin. Nurs.* **2014**, *23*, 2186–2195. [CrossRef] [PubMed]

4. Hogsnes, L.; Melin-Johansson, C.; Norbergh, K.G.; Danielson, E. The existential life situations of spouses of persons with dementia before and after relocating to a nursing home. *Aging Ment. Health* **2014**, *18*, 152–160. [CrossRef] [PubMed]

5. Dorell, A.; Sundin, K. Becoming visible—Experiences from families participating in family health conversations at residential homes for older people. *Geriatr. Nurs.* **2016**, *37*, 260–265. [CrossRef] [PubMed]

6. Gaugler, J.E. Family involvement in residential long-term care: A synthesis and critical review. *Aging Ment. Health* **2005**, *9*, 105–118. [CrossRef] [PubMed]

7. Whitaker, A. Family involvement in the institutional eldercare context. Towards a new understanding. *J. Aging Stud.* **2009**, *23*, 158–167. [CrossRef]

8. Gomes, B.; Calanzani, N.; Gysels, M.; Hall, S.; Higginson, I.J. Heterogeneity and changes in preferences for dying at home: A systematic review. *BMC Palliat. Care* **2013**, *12*, 7. [CrossRef] [PubMed]

9. Calanzani, N.; Moens, K.; Cohen, J.; Higginson, I.J.; Harding, R.; Deliens, L.; Toscani, F.; Ferreira, P.L.; Bausewein, C.; Daveson, B.A.; et al. Choosing care homes as the least preferred place to die: A cross-national survey of public preferences in seven european countries. *BMC Palliat. Care* **2014**, *13*, 48. [CrossRef] [PubMed]

10. Wiles, J.L.; Leibing, A.; Guberman, N.; Reeve, J.; Allen, R.E.S. The meaning of "aging in place" to older people. *Gerontologist* **2012**, *52*, 357–366. [CrossRef] [PubMed]

11. Ahlstrom, G.; Nilsen, P.; Benzein, E.; Behm, L.; Wallerstedt, B.; Persson, M.; Sandgren, A. Implementation of knowledge-based palliative care in nursing homes and pre-post post evaluation by cross-over design: A study protocol. *BMC Palliat. Care* **2018**, *17*, 52. [CrossRef] [PubMed]

12. National Board of Health and Welfare. *Care and Welfare for the Elderly, Progress Report (In Swedish: Vård och Omsorg om Äldre, Lägesrapport)*; National Board of Health and Welfare: Stockholm, Sweden, 2018.

13. Ersek, M.; Carpenter, J. Geriatric palliative care in long-term care settings with a focus on nursing homes. *J. Palliat. Med.* **2013**, *16*, 1180–1187. [CrossRef] [PubMed]

14. Van Soest-Poortvliet, M.C.; van der Steen, J.T.; Gutschow, G.; Deliens, L.; Onwuteaka-Philipsen, B.D.; de Vet, H.C.; Hertogh, C.M. Advance care planning in nursing home patients with dementia: A qualitative interview study among family and professional caregivers. *J. Am. Med. Dir. Assoc.* **2015**, *16*, 979–989. [CrossRef] [PubMed]

15. Bollig, G.; Gjengedal, E.; Rosland, J.H. They know!—Do they? A qualitative study of residents and relatives views on advance care planning, end-of-life care, and decision-making in nursing homes. *Palliat. Med.* **2016**, *30*, 456–470. [CrossRef] [PubMed]

16. Levine, S.; O'Mahony, S.; Baron, A.; Ansari, A.; Deamant, C.; Frader, J.; Leyva, I.; Marschke, M.; Preodor, M. Training the workforce: Description of a longitudinal interdisciplinary education and mentoring program in palliative care. *J. Pain Symptom Manag.* **2017**, *53*, 728–737. [CrossRef] [PubMed]

17. Nilsen, P.; Wallerstedt, B.; Behm, L.; Ahlstrom, G. Towards evidence-based palliative care in nursing homes in sweden: A qualitative study informed by the organizational readiness to change theory. *Implement. Sci.* **2018**, *13*, 1. [CrossRef] [PubMed]

18. Graneheim, U.H.; Lundman, B. Qualitative content analysis in nursing research: Concepts, procedures and measures to achieve trustworthiness. *Nurs. Educ. Today* **2004**, *24*, 105–112. [CrossRef] [PubMed]

19. Hsieh, H.F.; Shannon, S.E. Three approaches to qualitative content analysis. *Qual. Health Res.* **2005**, *15*, 1277–1288. [CrossRef] [PubMed]

20. QSR International Pty Ltd. Nvivo 11: Getting Started Guide. Available online: http://download.qsrinternational.com/Document/NVivo11/11.4.0/en-US/NVivo11-Getting-Started-Guide-Starter-edition.pdf (accessed on 31 March 2018).

21. Tong, A.; Sainsbury, P.; Craig, J. Consolidated criteria for reporting qualitative research (COREQ): A 32-item checklist for interviews and focus groups. *Int. J. Qual. Health Care* **2007**, *19*, 349–357. [CrossRef] [PubMed]

22. Scott, W.A. Structure of natural cognitions. *J. Pers. Soc. Psychol.* **1969**, *12*, 261–278. [CrossRef] [PubMed]

23. Gardner, P.L. Measuring ambivalence to science. *J. Res. Sci. Teach.* **1987**, *24*, 241–247. [CrossRef]

24. Priester, J.R.; Petty, R.E. Extending the bases of subjective attitudinal ambivalence: Interpersonal and intrapersonal antecedents of evaluative tension. *J. Pers. Soc. Psychol.* **2001**, *80*, 19–34. [CrossRef] [PubMed]

25. Zemborain, M.R.; Johar, G.V. Attitudinal ambivalence and openness to persuasion: A framework for interpersonal influence. *J. Consum. Res.* **2007**, *33*, 506–514. [CrossRef]

26. Hodson, G.; Maio, G.R.; Esses, V.M. The role of attitudinal ambivalence in susceptibility to consensus information. *Basic Appl. Soc. Psychol.* **2001**, *23*, 197–205. [CrossRef]

27. Van Hoof, J.; Verbeek, H.; Janssen, B.M.; Eijkelenboom, A.; Molony, S.L.; Felix, E.; Nieboer, K.A.; Zwerts-Verhelst, E.L.; Sijstermans, J.J.; Wouters, E.J. A three perspective study of the sense of home of nursing home residents: The views of residents, care professionals and relatives. *BMC Geriatr.* **2016**, *16*, 169. [CrossRef] [PubMed]

28. Irving, J. Beyond family satisfaction: Family-perceived involvement in residential care. *Australas. J. Ageing* **2015**, *34*, 166–170. [CrossRef] [PubMed]

29. Becker, G. *Disrupted Lives: How People Create Meaning in a Chaotic World*; University of California Press, Cop.: Berkeley, CA, USA, 1997.

30. Davies, S.; Nolan, M. 'Making the move': Relatives' experiences of the transition to a care home. *Health Soc. Care Commun.* **2004**, *12*, 517–526. [CrossRef] [PubMed]

31. Gladstone, J.W.; Dupuis, S.L.; Wexler, E. Changes in family involvement following a relative's move to a long-term care facility. *Can. J. Aging* **2006**, *25*, 93–106. [CrossRef] [PubMed]

32. Rowles, G.; High, D. Family involvement in nursing home facilities—A decision-making perspective. In *Gray Areas: Ethnographic Encounters with Nursing Home Culture*; Stafford, P.B., Ed.; School of American Research Press: Santa Fe, NM, USA, 2003; pp. 173–201.

33. Haesler, E.; Bauer, M.; Nay, R. Recent evidence on the development and maintenance of constructive staff-family relationships in the care of older people—A report on a systematic review update. *Int. J. Evid. Based Healthc.* **2010**, *8*, 45–74. [PubMed]

34. Fosse, A.; Schaufel, M.A.; Ruths, S.; Malterud, K. End-of-life expectations and experiences among nursing home patients and their relatives—A synthesis of qualitative studies. *Patient Educ. Couns.* **2014**, *97*, 3–9. [CrossRef] [PubMed]

35. Givens, J.L.; Lopez, R.P.; Mazor, K.M.; Mitchell, S.L. Sources of stress for family members of nursing home residents with advanced dementia. *Alzheimer Dis. Assoc. Dis.* **2012**, *26*, 254–259. [CrossRef] [PubMed]

36. Bollig, G.; Gjengedal, E.; Rosland, J.H. Nothing to complain about? Residents' and relatives' views on a "good life" and ethical challenges in nursing homes. *Nurs. Ethics* **2016**, *23*, 142–153. [CrossRef] [PubMed]

37. Dreyer, A.; Forde, R.; Nortvedt, P. Autonomy at the end of life: Life-prolonging treatment in nursing homes-relatives' role in the decision-making process. *J. Med. Ethics* **2009**, *35*, 672–677. [CrossRef] [PubMed]

38. Gjerberg, E.; Lillemoen, L.; Forde, R.; Pedersen, R. End-of-life care communications and shared decision-making in norwegian nursing homes—Experiences and perspectives of patients and relatives. *BMC Geriatr.* **2015**, *15*, 103. [CrossRef] [PubMed]

39. Brodtkorb, K.; Skisland, A.V.-S.; Slettebø, Å.; Skaar, R. Preserving dignity in end-of-life nursing home care: Some ethical challenges. *Nordic J. Nurs. Res.* **2017**, *37*, 78–84. [CrossRef]

40. Bernacki, R.; Hutchings, M.; Vick, J.; Smith, G.; Paladino, J.; Lipsitz, S.; Gawande, A.A.; Block, S.D. Development of the serious illness care program: A randomised controlled trial of a palliative care communication intervention. *BMJ Open* **2015**, *5*, e009032. [CrossRef] [PubMed]

41. Brighton, L.J.; Selman, L.E.; Gough, N.; Nadicksbernd, J.J.; Bristowe, K.; Millington-Sanders, C.; Koffman, J. 'Difficult conversations': Evaluation of multiprofessional training. *BMJ Support. Palliat. Care* **2018**, *8*, 45–48. [CrossRef] [PubMed]

42. Bone, A.E.; Morgan, M.; Maddocks, M.; Sleeman, K.E.; Wright, J.; Taherzadeh, S.; Ellis-Smith, C.; Higginson, I.J.; Evans, C.J. Developing a model of short-term integrated palliative and supportive care for frail older people in community settings: Perspectives of older people, carers and other key stakeholders. *Age Ageing* **2016**, *45*, 863–873. [CrossRef] [PubMed]

43. Forbat, L.; Chapman, M.; Lovell, C.; Liu, W.M.; Johnston, N. Improving specialist palliative care in residential care for older people: A checklist to guide practice. *BMJ Support. Palliat. Care* **2017**. [CrossRef] [PubMed]

44.   Frey, R.; Foster, S.; Boyd, M.; Robinson, J.; Gott, M. Family experiences of the transition to palliative care in aged residential care (ARC): A qualitative study. *Int. J. Palliat. Nurs.* **2017**, *23*, 238–247. [CrossRef] [PubMed]
45.   Lincoln, Y.S.; Guba, E.G. *Naturalistic Inquiry*; Sage: Beverly Hills, CA, USA, 1985.

## 5

Impact of Nurse Practitioner Practice Regulations on Rural Population Health Outcomes

Judith Ortiz [1,*], Richard Hofler [2], Angeline Bushy [3] 🔘, Yi-ling Lin [1], Ahmad Khanijahani [1] and Andrea Bitney [4]

[1] College of Health and Public Affairs, University of Central Florida, Orlando, FL 32816, USA; YLLin@knights.ucf.edu (Y.L.); khanijahani@knights.ucf.edu (A.K.)
[2] College of Business Administration, University of Central Florida, Orlando, FL 32816, USA; Richard.Hofler@ucf.edu
[3] College of Nursing, University of Central Florida, Orlando, FL 32816, USA; Angeline.Bushy@ucf.edu
[4] College of Sciences, University of Central Florida, Orlando, FL 32816, USA; andrea.bitney@cru.org
[*] Correspondence: Judith.Ortiz@ucf.edu

Abstract: *Background:* For decades, U.S. rural areas have experienced shortages of primary care providers. Nurse practitioners (NPs) are helping to reduce that shortage. However, NP scope of practice regulations vary from state-to-state ranging from autonomous practice to direct physician oversight. The purpose of this study was to determine if clinical outcomes of older rural adult patients vary by the level of practice autonomy that states grant to NPs. *Methods:* This cross-sectional study analyzed data from a sample of Rural Health Clinics (RHCs) (n = 503) located in eight Southeastern states. Independent *t*-tests were performed for each of five variables to compare patient outcomes of the experimental RHCs (those in "reduced practice" states) to those of the control RHCs (in "restricted practice" states). *Results:* After matching, no statistically significant difference was found in patient outcomes for RHCs in reduced practice states compared to those in restricted practice states. Yet, expanded scope of practice may improve provider supply, healthcare access and utilization, and quality of care (Martsolf et al., 2016). *Conclusions:* Although this study found no significant relationship between Advanced Registered Nurse Practitioner (ARNP) scope of practice and select patient outcome variables, there are strong indications that the quality of patient outcomes is not reduced when the scope of practice is expanded.

Keywords: nurse practitioners; rural; scope of practice; patient outcomes; rural workforce

1. Introduction

For decades, rural areas across the U.S. have experienced persistent shortages of primary care providers, leaving rural residents at greater risk for health problems and illness complications. Rural communities differ from each other; however, both rural and urban areas are becoming more culturally diverse. The Hispanic population, for example, as the fastest growing ethnic group in the U.S. [1,2] has dispersed across the 50 states to both rural and urban communities. Hispanics/Latinos, African Americans, and other subgroups differ from the majority population regarding their beliefs and preferences about health, illness, and their ability to access health care. These distinctions, in the absence of culturally sensitive healthcare, may contribute to health disparities of the subgroup as compared to the majority population.

Nurses make up the largest segment of the health care profession. They work in a wide variety of settings and provide care to diverse populations. As the healthcare system undergoes transformation due in part to the Affordable Care Act (ACA), the nursing profession has a significant role in delivering quality, patient-centered, accessible, and affordable care. The Institute of Medicine's (IOM's) [3] report entitled "The Future of Nursing: Leading Change, Advancing Health" made recommendations pertaining to the roles of nurses in the changing healthcare landscape.

Of relevance to rural areas are the IOM's recommendations for Removing Barriers to Practice and Care [4,5]. That is to say, if Advanced Practice Registered Nurses (including nurse practitioners) are permitted to practice to the full extent of their education and training, this could build the necessary workforce to satisfy the health care needs of an increasing number of people, especially those living in medically underserved regions. (Historically, in the literature the title nurse practitioner [NP] was used. Recently, the designated title is Advanced Registered Nurse Practitioner [ARNP]; hence, ARNP is used in this article.).

While steps have been taken at both federal and state levels to relax ARNP practice restrictions, many states inhibit ARNPs' ability to practice at the level for which they have been prepared. The IOM states: "Collaborative models of practice, in which all health professionals practice to the full extent of their education and training, optimize the efficiency and quality of care for patients and enhance the satisfaction of healthcare providers" [3] (p. 3). To facilitate formation of these models, and increase the accessibility of quality health care, the IOM recommends that the nursing community, other health professions groups, and policy makers, establish a common ground to remove scope of practice restrictions and increase interprofessional collaboration.

Relaxing scope of practice restrictions could help ARNPs meet the critical demand for primary care services in rural (and urban) areas. However, regulations vary from state-to-state regarding ARNPs' scope of practice and level of professional autonomy. Currently, the 50 states are categorized into the following three groups based on ARNP's practice regulations [6,7].

Full Practice: State practice and licensure laws provides for all nurse practitioners to evaluate patients, diagnose, order and interpret diagnostic tests, initiate and manage treatments—including prescribing medications and controlled substances—under the exclusive licensure authority of the state board of nursing. This is the model recommended by the National Academy of Medicine (formerly the IOM) and National Council of State Boards of Nursing.

Reduced Practice: State practice and licensure laws reduces the ability of nurse practitioners to engage in at least one element of ARNP practice. State law requires a career-long regulated collaborative agreement with another health provider in order for the ARNP to provide patient care; or, limits the setting of one or more elements of ARNP practice.

Restricted Practice: State practice and licensure laws restricts the ability of a nurse practitioner to engage in at least one element of NP practice. State law requires career-long supervision, delegation, or team-management by another health provider in order for the ARNP to provide patient care.

Research studies indicate that less restrictive ARNP scope of practice regulations can increase primary care access and utilization. In one study of persons residing in the full-practice states, 62% had higher geographic accessibility to primary care clinicians (including ARNPs), compared to only 35% in restricted practice states [8]. Furthermore, ARNPs' practice and prescriptive independence had a positive impact on physician referral, health education and counseling services, and the number of medications taken by patients [9]. These recent findings confirm Sakr's [10] early findings that ARNPs not only provided proper care of minor injuries, but performed better than 'novice" physicians at reading medical history records and planning patient follow-up care.

Several studies have examined outcomes of patients treated by ARNPs as compared to those treated by physicians. A systematic review found no differences in patient outcomes (as measured by emergency department (ED) or urgent care visits, rehospitalization rates, and mortality rates) of patients treated by ARNPs compared to those treated by medical doctors (MDs) [11]. However, there is a lack of consensus about the effects of ARNP practice regulatory policies on population health outcomes [12].

The current study concerned persons residing in rural areas of the U.S., many of whom are "vulnerable" to poor health, in particular older adults, low resource, and persons of minority groups.

The principal aim of the study was to determine how clinical outcomes of older adult patients vary by level of practice autonomy that states grant to ARNPs.

2. Materials and Methods

2.1. Study Design

This cross-sectional study included data from Rural Health Clinics (RHCs) providing health services in HHS Region 4 during 2013. Since the mid-1970s, ARNPs have played a significant role in the nation's RHCs. These approximately 4000 Medicare-certified clinics are intended to address the inadequate supply of physicians serving rural Medicare patients, and to increase the use of non-physician providers [13]. The RHC was the unit of analysis throughout the study. The study was approved by the Institutional Review Board of the University of Central Florida (IRB00001138).

The eight states that compose HHS Region 4 (Alabama, Florida, Georgia, Kentucky, Mississippi, South Carolina, Tennessee) have varying regulations regarding the scope of practice for ARNPs. By 2013, among these eight study states, three (AL, KY, and MS) had adopted reduced ARNP practice laws, and five states (FL, GA, NC, SC, and TN) had adopted restricted ARNP practice laws [8]. None had adopted full practice laws.

2.2. Data Sources

The secondary data used in this study included the Provider of Services (POS) files, Medicare beneficiaries' inpatient and outpatient claims, outpatient revenue center files, and the Centers for Medicare and Medicaid Services (CMS) Cost Reports for RHCs. Variables for each RHC's type (provider-based or independent) and location were constructed using data from the POS files. Patient outcome variables were constructed using the 2013 inpatient and outpatient claims and outpatient revenue center files. Finally, several RHC organizational characteristic variables were constructed using data from the 2013 CMS Cost Reports.

2.3. Variables

2.3.1. Outcome (Dependent) Variables

Five different patient outcomes were measured in this study: the 30-day readmission rate, and risk-adjusted rates of Ambulatory Care Sensitive Conditions for four principal diagnoses: COPD/Asthma, Congestive Heart Failure (CHF), Diabetes, and Pneumonia. The risk-adjustment statistical process controls for the potential effects of patient's gender, age, race, comorbidity (using the Charlson Comorbidity Index), and the claim year. All of the variables were analyzed and reported on the RHC level.

2.3.2. Independent Variables

The primary independent variable was the geographic "location" of the RHC. "Location" was defined as whether the RHC were located in a state with reduced (the experimental group) or restricted (the control group) ARNP scope of practice laws. Also included in the analysis were control variables for each RHC's characteristics, including the type of the RHC (independent or provider-based), "size" (measured as the total of physician + ARNP + PA FTEs), the percentage of ARNP FTEs (calculated as the number of ARNP FTEs divided by the "size"), and "rurality" (a measure of the RHC's geographic location.) RHCs were categorized by degrees of "rurality" using the Rural-Urban Commuting Area Code, or RUCA [14]. This method categorizes the rural status of each RHC's location based on Zip code.

2.4. Analysis

We constructed a panel of clinics continuously certified as Region 4 RHCs from 2007 through 2013 using the Provider of Services (POS) file. This process resulted in a panel of 503 RHCs. During the study period, an average of approximately 463 patients were assigned to each RHC in the study panel. In that patients often visit more than one medical facility, patients were assigned to the RHC that provided the plurality of his or her services during the year 2013. The patient outcome variables from the Medicare beneficiaries' claims were aggregated to the clinic level.

The study aimed to measure the effects of state regulatory laws regarding ARNP scope of practice on health outcomes. We attempted to eliminate (or at least, minimize) the effects of care provided by other clinicians with similar levels of authority—physicians and physician assistants of the RHCs. For this reason, only RHCs in which ARNPs accounted for 90% or more of a clinic's total FTEs (full-time equivalents) were included in the analysis. Of the 503 RHCs in the study panel, we found 77 where ARNPs made up 90% or more of their professional clinical staff.

Among the 77 RHCs with 90% of more ARNPs, two groups were created: RHCs in reduced practice states (the experimental group), and RHCs in restricted practice states (the comparison group.) The comparison group was constructed using the statistical technique "propensity score matching" (PSM) described in the next section.

2.4.1. Comparison Sample Construction

Propensity score matching (PSM) is used with secondary data to control for bias in the assignment to the experimental and control groups [15]. Variable selection for classic propensity score models consider only the exposure (for our study, RHCs in either reduced or restricted practice states). However, according to one study, variables unrelated to the exposure but related to outcomes can be included in a PSM model to increase the precision of the estimated exposure effect without increasing bias [16]. Thus, for the current study, variable selection for the propensity score models included three variables for RHC characteristics that are related to patient outcomes: "size," "rurality," and "type."

PSM was performed separately for each of the five patient outcome variables using radius matching. In each model, based on the structure of data, the specific caliper width was defined. To ensure good match quality, a caliper of one-fourth the standard deviation of each clinic's propensity scores was used, and bias balancing diagnostics such as standardized biased, variance ratio tests, *t*-tests, and Rubin's B and R statistics were evaluated.

2.4.2. Treatment of Missing Data

Some of the missing values in 2013 for variables in the propensity score models and patient outcomes were replaced using mean or linear estimation using the available data for the same variables in at least three years (from 2007–2012, and 2014). Since the number of study cases was limited, it was assumed that these replaced missing values could add to the quality of matching and further analysis by increasing the number of the valid observations (values). Table 1 shows the missing imputation method approaches and the imputation quality. We found no substantial differences in the means and standard deviations of the imputed variables before and after the imputation methods were applied.

Table 1. Frequency, Mean, and Standard Deviation before and after Missing Value Treatment.

Variable	Missing Imputation Method	Number of Valid Cases		Mean		Std. Deviation	
		Before	After	Before	After	Before	After
RHC Size	Mean	58	77	1.5278	1.4764	1.0533	0.95711
% NP FTEs	Mean	58	77	0.9859	0.9856	0.02847	0.02927
R_Readm13	Linear Regression	68	74	0.1760	0.1725	0.01971	0.02561
R_ACSCCOPD_Rate13	Linear Regression	63	72	0.0651	0.0631	0.03242	0.031
R_ACSCDiab_Rate13	Linear Regression	41	61	0.0293	0.0261	0.01916	0.01744
R_ACSCHF_Rate13	Linear Regression	50	65	0.1346	0.1271	0.04343	0.04149
R_ACSCPneu_Rate213	Mean	68	74	0.0093	0.0083	0.00359	0.00294

2.4.3. Independent *t*-Test

While performing the PSM technique, we controlled for three RHC-related variables: size, type, and "rurality." Since the effects of these factors were controlled for in the matching process, independent *t*-tests were then performed for each of the five outcome variables to compare the outcomes of the experimental RHCs (those in reduced practice states) to those of the control RHCs (those in restricted practice states).

3. Results

Table 2 shows characteristics of the experimental and control RHCs. Bivariate analysis of these characteristics was conducted, but no statistically significant differences were observed. Of the 77 RHCs, 32 (41.56%) were located in states with restricted ARNP practice law; and, 45 (58.44%) were in states with reduced ARNP practice law. More than 70% of the total RHCs were independent; less than 30% of them were provider-based. Most (34.4%) of the RHCs in restricted practice states belonged to RUCA category "urban," whereas more than half of the RHCs in reduced practice states were classified into RUCA categories "large" and "small" rural. The mean RHC "size" in restricted practice states was 1.42 FTEs, whereas for those in reduced practice states it was 1.52.

Table 2. Rural Health Clinic(RHC) Characteristics by Nurse Practitioner State Practice in Region 4

Characteristic	State with Restricted Practice (n = 32)		State with Reduced Practice (n = 45)		*p*-Value
	Mean/n	SD/%	Mean/n	SD/%	
RHC Type					0.196
Independent RHC	25	78.1%	29	64.4%	
Provided-Based RHC	7	21.9%	16	35.6%	
RUCA * Category					0.545
Urban	11	34.4%	9	20.0%	
Large Rural	7	21.9%	13	28.9%	
Small Rural	8	25.0%	12	26.7%	
Isolated	6	18.8%	11	24.4%	
RHC Size (No. of Physician + PA + NP FTEs)	1.42	0.81	1.52	1.05	0.649

* The Rural-Urban Commuting Area (RUCA) Code has four categories: 1 = Urban, 2 = Large rural, 3 = Small rural, and 4 = Isolated. This binary variable "rural" equals one for each RHC with a RUCA code equal to 4. We chose this specification for this binary variable because our analysis of survey responses we received showed that RHCs in isolated areas are less likely to join ACOs.

Table 3 shows the results of the bivariate analyses for the five patient outcomes. After matching, no statistically significant difference was found in patient outcomes for RHCs in the restricted practice states as compared to those in reduced practice states.

Table 3. Effect of the State's NP Practice Law on Patient Outcomes in 2013 in Region 4 Rural Health Clinic Using Independent *t*-test.

Patient Outcomes	State with Restricted Practice			State with Reduced Practice			*p*-Value
	n	Mean	SD	n	Mean	SD	
Readmission rate within 30 days	31	16.69%	2.64%	39	17.65%	2.51%	0.126
Hospitalization rate for COPD or Asthma	30	6.17%	3.68%	33	6.38%	2.91%	0.804
Hospitalization rate for Diabetes	25	2.24%	1.09%	28	2.68%	2.16%	0.349
Hospitalization rate for Heart Failure	27	12.48%	3.94%	29	13.31%	4.48%	0.467
Hospitalization rate for Pneumonia	31	0.86%	0.30%	39	0.79%	0.26%	0.303

4. Discussion

Nurse practitioners contribute to U.S. healthcare by providing health services individually and as a part of healthcare teams that include physicians, nurses and other health care professionals. Recruiting ARNPs and expanding their scope of practice to include providing diagnoses, prescriptions, treatments, consultations and other services could shift some of healthcare burden away from physicians. ARNPs functioning at the level for which they are prepared could help to improve healthcare access disparities in areas with severe physician shortages such as rural areas, where shortages have persisted and are anticipated for the foreseeable future.

This study compared healthcare outcomes of Medicare beneficiaries of RHCs located in states with reduced ARNP scope of practice laws to those with restricted laws. After controlling for individual patient-level confounders (using risk adjustment procedures), and RHC characteristics, no significant difference was observed between the two groups of RHCs for any of five patient outcomes. However, it is important to stress that populations derive other benefits when ARNP scope of practice is less restrictive.

According to the findings of a recent study by Graves and colleagues [8], restrictions on ARNPs' scope of practice were associated with up to 40% fewer primary care nurse practitioners (PCARNPs) in states with restricted ARNP practice environment compared to their full practice counterparts. These practice restrictions may contribute to limitations in access to primary healthcare services and perpetuate rural health disparities. Relaxing restrictions on ARNP scope of practice may also expand the capacity of primary care services in rural areas. Based on a review of 14 published articles focusing on ARNP scope of practice and its effect on quality of care, cost, health care utilization and outcomes, Martsolf and colleagues [17] suggest that expanded scope of practice improved the provider supply, healthcare access and utilization, and quality of care.

It is important to stress that professional and personal satisfaction is ideal for many ARNPs in rural practice, especially for those who have rural life experiences (i.e., having been raised, lived, or spent time in a rural setting) [18]. However, it is also important to note that a dichotomy exists in states having large rural and remote areas as well as less restrictive regulations regarding ARNP scope of practice. Specifically, many rural communities, particularly those in isolated regions, have the least restrictive APRN scope of practice regulations. Yet, these regions experience serious, consistent challenges in recruiting and retaining health professionals of all types—physicians, mental and behavioral health professionals, as well as ARNPs [19].

Several reasons are offered to explain why APRNs may choose *not* to practice in a state with the least restrictive scope of practice. Among others, there is an urban bias in the higher education system where professional clinical experiences tend to take place in an urban-based healthcare facility. Urban-based education contributes to minimal (if any) student exposure to rural populations, cultural preferences and practice environments. Another contributing factor is lower reimbursement by third party payers for primary care services coupled with disparate reimbursement for APRNs as well as rural healthcare providers.

Low population density in rural regions often can support only one or two providers; which, in turn, may lead to a sense of professional isolation for the ARNP (or physician) who chooses to practice in these more remote sites. This reality is often compounded by an expectation that the ARNP be available or "on call 24/7" to see patients with minimal backup support. Such professional community expectations and needs often conflict with an ARNP's personal and family roles. All too often, the result is a decision to relocate to a practice setting that better suits the ARNP's personal, professional and family preferences.

The findings of the current study should be viewed considering a few limitations. First, attributing changes in patient outcomes solely to the RHC's services may give an incomplete picture. The change in health status of a patient is a result of services provided by a group of healthcare providers, including ARNPs. Even after including only RHCs with 90% or more ARNP staff, the impact of care given by other healthcare providers such as physicians should not be ignored. Second, there is considerable variation in ARNP scope of practice among states within a scope of practice category (i.e., reduced, restricted). For example, one state may only restrict the ARNPs in prescribing medicine, but allow full authority to diagnose, treat, and consult patients, whereas another state may restrict ARNPs in all aspects of their practice. Finally, this study was limited to one year of data.

5. Conclusions

Although this study found no significant relationship between ARNP scope of practice and select patient outcome variables, there are strong indications that the quality of patient outcomes is not reduced when the scope of practice is expanded. Well-qualified and high-performing ARNPs may positively contribute to access and utilization of primary care services in rural areas (Institute of Medicine, 2010). The increased access and reduced costs may warrant expanded nurse practitioner autonomy, particularly in rural and other underserved areas. Further longitudinal research that includes additional patient outcome indicators may broaden our understanding of the patient experience with nurse practitioner services, as well as the relationship between their scope of practice and patient outcomes.

Author Contributions: Contribution of the authors can be summarized as follows: Conceptualization: J.O., R.H.; Data Acquisition: J.O.; Methodology: J.O., R.H.; Analyses: R.H., Y.L., A.K., A.B.; Interpretation of Findings: J.O., R.H., A.B.

Funding: The research for this paper was supported by the National Institute on Minority Health and Health Disparities of the National Institutes of Health under Award Number U24MD006954. The content is solely the responsibility of the authors and does not necessarily represent the official views of the National Institutes of Health.

References

1. Office of Minority Health. HHS Action Plan to Reduce Racial and Ethnic Health Disparities: Implementation Progress Report 2011–2014. 2015. Available online: https://www.minorityhealth.hhs.gov/assets/pdf/FINAL_HHS_Action_Plan_Progress_Report_11_2_2015.pdf (accessed on 12 June 2018).

2. Office of Minority Health. Minority Population Profile. 2017. Available online: https://www.minorityhealth.hhs.gov/omh/browse.aspx?lvl=2&lvlid=26 (accessed on 12 June 2018).

3. Institute of Medicine (IOM). The Future of Nursing: Leading Change, Advancing Health. 2010. Available online: https://www.ncbi.nlm.nih.gov/pubmed/24983041 (accessed on 12 June 2018).

4. Van Vleet, A.; Paradise, J. Tapping Nurse Practitioners to Meet Rising Demand for Primary Care. 2015. Available online: https://www.kff.org/medicaid/issue-brief/tapping-nurse-practitioners-to-meet-rising-demand-for-primary-care/ (accessed on 12 June 2018).

5. National Council of State Legislatures (NCSL). Meeting the Primary Care Needs of Rural America. Examining the Role of Non-Physician Providers. Available online: http://www.ncsl.org/research/health/meeting-the-primary-care-needs-of-rural-america.aspx (accessed on 12 June 2018).

6. American Association of Nurse Practitioners (AANP). Scope of Practice for Nurse Practitioners. 2015. Available online: https://www.aanp.org/images/documents/publications/scopeofpractice.pdf (accessed on 12 June 2018).

7. American Association of Nurse Practitioners (ARNP). State Practice Environment. 2018. Available online: https://www.aanp.org (accessed on 12 June 2018).

8. Graves, J.A.; Mishra, P.; Dittus, R.S.; Parikh, R.; Perloff, J.; Buerhaus, P.I. Role of geography and nurse practitioner scope-of-practice in efforts to expand primary care system capacity. *Med. Care* **2016**, *54*, 81–89. [CrossRef] [PubMed]

9. Kurtzman, E.T.; Barnow, B.S.; Johnson, J.E.; Simmens, S.J.; Infeld, D.L.; Mullan, F. Does the regulatory environment affect nurse practitioners' patterns of practice or quality of care in health centers? *Health Serv. Res.* **2017**, *52*, 437–458. [CrossRef] [PubMed]

10. Sakr, M.; Angus, J.; Perrin, J.; Nixon, C.; Nicholl, J.; Wardrope, J. Care of minor injuries by emergency nurse practitioners or junior doctors: a randomized controlled trial. *Lancet* **1999**, *354*, 1321–1326. [CrossRef]

11. Newhouse, R.P.; Stanik-Hutt, J.; White, K.M.; Johantgen, M.; Bass, E.B.; Zangaro, G.; Weiner, J.P. Advanced practice nurse outcomes 1990–2008: A systematic review. *Nurs. Econ.* **2011**, *29*, 230–250. [PubMed]

12. Sonenberg, A.; Knepper, H.J. Considering disparities: How do nurse practitioner regulatory policies, access to care, and health outcomes vary across four states? *Nurse Outlook* **2017**, *65*, 143–153. [CrossRef] [PubMed]

13.   Centers for Medicare and Medicaid Services.   Rural Health Clinic.   2018.   Available online:
       https://www.cms.gov/Outreach-and-Education/Medicare-Learning-Network-MLN/MLNProducts/
       downloads/RuralHlthClinfctsht.pdf (accessed on 12 June 2018).

14.   University of Washington. Rural Urban Community Area (RUCA) Codes Maps. Rural Health Research
       Center.   2014.   Available online: http://depts.washington.edu/uwruca/ruca-maps.php (accessed on
       12 June 2018).

15.   D'Agostino, R.B. Tutorial in biostatistics: propensity score methods for bias reduction in the comparison of a
       treatment to a non-randomized control group. *Stat. Med.* **1998**, *17*, 2265–2281. [CrossRef]

16.   Brookhart, M.A.; Schneeweiss, S.; Rothman, K.J.; Glynn, J.; Avorn, J.; Sturmer, T. Variable selection for
       propensity score models. *Am. J. Epidemiol.* **2006**, *163*, 1149–1156. [CrossRef] [PubMed]

17.   Martsolf, G.R.; Kandrack, R.; Gabbay, R.A.; Friedberg, M.W. Cost of transformation among primary care
       practices participating in a medical home pilot. *J. General Int. Med.* **2016**, *31*, 723–731. [CrossRef] [PubMed]

18.   Spetz, J.; Skillman, S.; Andrilla, C. Nurse practitioner autonomy and satisfaction in rural settings.
       Med. Res. Rev. **2017**, *74*, 227–235. [CrossRef] [PubMed]

19.   National Council of State Legislatures (NCSL). Closing the Gaps in Rural Primary Care Workforce.
       2018.   Available online: http://www.ncsl.org/research/health/closing-the-gaps-in-the-rural-primary-
       care-workfor.aspx (accessed on 12 June 2018).

6

The Patient Experience: Informing Practice through Identification of Meaningful Communication from the Patient's Perspective

Angela Grocott [1,*] and Wilfred McSherry [1,2,3] (iD)

1 The University Hospitals of North Midlands NHS NHS Trust, Newcastle Rd,
   Stoke-on-Trent ST4 6QG, UK; W.McSherry@staffs.ac.uk
2 Department of Nursing, School of Health and Social Care, Staffordshire University,
   Blackheath Lane, Stafford ST18 0YB, UK
3 VID vitenskapelige høgskole, Haraldsplass Bergen, Ulriksdal 10, 5009 Bergen, Norway
* Correspondence: Angela.Grocott@uhnm.nhs.uk

Abstract: (1) Background: There is limited empirical knowledge concerning aspects of healthcare that contribute to a good patient experience from the patient's perspective and how patient feedback informs service development. (2) Aim: To examine the issues that influence the effectiveness of communication on patient satisfaction, experience and engagement, in an acute National Health Service (NHS) setting, through identification of the patient's requirements and expectations. (3) Method: Data was gathered from a large teaching hospital using a Friends and Family Test (FFT) and a communication specific survey. Both surveys captured patient narrative to identify predominant influences to explain the quantitative responses. (4) Results: The key priorities for patients are involvement in their care and receiving the right amount of information to support this. However, the delivery of compassionate care was identified as having the most influence on the likelihood of patients to recommend an acute NHS Trust. (5) Conclusion: The findings support a broader understanding of the constituents of an all-encompassing patient experience from the patient's perspective. (6) Implications: healthcare organizations need to focus their resources on how to improve patient/provider communication to support patients to be true partners in their care.

Keywords: communication; patient experience; patient satisfaction; engagement; involvement

1. Introduction

Patient participation in healthcare decision-making is part of a wider trend towards a more bottom-up approach to service planning and delivery with patient experience increasingly conceptualised as a fundamental measurement of healthcare quality [1], patient safety and clinical effectiveness [2]. This has resulted in the introduction of politically driven surveys to measure patient satisfaction and to evaluate the degree to which care is patient-centred [3].

The development of patient/healthcare partnership through reciprocal communication has the potential to strengthen therapeutic bonds [4]. However, to achieve this, it is imperative that patient expectations are considered with an awareness that patient and provider definitions of meaningful communication are likely to differ [5]. As there is a global scarcity of empirical studies that examine influential encounters in an acute healthcare setting [6], an aim of this study was to explore the attributes of meaningful communication in an acute healthcare setting from the patient's perspective. The authors are aware that there is growing interest in the area of patient experience and this is reflected in the growing number of journals devoted specifically to this field, for example the *Journal of Patient Experience* (published by the Association for Patient Experience).

Communication continues to figure consistently as a significant theme in both patient satisfaction and complaints about care delivery [7]. Gaining an understanding of preferred communication from the patient's perspective has the potential to encompass the range of interactions that they prioritise and to take seriously the need for responsiveness to individuals [8]. Putting involvement at the forefront of policy and practice provides the opportunity not only to create an effective and sustainable health and care system, but also to contribute to a more equitable and healthier society [9]. The evidence shows that when patients feel they have a role to play in their care, decisions are better, health and health outcomes improve, and resources are targeted more efficiently [9].

Despite political drivers [10,11], to encourage patient feedback as a resource for the development of patient focused care delivery, National Health Service (NHS) patients continue to provide feedback indicating that they would like more information and greater opportunities to participate in decision making about their daily care and treatment [12,13]. There is limited evidence to indicate that this situation has improved over the last ten years demonstrating the need for further research [14].

As patient experience is multi-faceted, it is very difficult to develop an approach that suits all. However, learning what actually matters for patients during a time of acute illness provides a commonality, which has the potential to inform future practice [15] The majority of patients are naturally anxious about their illness and this is exacerbated when a trusting relationship has not been developed and the patient feels they are not provided with an opportunity for informed choice about treatment options [16].

It has long been argued that communication forms the foundation of all human interaction [17]. Gaining an understanding of preferred communication from the patient's perspective has the potential to encompass the range of interactions that take priority from their perspective and to take seriously the need for responsiveness to individuals [8].

2. Literature Review

A review of existing literature was undertaken to examine current findings relating to the impact of communication on the patient experience from the patient's perspective. The review revealed that there is a scarcity of available literature on this subject. From 2010 to 2012 the literature focused on the behaviours affecting a good patient experience. There was a shift in focus during 2014 as both [18,19] examined the characteristics of negative patient experiences.

The key words used for the search were "Communication" and "Patient Experience" in the title or abstract. As the initial search provided a large number of inappropriate hits the words "Acute Care" and "Research" were added to provide articles which were more relevant to the aims of the evaluation. The following databases were searched indicating the number of hits on each site:

- Cinahl plus with full text (hits – 46)
- BMJ Journals online (hits = 47)
- Cochrane Library (hits = 69)
- Medline (hits = 3)
- Pro Quest Nursing and Allied Health Source (hits = 300)
- RCN Journal (hits = 35)
- Wiley online library (hits = 38)
- Google Scholar (hits = 96)

An inclusion and exclusion criteria was systematically applied resulting in 12 research studies for an empirical literature review.

The search was restricted to papers published in English. Searches were also restricted to papers published from 2008 to date, to reflect relatively current experiences following the Lord Darzi report [20], which put patient experience on the Political agenda. The inclusion criteria specified that the article was a research paper which explored experience from the patient's perspective and the patients were adults who were providing feedback on their experience in an acute hospital setting. Scanning of the reference lists identified a further 3 papers.

As collecting feedback from NHS patients in England became routine during 2012, with the implementation of the Friends and Family Test (FFT) [21] there developed recognition that this feedback was often not shared or acted upon leading to research being conducted to identify how this could be encouraged [22]. Recognition of the benefits and importance of gaining patient feedback was driven by the introduction of the "Friends and Family Test" [21]. The Friends and Family Test (FFT) was piloted in many hospitals in April 2012 with at least ten percent of acute adult in-patients asked how likely they would be to recommend the hospital to their family and friends should they need similar treatment. The usefulness of the test, based on one used in the retail industry, has been challenged as inappropriate for use in a healthcare setting [23]. It has been suggested this quantitative data is not sophisticated enough to capture the specific personal issues that are important to the patients and it is argued data collected in this way is more meaningful to the provider than the patient [24,25].

The Picker Institute Europe [26] recently reviewed the FFT concluding that it is unsuitable to use as a performance indicator between Trusts with criticism of its methodology by researcher [27,28]. The combination of the varying collection methods used by individual Trusts (for example paper based, online, and text) and different patient demographic profiles of respondents has always had the potential to significantly skew the test's results. It is argued therefore that these factors mean that true comparisons between Trusts are impossible [29].

There is recognition that patient narrative is a powerful tool to drive improvement when staff can see patient responses in their own words [30]. Many Trusts have introduced the opportunity for patients to explain why they have chosen their response to the FFT question and this was rolled out as a national requirement from April 2015. The addition of qualitative patient feedback has the potential to provide a richer conceptualisation of both negative and positive interactions and how these may be developed as experience perceptions are subjective and individual [14–31].

Relationship-centred care remains a key theme in contemporary healthcare with recognition that patients who are listened to feel more involved in their care and retain a sense of control [32]. Patients who understand the information provided by the doctor (the term doctor has been used as opposed to physician because this is the term used in the questions) feel a greater sense of control over the treatment decision reducing anxiety and increasing hopefulness making adherence to treatment more likely as they have been motivated by the promise of a positive outcome through the development of a trusting relationship [18].

Contemporary studies suggest that, when patient's expectations and emotional needs are met, communication outcomes are enhanced [32]. However, it is difficult to determine the impact patient expectations have on the overall patient experience and the consequent feedback they provide. As patient experience is strongly linked to fulfilment of expectations, research is required to further examine how to measure expectations and their influences [33].

Limited resources feature highly in patient expectations with more patients reporting doctors and nurses often do not have sufficient time for communication affecting their ability to involve patients in their care and listen to their concerns [34]. As this is a subjective evaluation individual factors should be considered to accommodate individuality [35]. With recognition that people assign different weights to different experiences to arrive at an overall evaluation, customer satisfaction theoretical models have been successfully used to identify what matters most to patients through correlation of survey responses with the patient's numerical rating of the quality of the care they received and their willingness to recommend [36].

It is recognised that a caring environment promotes patients' awareness, resulting in reduced anxiety, improved self-esteem and feelings of being in control [6]. Caring behaviours have the most impact on patient satisfaction with the attributes of closeness, involvement, interaction and relationship being those most wanted by patients and interestingly these are the least observed [37].

A caring environment is the most influential when patients make judgements on their willingness to recommend the hospital [36]. The concept of caring staff incorporates a willingness to help and answer questions, responsiveness to requests, showing courteous behaviour, dignity and respect, providing clear explanations about medicines and how patients should care for themselves post discharge [36].

Authors have identified positive patient responses for older patients were around staff attitude and the most negative were food quality, noise and the inability to obtain help with poor communication cited as a contributing factor [34]. However, a high willingness to recommend score suggests that staff attitude may have the most influence on a good experience for older patients and the patients expect the nurses to have limited time to communicate as they are "too busy" reflecting the findings of [32] in relation to "busy" doctors.

3. Methods

The literature demonstrates that although there are a variety of survey tools, these may be inadequate for measurement of the effects of communication on patient experience and the actions that influence this. However, some positive recommendations were identified and utilised in this investigation especially around data collection and analysis. For example, a communication-specific survey was adopted with recognition that a focus on an individual theme (communication) has the potential to refine the data collection [22]. Furthermore, measuring the quality of communication alongside willingness to recommend has the potential to provide generalisations which may support a strategy to recognise and manage individual expectations [36,37].

A major observation in the literature is that data collection tools are predominantly quantitative (using surveys) therefore this investigation encouraged patient narrative to demonstrate why they chose their specific responses to the questions asked. This method supplemented the wealth of data collection and is more likely to influence staff engagement [22].

It is argued that carrying out studies while the patient is still in hospital is more likely to provide feedback on how the patient is feeling at the time [33] and gain information on those aspects of patient experience the patients themselves see as important [14]. Despite this the literature review identified that the majority of studies examining patient experience of acute care are based on retrospective data.

3.1. Aims

This investigation sought to go beyond what patients liked or did not like about their care in an attempt to identify how the experience made them feel and the contributing attributes of both a positive and negative experience. The aims were:

(1) Examine the issues that influence the effectiveness of communication on patient satisfaction, experience and engagement, in an acute National Health Service setting, through identification of the patient's requirements and expectations.

(2) Explore the attributes of meaningful communication in an acute healthcare setting from the patient's perspective.

3.2. Design

This investigation used a quantitative design comprising of two questionnaires each with free text boxes to encourage patient narrative. A key word analysis of patients' free text responses was carried out to provide a meaningful picture of their perceptions, feelings and experiences in acute care [38]. Identifying emotions involved looking for words or phrases that describe the emotional impact of the patient experience in the data collected. The resulting commonalities and the frequency that they occur were then compared with the quantitative responses of the FFT and communication surveys.

3.3. Sample and Settings

The data for this study was gathered from a large acute NHS Trust situated across two hospital sites Royal Stoke Hospital (Stoke-on-Trent) and County Hospital (Stafford). Between 5000 and 6000 adult inpatients are discharged each month all of whom should be provided with the opportunity to answer a short FFT satisfaction survey on the day of discharge. Encouragement to provide narrative is included within the survey by asking the responder, "What is the main reason for the answers you have chosen?" and "What could we do better?" The FFT survey responses were gathered via tablet or paper survey and the responses uploaded onto a secure data base (See Table 1). The responses from discharged patients throughout the month of September 2015 were analysed.

Table 1. Meridian Desktop, Friends and Family Test (FFT) Results.

1	How likely are you to recommend our ward to your family and friends if they need similar care or treatment?	Extremely likely	Likely	Neither likely nor unlikely	Extremely unlikely	Don't know	Comments
		1151	261	4	3	2	0
2	Do you feel your pain was kept under control?	Yes always	Yes sometimes	Not at all	Never had pain	Comments	
		1166	150	9	119	0	
3	Do you feel your privacy and dignity were respected?	All of the time	Most of the time	Some of the time	None of the time	Comments	
		1328	92	22	2	0	
4	Did you get enough help from staff to eat your meals?	Yes always	Yes sometimes	Not at all	Did not need help	Comments	
		761	45	7	630	0	
5	Were you involved as much as you wanted to be in decisions about your care and treatment?	Yes	Most of the time	Sometimes	Never	Not applicable	Comments
		1195	177	57	9	5	0
6	Did you feel that you were treated with compassion?	All of the time	Most of the time	Some of the time	None of the time	Not applicable	Comments
		1285	122	23	1	13	0
7	Did you feel you were involved in decisions about you discharge from hospital?	Yes definitely	Yes, to some extent	No	I did not need to be involved	Not applicable	Comments
		1065	248	41	26	64	0
8	Were you given enough notice about when you were going to be discharged?	Yes definitely	Yes, to some extent	No	Not applicable	Comments	
		1086	241	34	80	0	
9	What was the best thing about your experience today?	Comments					
		584					
10	What one thing could we have done better?	Comments					
		169					

The following link provides all the information and guidance about the Friends and Family Test https://www.england.nhs.uk/fft/

During the week commencing 15th September 2015, an additional survey containing 14 questions specifically about communication was hand delivered to all adult in-patients in the same acute Trust across both hospital sites. This survey also provided an opportunity for free text patient responses. The questions were adopted from the standard National Inpatient Survey questions designed by Picker Institute Europe, utilising a Likert scale for data analysis. The data generated using standardised National survey tools is generally of high quality, reliability and validity as these have been psychometrically tested [39].

3.4. Ethics

As this study was an evaluation of existing practices for capturing patient feedback, with no identifiable patient information, ethical approval was not required. This decision was confirmed by the local Research and Development Department at the University Hospitals of North Midlands NHS Trust who reviewed the proposal and associated documents.

3.5. Data Analysis

The dependent variables for this study are:

"How likely are you to recommend our ward to your friends and family if they needed similar care or treatment?"and, "Did you feel you were involved as much as you wanted to be in decisions about your care?"

The independent variable questions related to the characteristics most likely to influence the response were care and communication specific to enable the authors to identify the causal relationship between good communication and patient experience [40].

Optimum Contact Ltd., Meridian software was used to numerically weight the multiple-choice responses to each survey to identify the strength of agreement or disagreement with each question in line with the National Inpatient Survey methodology. Pearson's statistical correlation [41] was used to calculate the importance of each question to the patient's likelihood to recommend and feeling that they were involved in their care whilst in hospital (See Tables 2 and 3).

The narrative feedback from both surveys was reviewed to gain an initial impression of the content. This was followed by a more in-depth review and analysis conducted with the aid of the Meridian software tool. The most commonly cited key words (See Tables 4 and 5) were identified and used to classify and cluster the responses to summarise the data and identify categories.

Concentration was focused on identification of the key words most commonly used by those patients who scored highest and those who scored lowest in each survey to examine the variation of behaviour and effect identified in the data. This approach allowed the authors to revisit the data to refine their understanding of the context in which these words were used. As the narrative responses were predominantly positive, the researcher scanned for those words that scored at least equal to the average FFT weighted response score and occurred more than 20 times (Table 5). Scanning the narrative feedback for those words that scored less than the average 94% weighted score resulted in identification of the key words used most by those patients who are least satisfied about their hospital stay. Due to the predominantly positive weighted narrative feedback there were only 2 words identified as appearing at least 20 times: "better" scoring 89.51% and "nurses" scoring 86.51%. The researcher therefore scanned for words written in a negative context on 5 or more occasions (Table 4).

Table 2. Friends and Family Test questions most likely to influence a likely to recommend score.

Question Number	Question in Order of Importance	Score	Importance
6	Did you feel you were treated with compassion?	96.08	0.52
7	Did you feel you were involved in decisions about your discharge from hospital?	87.82	0.34
5	Were you involved as much as you wanted to be in decisions about your care and treatment?	92.69	0.34
2	Do you feel your pain was kept under control?	93.65	0.32
3	Do you feel your privacy and dignity were respected?	96.75	0.30
8	Were you given enough notice about when you were going to be discharged?	88.73	0.29
4	Did you get enough help from staff to eat your meals?	96.36	0.23

Table 3. Communication Survey questions most likely to influence patients feeling involved in decisions about their care.

Question Number	Question in Order of Importance (Patient to Staff)	Score	Importance (r)
11	How much information about your condition or treatment has been given to you?	99%	0.48
12	Has a member of staff answered your questions about the operation or procedure? (if applicable)	97%	0.46

Table 3. *Cont.*

Question Number	Question in Order of Importance (Patient to Staff)	Score	Importance (r)
14	Afterwards, did a member of staff explain the operation or procedure? (if applicable)	94%	0.41
4	Did you have confidence and trust in the doctors treating you?	99%	0.40
2	When you have important questions to ask a doctor do you get answers that you can understand?	99%	0.40
15	Do you feel you were given enough privacy when discussing your condition or treatment?	98%	0.40
13	Have you been told how you will feel after you had the operation or procedure? (if applicable)	88%	0.35
3	When you have important questions to ask a nurse do you get answers that you can understand?	99%	0.34
6	Do doctors talk in front of you as if you weren't there?	93%	0.29
5	Did you have confidence and trust in the nurses treating you?	100%	0.27
9	Does one member of staff say one thing and another say something different regarding your care?	93%	0.27
7	Do nurses talk in front of you as if you weren't there?	95%	0.21
8	In your opinion, are there enough nurses on duty to care for you in hospital?	80%	0.20

Table 4. Friends & Family Test Questionnaire, Words contributing towards the lowest scores.

Word	Word Count	Average Score	Negative Context
Discharge	17	82.86%	15
Waiting	7	82.36%	7
Communication	11	81.74%	8
Night	15	70.34%	10

Table 5. Friends & Family Test Questionnaire, Top scoring staff attributes.

Attribute	Word Count	Average Score
Professional	23	98.40%
Kind	28	95.99%
Friendly	61	95.41%
Caring	65	95.22%
Helpful	61	94.58%

4. Results

4.1. The Friends and Family Test (FFT) Survey Results

A total of 1444 adult patients, age 18 years or over and spending at least 1 night in hospital, responded to the FFT Survey (out of 5354 discharges) providing a 26.9% response rate against an average national response rate of 25% for the same period [42]. For a breakdown of the individual responses, please see Table 1. Maternity patients were excluded as these patients complete a different FFT survey, which is relevant to their circumstance.

The overall percentage satisfaction score demonstrated by patients likely or extremely likely to recommend the ward to their friends and family should they require similar care or treatment, was 98% exceeding the National score of 95% [42].

The scatter diagram (Figure 1) presents the correlation between Question 1 "How likely are you to recommend our ward to your family and friends should they need similar care or treatment?" and the other 7 questions in the FFT survey. Each square on the chart represents an individual question from the survey. The position of these squares identifies which questions have the most influence on the patient's likelihood to recommend the hospital.

The results suggest that questions 5, 6 and 7 have the highest influence on a positive likely to recommend score. Questions in the upper left quadrant have an above average score and a low importance to the patient. Questions in the bottom left quadrant have a below average score and low importance. Therefore, these questions are less likely to influence the patient's willingness to recommend the hospital.

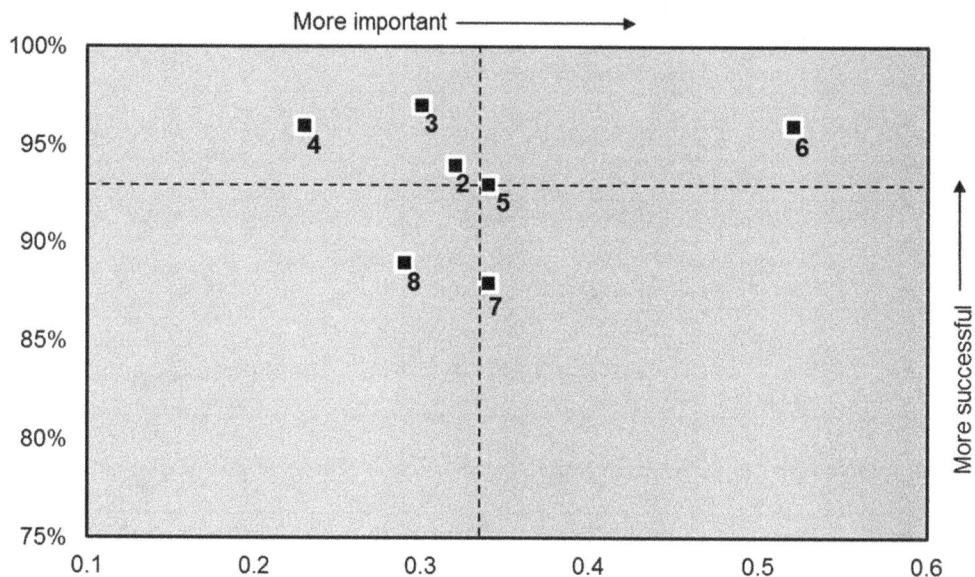

Figure 1. Scatter Diagram (FFT Survey).

The question results are displayed in Table 2 show the co-ordinates used to plot the scatter diagram (Figure 1)

4.2. The Friends and Family Test (FFT) Narrative Analysis

Analysis of the narrative feedback resulted in the identification of the 5 key words that contributed to the overall FFT likely to recommend score (Table 2) and the 4 words that contributed towards the lowest scores (Table 5).

4.3. The Communication Survey Results

The Communication Survey generated a 39% response rate, with 1510 surveys distributed and 591 returned.

Question 10 "Did you feel you were involved as much as you wanted to be in decisions about your care?" was used as the independent variable on which to measure the relationship between the other 13 questions and the patient's perception of feeling involved in their care.

The results suggest that questions 2, 4, 11, 12, 13, 14 and 15 have the highest patient priority when measured against their perceived involvement in their care (Figure 2).

Table 4 shows the patient to staff communication results in order of importance to the patient and the coordinates used to plot the diagram.

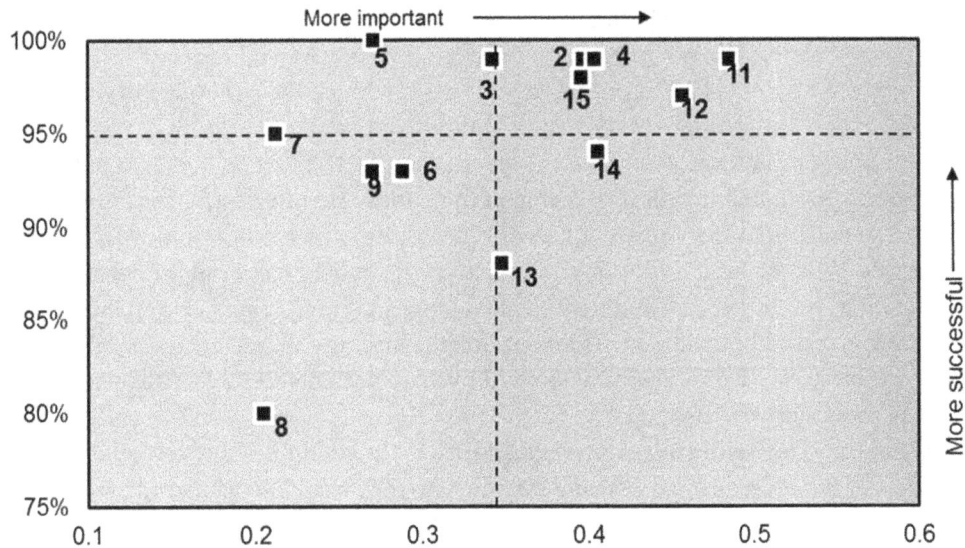

Figure 2. Scatter Diagram (patient-to-staff communication).

4.4. The Communication Survey Narrative Analysis

Analysis of the narrative feedback—provided in the Communication survey—identified that the word "communication" was used 27 times. Twelve of these were in a negative context with patients either stating they would have liked more communication with the health professional or better quality communication.

Analysis of both surveys:

An in-depth analysis of the negative comments/suggestions for improvement in both surveys resulted in the emergence of 3 key themes:

- 21 patients suggested that more staff were needed on the wards as they felt that the staff caring for them were too busy.
- 42 patients felt there was too little or inconsistent communication about their condition and/or hospital stay
- 22 patients described frustrations with delays resulting in a longer hospital stay after they had been told they could go home.

5. Discussion

The words "compassion" and "compassionate" were used positively in 15 responses and the words "care" or "caring" used positively 133 times in the patient narrative of both surveys. This study has identified positive attributes of staff described as "professional," "kind," "friendly" and "helpful" alongside "caring." It may therefore be presumed that these are the key characteristics which lead to patients feeling they have been treated with compassion.

It has been argued that patient experience measures the structures and processes of care based on expectations [43]. Consistent with the findings of [34] the written narrative of respondents identified an impression of limited resources in the NHS. However, this does not affect their overall likely to recommend score. The FFT scatter diagram (Figure 1) suggests patients may have a preconceived expectation that, as they are likely to be cared for in a shared room, their privacy and dignity is at risk of compromise. This is demonstrated by the fact that although question 3—"Do you feel your privacy and dignity was respected?"—scores relatively high, it is situated 5th in the importance ranking and in the left quadrant, and is therefore less influential on the FFT score than may be expected.

Questions 5 and 7 are situated in the right-hand quadrant (Figure 1), indicating that patients do want more involvement in decisions about their care, treatment and discharge. Despite their ranking as

2nd and 3rd importance and the position on the chart indicating these two subjects should be the main focus for improvement, this has not influenced the overall "likely to recommend" score. Interestingly, this does influence the National Inpatient Survey results on which the communication survey results are based [13].

Although a specific question is not asked about the numbers of staff on the ward in the FFT survey a perception of too few staff emerges as a theme in the patient narrative. The communication scatter diagram (Figure 2) identifies question 8, "In your opinion were there enough nurses on duty to care for you in hospital?" as the least important influence on the patient's overall impression of receiving enough information about their care and treatment and being involved as much as they wanted to be in decisions about their care and treatment. This supports the findings of References [32,34]—that patients expect clinicians not to have the time to listen and involve patients in their care, perpetuating their reluctance to become actively engaged.

Rapport-building can be difficult as time constraints for busy clinicians often dictate a task focused approach with concentration on diagnosis and treatment to the detriment of ensuring individual patient concerns are addressed [44]. The high "likely to recommend" score suggests patients interpret this as expected behaviour. However, an environment where patients and relatives perceive staff are not readily available to respond to questions or requests leads to a loss of opportunity for partnership working by presenting a barrier to initiating communication [45]. The long-held belief that time is essential for meaningful conversation is challenged with the findings of this study that patients put more importance on a caring manner and a willingness to communicate demonstrated by kind, friendly staff.

Although 73% of patients and carers responded that they always received answers to important questions from the doctor in a way they could understand the 26% "sometimes" responses suggest that a number of patients are seeking more or clearer information. Doctors talking about the patient as if they were not there is a missed opportunity for information sharing with only 66% of patients reporting that they were always included in conversation with their doctor and 77% receiving enough information about their condition or treatment. Although there are some studies that suggest the time spent during communication between clinician and patient has a direct influence on the quality of the information receive [46] there are studies which argue that the content of the communication and the ability to listen outweighs any benefit which may be gained through time spent [19].

Of the FFT respondents, 83% were involved as much as they wanted to be in decisions about their care and this reduced further to 77% for involvement in discharge decisions. Although this did not affect the likely to recommend score it highlights a need for improved engagement and communication with patients.

The scatter diagrams (s 1 and 2) demonstrate key priorities for patients who expect and want to be involved in their care and receive the right amount of information to enable this. They want to receive answers to their questions in a way they can understand, have any tests and/or procedures explained and have confidence and trust in the doctors treating them. These results suggest patients want to be provided with the opportunity to be actively engaged contrary to the belief of many clinicians [47].

With a political drive to encourage and support the public to be more actively engaged in decisions about their own health [10], it is important to ensure their expectations are realistic and opportunities for communication are sought without creating barriers to potential patient led improvements [48]. An ability to communicate in a manner, which identifies the situation from the patient's perspective, is arguably the pivotal skill required to enable this [49] with recognition this is particularly difficult when personal characteristics or beliefs differ.

This study suggests that patients want to be afforded the opportunity to be actively engaged however their expectations are often linked to past experience of self or others. They are understandably often anxious, finding themselves in strange surroundings reliant on unfamiliar staff and are reluctant to ask questions for fear of being considered a difficult patient [50], with an expectation that the healthcare professionals will be too busy to answer their questions.

Encouraging patients to share decision-making, alongside the professionals caring for them, requires interventions aimed at changing long established behaviours and perceptions of both staff and patients [47]. Contemporary healthcare is evolving with a change in attitudes from a paternalistic approach which some patients and staff find difficult [51]. Health Professionals who provide tools to support understanding and encourage patients to ask questions are more likely to tailor information sharing to individual needs [10]. Patients who have the opportunity to communicate are more likely to have realistic expectations around their care and prognosis. However, to reduce barriers, this must be at the patient's own level of understanding and at the most appropriate time [52] with consideration for the effect of acute illness on engagement.

6. Conclusions

The findings indicate that it is the responsibility of all healthcare providers to improve their communication skills, demonstrating a willingness to communicate by proactively encouraging patients to ask questions. Providers may also need to promote extended visiting hours to support more opportunity for communication. Finally, there is a need to ensure patient information leaflets are written to comply with national guidance to promote understanding [52]. As long as the patient remains dissatisfied with the communication they have received there will remain opportunity for improvement through a patient-centred approach. This will only be achieved when the caring encounter is experienced as a meaningful encounter. Patients who understand the information given to them and are given a sense of control in the decision-making process are likely to be less anxious and comply with treatment recommendations [18] with potential to reduce the length of stay and risk of readmission. Despite the limitations of this study, it has provided a foundation for future research in this field through the identification of influencing factors that contribute to overall patient satisfaction and the difficulties surrounding patient understanding and engagement.

7. Implications for Practice

The results from this evaluation can be used to develop a culture that encourages patients to ask questions by:

- Developing an inpatient leaflet which explains the concept of shared decision making and why it is important. Provides an explanation that their knowledge about their health and lifestyle is as important as the clinician's expertise with each complimenting each other.
- Creating a communication drive to encourage patients to ask questions providing suggested questions as examples on electronic posters, notice boards and hospital websites
- Introducing a paper at the bedside for question prompt lists to enable questions to be written down as the patient and/or relative thinks of them in preparation of ward rounds
- Exploring the use of the internet as a patient information tool to generate questions.
- Supporting clinicians to improve their communication skills—Develop a training programme for introduction of "teach back" methodology
- Promoting extended visiting hours to support more opportunity for communication.
- Ensure patient information leaflets are written to the recommended reading age to facilitate understanding by the majority of the population.

8. Recommendations for Future Evaluations/Research

A significant limitation of this research is its cross-sectional nature, meaning that the patient's experiences were captured at a single time point and with a specific cohort or group of patients. This type of evaluation may be better conducted more longitudinally. Similarly, patients may report more positive experiences when completing surveys while in hospital, just prior to discharge.

- Conduct the evaluation for planned and emergency admissions separately to identify if there are any variances in results

- Repeat at ward level to identify examples of good practice for dissemination across the organisation
- Repeat with inclusion of demographic detail to identify if there are any variances in results.
- Repeat for individual demographic patient groups to identify specific communication strategies and needs.

Author Contributions: A.G. and W.M. conceived and designed the investigation. A.G. conducted the investigation; A.G. and W.M. analyzed the data; A.G. and W.M. wrote the paper.

References

1. Wiig, S.; Storm, M.; Aase, K.; Gjestsen, M.; Solhelm, M.; Harthug, S.; Robert, G.; Fulop, N. QUASER Team. Investigating the use of patient involvement and patient experience in quality improvement in Norway: Rhetoric or reality? *BMC Health Serv. Res.* **2013**, *13*, 206. [CrossRef] [PubMed]
2. Ahmed, F.; Burt, J.; Roland, M. Measuring Patient Experience: Concepts and Methods. *Patient* **2014**, *7*, 235–241. [CrossRef] [PubMed]
3. Price, R.; Elliott, M.; Zaslavsky, A.; Hays, R.; Lehrman, W.; Rybowski, L.; Edgman-Levitan, S.; Clearly, P. Examining the role of patient experience surveys in measuring healthcare quality. *Med. Care Res. Rev.* **2014**, *71*, 522–554. [CrossRef] [PubMed]
4. Juve-Udina, M.; Perez, E.; Padres, N.; Samartino, M.; Garcia, M.; Creus, M.; Batilori, N.; Calvo, C. Basic Nursing Care: Retrospective evaluation of communication and psychosocial interventions documented by nurses in the acute care setting. *J. Nurs. Scholarsh.* **2014**, *46*, 65–72. [CrossRef] [PubMed]
5. Snellman, I.; Gustafsson, C.; Gustafsson, L. Patients' and Caregivers' Attributes in a Meaningful Care Encounter: Similarities and Notable Differences. *Int. Sch. Res. Netw. Nurs.* **2012**, *2012*, 320145. [CrossRef] [PubMed]
6. Gustafsson, C.; Gustafsson, L.; Snellman, I. Trust leading to hope—The signification of meaningful encounters in Swedish healthcare. The narratives of patients, relatives and healthcare staff. *Int. Pract. Dev. J.* **2013**, *3*, 1–13.
7. Newell, S.; Jordan, Z. The patient experience of patient-centred communication with nurses in the hospital setting: A qualitative systematic review protocol. *JBI Database Syst. Rev. Implement. Rep.* **2015**, *13*, 76–87. [CrossRef] [PubMed]
8. Entwistle, V.; Firnigl, D.; Ryan, M.; Francis, J.; Kinghorn, P. Which experiences of healthcare delivery matter to service users and why? A critical interpretive synthesis and conceptual map. *J. Health Serv. Res. Policy* **2012**, *17*, 70–78. [CrossRef] [PubMed]
9. Foot, C.; Gilbert, H.; Dunn, P.; Jabbal, J.; Seale, B.; Goodrich, J.; Buck, D.; Taylor, J. *People in Control of Their Own Health and Care: The State of Involvement*; The Kings Fund: London, UK, 2014.
10. Department of Health. *Liberating the NHS: No Decision About Me Without Me*; The Stationary Office: London, UK, 2012.
11. Francis, R. *Report of the Mid Staffordshire NHS Foundation Trust Public Inquiry: Executive Summary*; The Stationary Office: London, UK, 2013.
12. Keogh, B. Review into the Quality of Care and Treatment Provided by 14 Hospital Trusts In England: Overview Report. 2013. Available online: http://www.nhs.uk/nhsengland/bruce-keogh-review/documents/outcomes/keogh-review-final-report.pdf (accessed on 1 February 2018).
13. Care Quality Commission. Adult Inpatient Survey. 2015. Available online: http://www.cqc.org.uk/content/adult-inpatient-survey-2015 (accessed on 1 February 2018).
14. Ponsignon, F.; Smart, A.; Williams, M.; Hall, J. Healthcare experience quality: An empirical exploration using content analysis techniques. *J. Serv. Manag.* **2015**, *26*, 460–485. [CrossRef]
15. Fredericks, S.; Lapum, J.; Hui, G. Examining the effect of patient-centred care on outcomes. *Br. J. Nurs.* **2015**, *24*, 394–400. [CrossRef] [PubMed]
16. Levinson, W.; Hudak, P.; Tricco, A. A systematic review of surgeon-patient communication: Strengths and opportunities for improvement. *Patient Educ. Couns.* **2013**, *93*, 3–17. [CrossRef] [PubMed]

17. Mortensen, D. *Communication: The Study of Human Interaction*; McGraw-Hill Book Company: New York, NY, USA, 1972.

18. Legg, A.; Andrews, S.; Huynh, H.; Ghane, A.; Tabuenca, A.; Sweeny, K. Patients' anxiety and hope: Predictors and adherence intensions in an acute care context. *Health Expect.* **2014**, *18*, 3034–3043. [CrossRef] [PubMed]

19. Saunders, C.; Abel, G.; Lyratzopoulos, G. What explains worse patient experience in London? Evidence from secondary analysis of the cancer patient experience survey. *BMJ Open* **2014**, *4*. [CrossRef] [PubMed]

20. Department of Health. *High Quality Care for All: NHS Next Stage Review Final Report*; The Stationary Office: London, UK, 2008.

21. Department of Health & NHS Midlands and East. NHS Friends and Family Test Implementation Guidance. 2012. Available online: http://www.england.nhs.uk/wp-content/uploads/2013/07/fft-imp-guid.pdf (accessed on 1 February 2018).

22. Reeves, R.; West, E.; Barron, D. Facilitated patient experience feedback can improve nursing care: A pilot study for a phase III cluster randomised controlled trial. *BMC Health Serv. Res.* **2013**, *13*, 259. [CrossRef] [PubMed]

23. Graham, C.; McCormick, S. *Overarching Questions for Patient Surveys: Development Report for the Care Quality Commission*; National Patient Survey Coordination Centre: Oxford, UK, 2012.

24. Dawood, M.; Gallini, A. Using discovery interviews to understand the patient experience. *Nurs. Manag.* **2010**, *17*, 26–31. [CrossRef] [PubMed]

25. Manacorda, T.; Erens, B.; Black, N.; Mays, N. The Friends and Family Test in General Practice in England: A qualitative study of the views of staff and patients. *Br. J. Gen. Pract.* **2017**, *67*, 370–376. [CrossRef] [PubMed]

26. Picker Institute Europe. *Policy Briefing: The Friends and Family Test*; Picker Institute Europe: Oxford, MI, USA, August 2014.

27. Lynn, P. The Friends and Family Test Is Unfit for Purpose. *The Guardian*, 2013. Available online: http://www.theguardian.com/healthcare-network/2013/apr/09/friends-family-test-unfit-forpurpose(accessed on 1 February 2018).

28. Reeves, R. Why the Friends and Family Test Won't Work. *Health Serv. J.* 2012. Available online: http://www.hsj.co.uk/comment/columnists/why-the-friends-and-family-testwont-work/5052423.article (accessed on 1 February 2018).

29. Sizmur, S.; Graham, C.; Walsh, J. Influence of patients' age and sex and the mode of administration on results from the NHS Friends and Family Test of patient experience. *J. Health Serv. Res. Policy* **2014**, *20*, 5–10. [CrossRef] [PubMed]

30. Graham, C. The Friends and Family Test Can Make the Grade. *Health Serv. J.* 2013. Available online: http://www.hsj.co.uk/comment/the-friends-andfamily-test-can-make-thegrade/5062422.article (accessed on 1 February 2018).

31. Lemke, F.; Clark, M.; Wilson, H. Customer experience quality: An exploration in business and consumer contexts using repertory grid technique. *J. Acad. Mark. Sci.* **2011**, *39*, 846–869. [CrossRef]

32. Ross, L.; Petersen, A.; Johnsen, A.; Lundstrom, L.; Groenvold, M. Cancer patients' evaluation of communication: A report from the population based study "The Cancer Patient's World". *Support. Care Cancer* **2013**, *21*, 235–244. [CrossRef] [PubMed]

33. Bjertnaes, O.; Sjetne, I.; Iversen, H. Overall patient satisfaction with hospitals: Effects of patient reported experiences and fulfilment of expectations. *Br. Med. J. Qual. Saf.* **2012**, *21*, 39–49. [CrossRef] [PubMed]

34. Dicks, S.; Chaplin, R.; Hood, C. Factors affecting care on acute hospital wards. *Nurs. Older People* **2013**, *25*, 18–23. [CrossRef] [PubMed]

35. Vinagre, M.; Neves, J. The influence of service quality and patients' emotions on satisfaction. *Int. J. Health Care Qual. Assur.* **2008**, *21*, 87–103. [CrossRef] [PubMed]

36. Otani, K.; Waterman, B.; Claiborne, W.; Ehinger, S. Patient satisfaction: How patient health conditions influence their satisfaction. *J. Healthc. Manag.* **2012**, *57*, 276–293. [CrossRef] [PubMed]

37. Palese, A.; Tornietto, M.; Suhonen, R.; Efstathiou, G.; Tsangari, H.; Merkouris, A.; Jarosova, D.; Leino-Kilpi, H.; Patiraki, E.; Kariou, C.; et al. Surgical patient satisfaction as an outcome of nurses' caring behaviours: A descriptive and correlational study in six European countries. *J. Nurs. Scholarsh.* **2011**, *43*, 341–350. [CrossRef] [PubMed]

38. LaVela, S.L.; Gallan, A.S. Evaluation and Measurement of Patient Experience. *Patient Exp. J.* **2014**, *1*, 28–36.

39. Al-Abri, R.; Al-Balushi, A. Patient Satisfaction Survey as a Tool towards Quality Improvement. *Oman Med. J.* **2014**, *29*, 3–7. [CrossRef] [PubMed]

40. Hart, C. *Doing Your Masters Dissertation*; Sage Publications Limited: London, UK, 2005.

41. Deviant, S. *The Practically Cheating Statistics Handbook*, 2nd ed.; The Sequel; Andale LLC: Orlando, FL, USA, 2010.

42. NHS England. Organisational Level Tables (Historic). FFT Inpatient—September 2015. 2015. Available online: https://www.england.nhs.uk/ourwork/pe/fft/friends-and-family-test-data/fft-data-historic/ (accessed on 1 February 2018).

43. Coulter, A.; Fitzpatrick, R.; Cornwell, J. *The Point of Care. Measures of Patients' Experience in Hospital: Purpose, Methods and Uses*; The Kings Fund: London, UK, 2009.

44. Angus, D.; Watson, B.; Smith, A.; Gallois, C.; Wiles, J. Visualising Conversation Structure across Time: Insights into Effective Doctor-Patient Consultations. *PLoS ONE* **2012**, *7*, e38014. [CrossRef] [PubMed]

45. McGilton, K.; Boscart, V.; Fox, M.; Sidani, S.; Rochon, E.; Sorin-Peters, R. A Systematic Review of the Effectiveness of Communication Interventions for Health Care Providers Caring for Patients in a Residential Setting. *World Views Evid. Based Nurs.* **2009**, *6*, 149–159. [CrossRef] [PubMed]

46. European Commission. *Eurobarometer Qualitative Study: Patient Involvement*. Aggregate Report. May 2012. Available online: http://ec.europa.eu/public_opinion/archives/quali/ql_5937_patient_en.pdf (accessed on 1 February 2018).

47. Joseph-Williams, N.; Edwards, A.; Elwyn, A. Power imbalance prevents shared decision making. *Br. Med. J.* **2014**, *348*, g3178. [CrossRef] [PubMed]

48. Legare, F.; Shemilt, M.; Stacey, D. Can Shared Decision Making Increase the Uptake of Evidence Based Practice? *Frontline Gastroenterol.* **2011**, *2*, 176–181. [CrossRef] [PubMed]

49. Grossman, V. Hot topics: Do we make the difficult patient more difficult? *J. Radiol. Nurs.* **2012**, *31*, 27–28. [CrossRef]

50. Judson, T.; Detsky, A.; Press, M. Encouraging Patients to Ask Questions. How to Overcome "White-Coat Silence". *J. Am. Med. Assoc.* **2013**, *309*, 2325–2326. [CrossRef] [PubMed]

51. Zahedi, F. The challenge of truth telling across cultures: A case study. *J. Med. Ethics Hist. Med.* **2011**, *4*, 11. [PubMed]

52. NHS England. *Accessible Information Standard. Making Health and Social Care Information Accessible*. 2016. Available online: https://www.england.nhs.uk/ourwork/accessibleinfo/ (accessed on 1 February 2018).

## 7

Defining the Optimal Dietary Approach for Safe, Effective and Sustainable Weight Loss in Overweight and Obese Adults

Chrysi Koliaki [1,*], Theodoros Spinos [2], Marianna Spinou [2], Maria-Eugenia Brinia [2], Dimitra Mitsopoulou [2] and Nicholas Katsilambros [1,3]

[1] First Department of Propaedeutic Medicine, National Kapodistrian University of Athens, Laiko University Hospital, Athens 11527, Greece; nicholaskatsilambros@gmail.com

[2] Medical School, National Kapodistrian University of Athens, Athens 11527, Greece; thspinos@otenet.gr (T.S.); mspinou@otenet.gr (M.S.); mairyjane1054@gmail.com (M.-E.B.); dimits96@gmail.com (D.M.)

[3] Research Laboratory Christeas Hall, Medical School, National Kapodistrian University of Athens, Athens 11527, Greece

* Correspondence: ckoliaki@yahoo.com

Abstract: Various dietary approaches with different caloric content and macronutrient composition have been recommended to treat obesity in adults. Although their safety and efficacy profile has been assessed in numerous randomized clinical trials, reviews and meta-analyses, the characteristics of the optimal dietary weight loss strategy remain controversial. This mini-review will provide general principles and practical recommendations for the dietary management of obesity and will further explore the components of the optimal dietary intervention. To this end, various dietary plans are critically discussed, including low-fat diets, low-carbohydrate diets, high-protein diets, very low-calorie diets with meal replacements, Mediterranean diet, and diets with intermittent energy restriction. As a general principle, the optimal diet to treat obesity should be safe, efficacious, healthy and nutritionally adequate, culturally acceptable and economically affordable, and should ensure long-term compliance and maintenance of weight loss. Setting realistic goals for weight loss and pursuing a balanced dietary plan tailored to individual needs, preferences, and medical conditions, are the key principles to facilitate weight loss in obese patients and most importantly reduce their overall cardiometabolic risk and other obesity-related comorbidities.

Keywords: obesity; weight loss diets; macronutrient composition; safety; efficacy

1. Introduction

Identifying safe and effective strategies for long-term weight control is critical to reduce the alarming prevalence of overweight and obesity in adults and adolescents worldwide and mitigate obesity-associated health risks [1]. Obesity and overweight affect together over a third of the world's population today, and if current trends continue, an estimated 38% of the world's adult population will be overweight and another 20% will be obese by 2030 [2]. Although obesity is a complex and multifactorial disease with genetic, behavioral, socioeconomic, and environmental origins, it is also preventable and treatable to a great extent [3]. There is no doubt that the first-line treatment of obesity is dietary management combined with behavior modification, and secondarily, increased physical activity [4]. Weight loss medication and bariatric surgery are further recommended for specific subgroups of obese patients [5].

Dietary guidelines for weight loss vary greatly between different scientific societies and have been revised many times, reflecting the uncertainty in the field of nutritional management of obesity and the difficulty to generate uniform recommendations for all patients [5,6]. Although there are dozens of weight loss diets promising to reduce body weight [7], the characteristics of the optimal strategy remain controversial, and no single dietary strategy is uniformly superior to others in terms of weight loss and maintenance for the general population.

The optimal macronutrient ratio of a diet, or else the proportion of calories contributed by fat, carbohydrate, and protein, has received significant attention in the past decades for its potential relevance in weight loss [8], but remains still elusive. Some researchers emphasize the role of energy deficit irrespective of macronutrient composition [9], some others highlight the role of macronutrient composition irrespective of caloric count [10,11], and finally others underscore the role of diet quality by means of naturally cooked and unprocessed healthy foods irrespective of macronutrient composition or energy intake [12,13], to achieve weight loss and other health benefits. All these approaches have their own rationale and are all evidence-based and partly correct. However, the key to successful weight loss lies in the prudent combination of all these approaches in the context of a healthy and balanced diet without severe restrictions or nutritional exaggerations.

The present review aims to provide general principles and practical recommendations for the dietary management of obesity, and further explore the components of the optimal dietary intervention. To this end, various dietary plans are critically discussed, such as low-fat diets, low-carbohydrate diets, high-protein diets, formula diets, Mediterranean diet, and diets with intermittent energy restriction, to define the optimal dietary approach for a safe, effective, and sustainable weight loss in overweight and obese adults.

2. General Principles

Generally, it is not possible to lose weight without a negative energy balance [14]. It is, therefore, necessary that energy intake is consistently lower than energy expenditure to achieve weight loss [14]. In addition to energy restriction, the macronutrient composition of a diet was originally thought to play an important role for weight loss, on the grounds that diets with specific macronutrient ratios may be more appropriate to facilitate weight loss than others based on their differential potential to promote satiety, burn fat, and preserve metabolically active lean body mass [15]. However, the relevance of macronutrient-centered weight loss diets has been mainly substantiated by short-term studies [16–18], and results may be influenced by inter-individual biological and behavioral differences as well as different adherence rates. Of note, longer-term studies fail to provide any robust evidence in support of modulating dietary macronutrient composition to achieve a better weight loss outcome [19,20]. Although literature in the field remains inconclusive, the current state of evidence suggests that modification of dietary macronutrient composition is not as effective and clinically relevant for long-term weight management as originally believed [8,21].

Setting realistic goals for weight loss is extremely important since the adoption of strict and difficult to reach goals may often lead to failure and discouragement [22]. Aiming to lose 5–10% of initial body weight within the first six months is a realistic approach, which is furthermore paralleled by a significant improvement in cardiometabolic risk factors [5,6]. Beyond setting realistic goals, long-term adherence to dietary interventions represents also a great challenge, since many diets are pursued for only short periods of time-especially those with extreme restrictions-, leading to suboptimal long-term weight control [23].

An even more important goal than weight loss is weight loss maintenance and prevention of weight regain. The physiological response to weight loss is resistance to further weight loss through a compensational biological adaptation expressed as a shift in hormone balance related to appetite regulation, a decline of resting energy expenditure and a reduction of diet-induced thermogenesis [24,25]. Diet-induced weight loss has been associated with increased levels of orexigenic hormones (ghrelin) and reduced levels of anorexigenic hormones (leptin, peptide YY, cholecystokinin) [26]. The effects of weight loss on postprandial secretion of gastrointestinal satiety hormones remain controversial [26]. Furthermore, it has been shown that a weight loss of 10% may lead to a reduction of total energy expenditure by 550 kcal/d [27]. Among all the implicated mechanisms, the increased drive to eat after weight loss is, in fact, several-fold larger than the corresponding adaptations in total energy expenditure, and potentially represents the main driver of weight regain [28,29]. Of note, these adaptations may persist for up to a year after the initial weight loss and may often lead to relapse [30]. As a result, only around 20% of obese patients can preserve and stabilize the weight loss effect in the long-term (data from National Weight Control Registry) [31]. In detail, more than half of dieters regain most of their weight loss within the first 12 months and less than one-third can avoid weight regain over a three-year period [32,33].

The ideal weight loss maintenance diet should be continuous, easy to comply with, and of low energy density [34,35]. Predictors of successful long-term weight maintenance after initial weight loss involve frequent self-monitoring of body weight [36], medical supervision for psychological support and positive feedback [37], consistency of food intake [38], eating breakfast [39,40], low-fat intake [35], low intake of unhealthy snacks [41], and high levels of regular physical activity [42]. It has been further suggested by preliminary evidence that the space of a meal consumption (fast vs. slow) may also affect body weight control and maintenance [43]. It has been shown in healthy volunteers that consuming slowly a standardized meal may lead to a sharper rise in anorexigenic hormones and promote more a feeling of fullness compared to a faster rate of meal consumption [44]. These preliminary findings warrant, however, further investigation.

3. Conventional Hypocaloric Diets

Conventional hypocaloric diets typically aim at reducing daily energy intake by 500–750 kcal. This energy restriction is usually achieved by diets of 1200–1500 kcal/d for females and 1500–1800 kcal/d for males [45]. Conventional diets are generally low-fat diets and most of them have the following macronutrient composition: 30% fat, 50% carbohydrate and 20% protein [45]. A particular emphasis is placed on reducing intake of saturated (animal-derived) fat and increasing intake of fiber-rich foods such as fruit and vegetables [45]. The latter can both promote satiety and provide a great variety of beneficial micronutrients. Reducing daily energy intake by 500–600 kcal can lead to a modest weight loss of approximately 0.5 kg per week or else 2 kg per month. This weight loss is usually seen only in the first months, since the rate of weight loss is expected to slow down because of the hormonal adaptations resisting weight loss, as described above [24]. It is essential that conventional diets are individualized based on the weight loss course of each subject, and individual food preferences need to be considered, since these diets are usually followed for long periods of time to achieve a clinically meaningful weight loss [45]. Although energy-restricted diets are modestly effective for short-term weight loss [46], individual response to hypocaloric diets is heterogeneous and long-term adherence to these diets is difficult to accomplish [47].

4. Low-Fat Diets

Low-fat diets have been recommended as safe and effective weight loss strategies for many decades on the basis of several observations: (1) energy from fat is less satiating than energy from carbohydrate, and a high fat/carbohydrate ratio in the diet can promote passive overconsumption, positive energy balance and weight gain in susceptible individuals [48–50]; (2) fat is more readily absorbed from the intestine than carbohydrate and fecal energy loss is much lower with a high dietary fat/carbohydrate ratio; (3) carbohydrate is more thermogenic than fat and energy expenditure is lower during a diet with a high fat/carbohydrate ratio than during a diet with a low fat/carbohydrate ratio [51,52]; and (4) a high-fat diet may damage the intestinal barrier and cause intestinal dysbiosis with an adverse impact on body weight and metabolic variables [53]. Another reason for lowering the proportion of calories consumed from fat is that a single gram of fat contains more than twice the calories of a gram of carbohydrates or protein (9 kcal/gram vs. 4 kcal/gram). Thus, reducing total fat intake may theoretically lead to a considerable effect on total amount of calories consumed.

Despite the above theoretical considerations, randomized trials have failed to consistently demonstrate that reducing fat intake may be superior to other dietary interventions in terms of long-term weight loss. In a meta-analysis comparing several popular weight loss diets, low-fat diets were found to be equally effective as other diets in terms of weight loss, without however reporting any differences between diets in qualitative aspects, compliance rates and adverse events [54]. Another study has shown that both low-fat and higher-fat diets have similar effects on weight loss, total and visceral fat loss, and lean body mass preservation [8]. In this study, both diets were characterized by low intake of saturated fat and foods of high glycemic index and an increased intake of fiber-rich foods, suggesting that when standards of a high-quality diet are met, variations in macronutrient composition play a secondary role for weight loss [8]. In another systematic review and meta-analysis comparing low-fat diets with other dietary interventions, it was found that the long-term effect of low-fat diets on body weight depends primarily on the intensity of diet intervention in the comparison group [55]. When compared to usual diets, low-fat diets are indeed more effective in weight reduction with a slight to modest effect [55]. However, when compared to other higher-fat dietary interventions of similar intensity such as low-carbohydrate diets and especially when high adherence rates are achieved, low-fat diets are equally or less effective in achieving significant long-term weight control [55].

5. Low-Carbohydrate Diets

Low-carbohydrate diets originated from the old ketogenic Atkins diet [56], which was based on a severe restriction of carbohydrate intake (<30 g/d) and was characterized thus by poor dietary quality [57]. In the current versions of low-carbohydrate diets, carbohydrate restrictions are less severe compared to Atkins diet but still quite substantial, and there is also an increased fiber intake [45]. Long-term compliance to low-carbohydrate diets is both difficult and potentially hazardous since a significant reduction of carbohydrate intake in combination with high fat intake may lead to increased low-density lipoprotein (LDL) cholesterol levels and an elevated mortality risk [58]. Meta-analyses have shown that very low carbohydrate ketogenic diets are more effective short-term than other dietary strategies in terms of weight loss and improvement of metabolic variables in patients with diabetes [10]. Regarding low-carbohydrate diets, meta-analyses of randomized clinical trials provide conflicting evidence. Some meta-analyses have suggested that low-carbohydrate diets provide better weight loss outcomes than low-fat diets, but weight loss benefits should be weighed against potential risks associated with LDL-cholesterol increase [59]. On the other hand, other meta-analyses have shown that low-carbohydrate diets confer equal weight loss short-term as isoenergetic balanced [60] or low-fat diets [61]. Some other meta-analyses have suggested that low-carbohydrate diets without energy restriction are as effective as energy-restricted low-fat diets in weight loss, emphasizing potential favorable effects on triglycerides and high-density-lipoprotein (HDL) cholesterol levels [62]. Of note, data on the long-term (beyond one year) safety and efficacy of these diets are currently limited, so there is insufficient evidence to support their long-term use.

A low-carbohydrate diet program has been recently introduced and successfully applied in Greece. This intervention is named Eurodiet and is based on the progressive reduction and reintroduction of carbohydrates in four consecutive stages [63]. At the last stage, patients apply a healthy balanced diet with characteristics of a Mediterranean diet and a modest restriction of carbohydrate intake. When this program is further accompanied by a frequent monitoring of psychological parameters and intense behavior modification, the effects are even greater [63].

6. High-Protein Diets

In high-protein diets, protein contributes by 20–30% to the total daily energy intake [64]. It has been suggested that such diets may deliver a greater weight loss than lower-protein diets (15–20%) due to their satiety-promoting effects and lean body mass preservation, in addition to relatively increased diet-induced thermogenesis [65,66]. Clinical intervention studies have shown that an ad libitum high-protein diet in overweight people may lead to a weight loss of 3.8 kg in a six-month weight loss program by enhancing satiety, as opposed to a high-carbohydrate diet [67]. It has been also demonstrated that an energy-restricted, high-protein diet may provide equal or even greater weight loss and metabolic benefits compared to a high-carbohydrate diet in obese women [68]. Furthermore, weight loss studies in overweight women have shown that diets with a high dietary protein to carbohydrate ratio may exert beneficial effects on body composition, blood lipid profile, and glucose homeostasis. These benefits may be partly mediated by effects on satiety and a lower glycemic load due to lower carbohydrate intake [69,70]. A higher protein intake during weight loss may also prevent some of the inevitable loss of lean body mass and may thus enhance insulin sensitivity [71,72], although this has not been observed at a very low energy intake [73]. In overweight men and women with either insulin resistance or type 2 diabetes, a high-protein weight loss diet (28–30% protein from mixed sources) was shown to enhance fat loss by 1–2 kg over 12 weeks, particularly in women, compared with an isocaloric high-carbohydrate diet [74,75]. Taken together, higher-protein diets may facilitate weight loss when compared to lower-protein diets in the short-term (up to 6 months), but longer-term data are limited and inconsistent [66]. The optimal amount and sources of dietary protein remain also controversial. Animal-derived proteins may be positively associated with obesity and weight gain as shown in longitudinal prospective studies, while plant-derived proteins may be protective for the development of obesity [19,20]. Furthermore, dietary patterns high in protein may vary in saturated fat and nutritional composition, and concerns have been raised regarding the effects of high-protein diets on serum lipids and subsequent cardiovascular disease risk [76]. In addition, high-protein diets and especially animal-derived proteins may pose an increased risk of nephrolithiasis, diabetes mellitus and atherosclerosis, as well as progressive kidney damage in susceptible individuals [77]. Based on the above, a prudent recommendation in dietary practice would be to partially replace refined carbohydrates with protein sources that are low in saturated fat [66]. An example of high-protein diets are formula diets, which are analytically described below.

7. Formula Diets

Formula diets represent an additional evidence-based intervention in the weight management tool box. They provide a greater energy deficit than conventional hypocaloric diets and are also referred to as very-low-calorie diets (VLCD, <800 kcal/d) or low-calorie diets (LCD, 800–1200 kcal/d). They comprise ready-to-ingest meal replacements in the form of nutrient-enriched bars, soups, and drinks, which are low in carbohydrate and fat and rich in vitamins, minerals, and proteins of high biological value. As a result of drastic energy restriction, formula diets promote a substantial weight loss of 10–20 kg within 8–12 weeks [78]. After the initial phase of rapid weight loss, several strategies have been proposed to ensure weight loss maintenance and prevent weight regain, including high-protein diets, anti-obesity drugs, partial use of meal replacements, and most importantly, high levels of physical activity [79]. It has been shown that if the above strategies are pursued, weight loss maintenance is feasible after VLCDs [79]. After the desired weight loss is achieved, food is gradually reintroduced, and patients return to a healthy and balanced dietary plan. In pathophysiological terms, the reduced caloric and in particular the reduced carbohydrate content of formula diets increases circulating blood ketones and may thus reduce hyperinsulinemia of obese patients leading to sustained suppression of hunger and thus to better compliance [80]. The profound initial weight loss experienced by severely obese patients may further motivate them and promote thus adherence to the diet [78,81].

It is important to note that formula diets are intended for short-term use of maximum 12 weeks and should be always applied in carefully selected patients under continuous medical supervision and accompanied by sufficient education and psychological support. If the above requirements are met, formula diets may deliver significant weight loss and maintenance with concomitant health benefits in terms of metabolic profile and symptomatic improvement in several subgroups of patients, such as patients with diabetes [82], osteoarthritis [83], obstructive sleep apnea [84], psoriasis [85], and more commonly, in the pre-operative period of morbidly obese patients who are planned to undergo bariatric surgery, since the reduction of liver size achieved by VLCDs may facilitate surgical manipulations [86].

8. Mediterranean Diet

DIRECT study (Dietary Intervention Randomized Controlled Trial) compared a Mediterranean diet to a low-carbohydrate and a low-fat diet in 322 obese subjects (mean BMI 31 kg/m^2, 86% males) in a controlled workplace setting [87]. At two years, mean weight loss was 2.9 kg for the low-fat, 4.4 kg for the Mediterranean diet and 4.7 kg for the low-carbohydrate group. Predictors of successful weight loss at six months were an increased intake of vegetables and a reduced intake of sweets and cakes [87]. At six years after study initiation, total weight loss was 0.6 kg in the low-fat, 3.1 kg in the Mediterranean diet and 1.7 kg in the low-carbohydrate group. Of note, Mediterranean and low-carbohydrate groups were not different from each other, but they were both superior to low-fat diet in terms of long-term weight maintenance [88]. In addition, it has been suggested that adherence to Mediterranean diet may be associated with reduced total and cause-specific mortality and promote thus longevity [89]. Furthermore, other data suggest that a diet supplemented by Mediterranean food products such as extra-virgin olive oil and nuts and resembling thus Mediterranean diet, may reduce the incidence of major cardiovascular events [90]. It may also reduce fasting glucose, lipids, and stroke incidence in a genetically susceptible high-risk population for cardiovascular events (PREDIMED study; PREvención con DIeta MEDiterránea) [91]. However, the cardioprotective properties of the Mediterranean diet need to be confirmed in other populations as well (outside Spain). Although epidemiological evidence regarding the overall health benefits of the Mediterranean diet is solid, the effect of this dietary pattern on long-term weight control remains to be investigated with additional randomized clinical trials conducted over longer periods of time in diverse cultures and populations. Furthermore, there is still no definitive data as to whether a specific component of Mediterranean diet is mainly responsible for the beneficial effects, or it is rather the combination and interaction of single ingredients which makes Mediterranean diet a healthy diet.

9. Intermittent Diets

Intermittent energy restriction (IER) is based on the intermittent restriction of food intake, with shifts between periods of reduced energy intake and periods of unrestricted feeding [92,93]. The most commonly studied regimens of IER are those of energy restriction on two consecutive days per week, alternate day energy restriction by 60–70%, and complete fasting on alternate days (intermittent fasting, IF) [92]. Reviews in the field of intermittent dieting reveal the lack of high-quality evidence to support the superior or equal long-term safety and efficacy of intermittent diets compared to conventional diets with continuous energy restriction [94]. The few available randomized studies comparing intermittent with continuous hypocaloric diets in overweight and obese patients, report equal efficacy in terms of weight loss for a period up to 6 months [95–97]. To date, no studies suggest that intermittent diets can prevent weight gain in normal-weight individuals. Furthermore, data regarding the impact of intermittent diets on ectopic fat stores, adipocyte size and adipose tissue function, fat-free mass, insulin resistance and metabolic flexibility in humans, are scarce and heterogeneous [98]. Of note, some studies in animal models and normal-weight humans have shown detrimental effects of intermittent diets on metabolic homeostasis, raising safety concerns and the need for further investigation [96,99]. IER is generally preferable compared to complete intermittent fasting, due to its higher compliance, lower stress response and milder metabolic fluctuations (free fatty acid and ketone fluxes) [92].

At present, the optimal pattern and severity of energy restriction (e.g., two consecutive days per week i.e., 5:2, alternate days, five consecutive days per month, energy restriction by 60–70% or complete fasting) remains controversial. It remains also unclear which would be the optimal macronutrient composition of such intermittent diets. Taken together, in view of the multiple knowledge gaps and unaddressed questions in the field of intermittent dieting, the increasing popularity of these diets underscores the vital need for rigorous future research with appropriately designed, long-term, randomized studies in several subgroups of patients. In any case, an individualized critical appraisal is warranted to inform and guide the decision about which subjects might benefit from an intermittent diet for a short period of time, based on their social and personal contexts and coexisting clinical conditions.

10. Diet-Induced Weight Loss: A Matter of Quality or Quantity?

The general rule that weight loss requires a negative energy balance with energy intake being lower than energy expenditure is both well-established and widely accepted. However, whether counting calories and limiting portion sizes is necessary to achieve weight loss has been disputed. The critical question of whether diet quantity or rather quality plays the most crucial role for long-term weight loss and maintenance was recently addressed in a randomized clinical trial (DIETFITS trial) conducted in Stanford University [13]. In this study, 609 overweight/obese and non-diabetic adults (age 18–50 years, BMI 28–40 kg/m^2) were randomized to either a healthy low-fat or a healthy low-carbohydrate diet. All participants underwent an intensive dietician-guided training to eat healthy, minimally processed, whole foods cooked at home, without any caloric limits. The major finding of this study was that both diets delivered a significant weight loss of 5.3 kg for low-fat and 6 kg for low-carbohydrate over 12 months with similar improvement in waist circumference, body fat, fasting glucose and blood pressure. Interestingly, this effect was independent of genotype patterns or carbohydrate tolerance assessed by insulin secretion [13]. The authors concluded that diet quality defined as low intake of added sugars and highly processed foods and high intake of fruit, vegetables and whole-grain products, independent of energy intake, is fundamental for weight loss in overweight and obese adults, and furthermore, that predicting which diets are most effective based on genetics or insulin response to carbohydrates is not possible at the moment based on the limited number of candidate genes which were assessed [13]. Further research is warranted to explore in depth potential diet-genome interactions and possible epigenetic effects, to conclusively suggest that genetics or insulin response do not play a role in the effectiveness of particular diets. The finding that diet quality is essential for weight loss independent of energy intake is certainly stimulating, but several issues need to be considered. First, the long-term sustainability of newly-adopted dietary habits was not assessed in this study. Second, both groups ended up consuming fewer calories on average (daily energy deficit of 500–600 kcal) even though they were instructed not to count calories. Finally, the relatively modest weight loss effect of 6 kg within a year was not achieved without a cost, since multiple time-demanding educational sessions were required by highly-qualified healthcare professionals who emphasized behavior modification to support weight loss.

11. Conclusions and Recommendations

The ideal diet for treatment of overweight and obesity is defined as being safe, efficacious, healthy, nutritionally adequate, culturally acceptable, and economically affordable. It should further ensure long-term compliance and maintenance of weight loss effect. Various dietary plans with different caloric content and macronutrient composition have been assessed in randomized clinical trials, reviews, and meta-analyses, and found to be promising in promoting weight loss in adults. Nevertheless, the optimal diet remains still under debate. Only general principles and recommendations can be provided, and no single diet can be prescribed to all people with obesity or recommended as the best fit-for-all diet without strict individualization.

Conventional hypocaloric diets are safe, healthy, and modestly effective. There is insufficient evidence to support the superiority of low-fat diets over other higher-fat dietary interventions of similar intensity to achieve long-term weight loss and maintenance. Low-carbohydrate diets are effective and metabolically beneficial in the short-term, but long-term adherence is an issue. There might also be some health risks associated with long-term consumption of these diets, depending on their nutrient content as well as the individual's health status and risk factor profile. High-protein diets may promote satiety and prevent loss of muscle mass but can be also difficult to adhere to in the long-term and potentially hazardous for subgroups of patients with impaired kidney function or other health problems. Formula diets are the most effective strategy to achieve substantial and rapid weight loss but are indicated for specific subgroups of patients and intended for short-term use. The Mediterranean diet is as effective as low-carbohydrate diets in weight loss and can also provide benefits for overall health due to its balanced composition and diversity of health-promoting micronutrients. Intermittent diets are promising, but long-term safety and efficacy data are lacking, and the optimal pattern and severity of energy restriction remain controversial. As to the question of whether diet quality or quantity is more important, energy intake does certainly play a role, but the most effective strategy to achieve long-term weight loss and good cardiometabolic health is shifting to a healthy dietary pattern, compatible with individual food preferences and lifestyle habits. This dietary pattern should have restrictions in added sugars, refined grains and highly processed foods and include instead fruit, vegetables, whole-grain foods, and low-fat dairy products, without necessarily counting calories daily. The dietary pattern described above should be further combined with intensive education, motivation, and behavior modification, to obtain slow but steady weight loss and other health benefits.

Setting realistic goals for weight loss is important. Successful diets involve slow and steady changes. An even more important goal is weight loss maintenance and prevention of weight regain. The ideal weight loss maintenance diet should be continuous and easy to comply with. Eating high-quality fats and carbohydrates in the setting of a balanced diet cannot only promote weight loss, but also prevent coronary heart disease, diabetes, and other diseases.

In general, scientific evidence about what constitutes a healthy diet is both consistent and straightforward: a healthy diet is a varied diet rich in fruits, vegetables, whole-grain products and high-quality proteins and poor in added sugar, refined grains, and highly-processed foods. People who make the above dietary choices may find it easier to control their body weight without necessarily counting calories or limiting portion sizes daily. Physical activity and energy expenditure play also an important role in weight loss since sedentary individuals need to reduce their energy intake even when consuming a healthy diet to achieve and maintain weight loss. Most importantly, the best diet is a diet that people can comply with for a long period of time without significant weight regain, so whatever facilitates this effort is greatly appreciable.

Author Contributions: C.K. reviewed literature and wrote the manuscript; T.S., M.S., M.-E.B. and D.M. reviewed literature; N.K. edited the manuscript, provided critical input, and coordinated the other authors.

Funding: This research received no external funding.

References

1. Malik, V.S.; Willett, W.C.; Hu, F.B. Global obesity: Trends, risk factors and policy implications. *Nat. Rev. Endocrinol.* **2013**, *9*, 13–27. [CrossRef] [PubMed]
2. Kelly, T.; Yang, W.; Chen, C.S.; Reynolds, K.; He, J. Global burden of obesity in 2005 and projections to 2030. *Int. J. Obes. (Lond.)* **2008**, *32*, 1431–1437. [CrossRef] [PubMed]
3. Hruby, A.; Hu, F.B. The Epidemiology of obesity: A big picture. *PharmacoEconomics* **2015**, *33*, 673–689. [CrossRef] [PubMed]
4. Mozaffarian, D.; Hao, T.; Rimm, E.B.; Willett, W.C.; Hu, F.B. Changes in diet and lifestyle and long-term weight gain in women and men. *N. Engl. J. Med.* **2011**, *364*, 2392–2404. [CrossRef] [PubMed]
5. National Heart, Lung and Blood Institute (NHLBI) Obesity Education Initiative Expert Panel on the Identification, Evaluation, and Treatment of Obesity in Adults (US). Clinical guidelines on the identification, evaluation, and treatment of overweight and obesity in adults: Executive summary. *Am. J. Clin. Nutr.* **1998**, *68*, 899–917.
6. Jensen, M.D.; Ryan, D.H.; Apovian, C.M.; Ard, J.D.; Commuzzie, A.G.; Donato, K.A.; Hu, F.B.; Hubbard, V.S.; Jakicic, J.M.; Kushner, R.F.; et al. 2013 American Heart Association/American College of Cardiology/Task force on Practice Guidelines and the Obesity Society guideline for the management of overweight and obesity in adults: A report of the American College of Cardiology/American Heart Association Task Force on Practice Guidelines and the Obesity Society. *Circulation* **2014**, *129*, S102–S138. [PubMed]

7.   Clifton, P. Assessing the evidence for weight loss strategies in people with and without type 2 diabetes. *World J. Diabetes* **2017**, *8*, 440–454. [CrossRef] [PubMed]

8.   Sacks, F.M.; Bray, G.A.; Carey, V.J.; Smith, S.R.; Ryan, D.H.; Anton, S.D.; McManus, K.; Champagne, C.M.; Bishop, L.M.; Laranjo, N.; et al. Comparison of weight-loss diets with different compositions of fat, protein, and carbohydrates. *N. Engl. J. Med.* **2009**, *360*, 859–873. [CrossRef] [PubMed]

9.   Van Horn, L. A diet by any other name is still about energy. *JAMA* **2014**, *312*, 900–901. [CrossRef] [PubMed]

10. Bueno, N.B.; de Melo, I.S.; de Oliveira, S.L.; da Rocha Ataide, T. Very-low-carbohydrate ketogenic diet v. low-fat diet for long-term weight loss: A meta-analysis of randomised controlled trials. *Br. J. Nutr.* **2013**, *110*, 1178–1187. [CrossRef] [PubMed]

11. Bazzano, L.A.; Hu, T.; Reynolds, K.; Yao, L.; Bunol, C.; Liu, Y.; Chen, C.S.; Klag, M.J.; Whelton, P.K.; He, J. Effects of low-carbohydrate and low-fat diets: A randomized trial. *Ann. Intern. Med.* **2014**, *161*, 309–318. [CrossRef] [PubMed]

12. Atkins, J.L.; Whincup, P.H.; Morris, R.W.; Lennon, L.T.; Papakosta, O.; Wannamethee, S.G. High diet quality is associated with a lower risk of cardiovascular disease and all-cause mortality in older men. *J. Nutr.* **2014**, *144*, 673–680. [CrossRef] [PubMed]

13. Gardner, C.D.; Trepanowski, J.F.; Del Gobbo, L.C.; Hauser, M.E.; Rigdon, J.; Ioannidis, J.P.A.; Desai, M.; King, A.C. Effect of Low-Fat vs. Low-carbohydrate diet on 12-month weight loss in overweight adults and the association with genotype pattern or insulin secretion: The DIETFITS (Diet Intervention Examining The Factors Interacting with Treatment Success) randomized clinical trial. *JAMA* **2018**, *319*, 667–679. [PubMed]

14. Hill, J.O.; Wyatt, H.R.; Peters, J.C. Energy balance and obesity. *Circulation* **2012**, *126*, 126–132. [CrossRef] [PubMed]

15. Wilkinson, D.L.; McCargar, L. Is there an optimal macronutrient mix for weight loss and weight maintenance? *Best Pract. Res. Clin. Gastroenterol.* **2004**, *18*, 1031–1047. [CrossRef]

16. Samaha, F.F.; Iqbal, N.; Seshadri, P.; Chicano, K.L.; Daily, D.A.; McGrory, J.; Williams, T.; Williams, M.; Gracely, E.J.; Stern, L. A low-carbohydrate as compared with a low-fat diet in severe obesity. *N. Engl. J. Med.* **2003**, *348*, 2074–2081. [CrossRef] [PubMed]

17. Yancy, W.S., Jr.; Olsen, M.K.; Guyton, J.R.; Bakst, R.P.; Westman, E.C. A low-carbohydrate, ketogenic diet versus a low-fat diet to treat obesity and hyperlipidemia: A randomized, controlled trial. *Ann. Intern. Med.* **2004**, *140*, 769–777. [CrossRef] [PubMed]

18. Layman, D.K.; Evans, E.M.; Erickson, D.; Seyler, J.; Weber, J.; Bagshaw, D.; Griel, A.; Psota, T.; Kris-Etherton, P. A moderate-protein diet produces sustained weight loss and long-term changes in body composition and blood lipids in obese adults. *J. Nutr.* **2009**, *139*, 514–521. [CrossRef] [PubMed]

19. Bujnowski, D.; Xun, P.; Daviglus, M.L.; Van Horn, H.L.; He, K.; Stamler, J. Longitudinal association between animal and vegetable protein intake and obesity among men in the United States: The Chicago western electric study. *J. Am. Diet. Assoc.* **2011**, *111*, 1150–1155. [CrossRef] [PubMed]

20. Halkjaer, J.; Olsen, A.; Overvad, K.; Jakobsen, M.U.; Boeing, H.; Buijsse, B.; Palli, D.; Tognon, G.; Du, H.; van der, A.D.L.; et al. Intake of total, animal and plant protein and subsequent changes in weight or waist circumference in European men and women: The Diogenes project. *Int. J. Obes. (Lond.)* **2011**, *35*, 1104–1113. [CrossRef] [PubMed]

21. Boaz, M. Macronutrient composition in weight loss diets—A meta-analysis. *J Obes. Weight Loss Ther.* **2015**, *5*, 3. [CrossRef]

22. Byrne, S.; Cooper, Z.; Fairburn, C. Weight maintenance and relapse in obesity: A qualitative study. *Int. J. Obes. Relat. Metab. Disord.* **2003**, *27*, 955–962. [CrossRef] [PubMed]

23. Alhassan, S.; Kim, S.; Bersamin, A.; King, A.C.; Gardner, C.D. Dietary adherence and weight loss success among overweight women: Results from the A TO Z weight loss study. *Int. J. Obes. (Lond.)* **2008**, *32*, 985–991. [CrossRef] [PubMed]

24. MacLean, P.S.; Bergouignan, A.; Cornier, M.A.; Jackman, M.R. Biology's response to dieting: The impetus for weight regain. *Am. J. Physiol. Regul. Integr. Comp. Physiol.* **2011**, *301*, R581–R600. [CrossRef] [PubMed]

25. Sumithran, P.; Proietto, J. The defence of body weight: A physiological basis for weight regain after weight loss. *Clin. Sci.* **2013**, *124*, 231–241. [CrossRef] [PubMed]

26. Coutinho, S.R.; Rehfeld, J.F.; Holst, J.J.; Kulseng, B.; Martins, C. Impact of weight loss achieved through a multidisciplinary intervention on appetite in patients with severe obesity. *Am. J. Physiol. Endocrinol. Metab.* **2018**. [CrossRef] [PubMed]

27. Leibel, R.L.; Rosenbaum, M.; Hirsch, J. Changes in energy expenditure resulting from altered body weight. *N. Engl. J. Med.* **1995**, *332*, 621–628. [CrossRef] [PubMed]

28. Polidori, D.; Sanghvi, A.; Seeley, R.J.; Hall, K.D. How strongly does appetite counter weight loss? Quantification of the feedback control of human energy intake. *Obesity* **2016**, *24*, 2289–2295. [CrossRef] [PubMed]

29. Rosenbaum, M.; Kissileff, H.R.; Mayer, L.E.; Hirsch, J.; Leibel, R.L. Energy intake in weight-reduced humans. *Brain Res.* **2010**, *1350*, 95–102. [CrossRef] [PubMed]

30. Sumithran, P.; Predergast, L.A.; Delbridge, E.; Purcell, K.; Shulkes, A.; Kriketos, A.; Proietto, J. Long-term persistence of hormonal adaptations to weight loss. *N. Engl. J. Med.* **2011**, *365*, 1597–1604. [CrossRef] [PubMed]

31. Wing, R.R.; Hill, J.O. Successful weight loss maintenance. *Annu. Rev. Nutr.* **2001**, *21*, 323–341. [CrossRef] [PubMed]

32. Crawford, D.; Jeffery, R.W.; French, S.A. Can anyone successfully control their weight? Findings of a three year community-based study of men and women. *Int. J. Obes. Relat. Metab. Disord.* **2000**, *24*, 1107–1110. [CrossRef] [PubMed]

33. Serdula, M.K.; Mokdad, A.H.; Williamson, D.F.; Galuska, D.A.; Mendlein, J.M.; Heath, G.W. Prevalence of attempting weight loss and strategies for controlling weight. *JAMA* **1999**, *282*, 1353–1358. [CrossRef] [PubMed]

34. Vogels, N.; Diepvens, K.; Westerterp-Plantenga, M.S. Predictors of long-term weight maintenance. *Obes. Res.* **2005**, *13*, 2162–2168. [CrossRef] [PubMed]

35. Raynor, H.A.; Van Walleghen, E.L.; Bachman, J.L.; Looney, S.M.; Phelan, S.; Wing, R.R. Dietary energy density and successful weight loss maintenance. *Eat. Behav.* **2011**, *12*, 119–125. [CrossRef] [PubMed]

36. Butryn, M.L.; Phelan, S.; Hill, J.O.; Wing, R.R. Consistent self-monitoring of weight: A key component of successful weight loss maintenance. *Obesity* **2007**, *15*, 3091–3096. [CrossRef] [PubMed]

37. Sherwood, N.E.; Crain, A.L.; Martinson, B.C.; Anderson, C.P.; Hayes, M.G.; Anderson, J.D.; Senso, M.M.; Jeffery, R.W. Enhancing long-term weight loss maintenance: 2 year results from the keep it off randomized controlled trial. *Prev. Med.* **2013**, *56*, 171–177. [CrossRef] [PubMed]

38. Soeliman, F.A.; Azadbakht, L. Weight loss maintenance: A review on dietary related strategies. *J. Res. Med. Sci.* **2014**, *19*, 268–275. [PubMed]

39. Brikou, D.; Zannidi, D.; Karfopoulou, E.; Anastasiou, C.A.; Yannakoulia, M. Breakfast consumption and weight-loss maintenance: Results from the MedWeight study. *Br. J. Nutr.* **2016**, *115*, 2246–2251. [CrossRef] [PubMed]

40. Koliaki, C.; Katsilambros, N. The timing of meals and obesity: An emerging association with clinical implications. *Arch. Hell. Med.* **2016**, *33*, 1–6.

41. Ball, K.; Brown, W.; Crawford, D. Who does not gain weight? Prevalence and predictors of weight maintenance in young women. *Int. J. Obes. Relat. Metab. Disord.* **2002**, *26*, 1570–1578. [CrossRef] [PubMed]

42. Carels, R.A.; Konrad, K.; Young, K.M.; Darby, L.A.; Coit, C.; Clayton, A.M.; Oemig, C.K. Taking control of your personal eating and exercise environment: A weight maintenance program. *Eat. Behav.* **2008**, *9*, 228–237. [CrossRef] [PubMed]

43. Karfopoulou, E.; Brikou, D.; Mamalaki, E.; Bersimis, F.; Anastasiou, C.A.; Hill, J.O.; Yannakoulia, M. Dietary patterns in weight loss maintenance: Results from the MedWeight study. *Eur. J. Nutr.* **2017**, *56*, 991–1002. [CrossRef] [PubMed]

44. Kokkinos, A.; Le Roux, C.W.; Alexiadou, K.; Tentolouris, N.; Vincent, R.P.; Kyriaki, D.; Perrea, D.; Ghatei, M.A.; Bloom, S.R.; Katsilambros, N. Eating slowly increases the postprandial response of the anorexigenic gut hormones, peptide YY and glucagon-like peptide-1. *J. Clin. Endocrinol. Metab.* **2010**, *95*, 333–337. [CrossRef] [PubMed]

45. Katsilambros, N.L. Nutritional treatment of obesity in adults. What is certain and what uncertain. *Arch. Hell. Med.* **2015**, *32*, 340–343.

46. Langeveld, M.; DeVries, J.H. The long-term effect of energy restricted diets for treating obesity. *Obesity* **2015**, *23*, 1529–1538. [CrossRef] [PubMed]

47. Heymsfield, S.B.; Harp, J.B.; Reitman, M.L.; Beetsch, J.W.; Schoeller, D.A.; Erondu, N.; Pietrobelli, A. Why do obese patients not lose more weight when treated with low-calorie diets? A mechanistic perspective. *Am. J. Clin. Nutr.* **2007**, *85*, 346–354. [CrossRef] [PubMed]

48. Holt, S.H.; Delargy, H.J.; Lawton, C.L.; Blundell, J.E. The effects of high-carbohydrate vs high-fat breakfasts on feelings of fullness and alertness, and subsequent food intake. *Int. J. Food Sci. Nutr.* **1999**, *50*, 13–28. [CrossRef] [PubMed]

49. Rolls, B.J. The role of energy density in the overconsumption of fat. *J. Nutr.* **2000**, *130*, 268S–271S. [CrossRef] [PubMed]

50. Green, S.M.; Burley, V.J.; Blundell, J.E. Effect of fat- and sucrose-containing foods on the size of eating episodes and energy intake in lean males: Potential for causing overconsumption. *Eur. J. Clin. Nutr.* **1994**, *48*, 547–555. [PubMed]

51. Quatela, A.; Callister, R.; Patterson, A.; MacDonald-Wicks, L. The energy content and composition of meals consumed after an overnight fast and their effects on diet induced thermogenesis: A systematic review, meta-analyses and meta-regressions. *Nutrients* **2016**, *8*, 670. [CrossRef] [PubMed]

52. Horton, T.J.; Drougas, H.; Brachey, A.; Reed, G.W.; Peters, J.C.; Hill, J.O. Fat and carbohydrate overfeeding in humans: Different effects on energy storage. *Am. J. Clin. Nutr.* **1995**, *62*, 19–29. [CrossRef] [PubMed]

53. Murphy, E.A.; Velazquez, K.T.; Herbert, K.M. Influence of high-fat diet on gut microbiota: A driving force for chronic disease risk. *Curr. Opin. Clin. Nutr. Metab. Care* **2015**, *18*, 515–520. [CrossRef] [PubMed]

54. Johnston, B.C.; Kanters, S.; Bandayrel, K.; Wu, P.; Naji, F.; Siemieniuk, R.A.; Ball, G.D.; Busse, J.W.; Thorlund, K.; Guyatt, G.; et al. Comparison of weight loss among named diet programs in overweight and obese adults: A meta-analysis. *JAMA* **2014**, *312*, 923–933. [CrossRef] [PubMed]

55. Tobias, D.K.; Chen, M.; Manson, J.E.; Ludwig, D.S.; Willett, W.; Hu, F.B. Effect of low-fat diet interventions versus other diet interventions on long-term weight change in adults: A systematic review and meta-analysis. *Lancet Diabetes Endocrinol.* **2015**, *3*, 968–979. [CrossRef]

56. Atkins, R.C. *Dr. Atkins' New Diet Revolution*; Simon & Schuster: New York, NY, USA, 1998.

57. Astrup, A.; Meinert Larsen, T.; Harper, A. Atkins and other low-carbohydrate diets: Hoax or an effective tool for weight loss? *Lancet* **2004**, *364*, 897–899. [CrossRef]

58. Noto, H.; Goto, A.; Tsujimoto, T.; Noda, M. Low carbohydrate diets and all-cause mortality: A systematic review and meta-analysis of observational studies. *PLoS ONE* **2013**, *8*, e55030. [CrossRef] [PubMed]

59. Mansoor, N.; Vinknes, K.J.; Veierød, M.B.; Retterstøl, K. Effects of low-carbohydrate diets v. low-fat diets on body weight and cardiovascular risk factors: A meta-analysis of randomised controlled trials. *Br. J. Nutr.* **2016**, *115*, 466–479. [CrossRef] [PubMed]

60. Naude, C.E.; Schoonees, A.; Senekal, M.; Young, T.; Garner, P.; Volmink, J. Low carbohydrate versus isoenergetic balanced diets for reducing weight and cardiovascular risk: A systematic review and meta-analysis. *PLoS ONE* **2014**, *9*, e100652. [CrossRef] [PubMed]

61. Hu, T.; Mills, K.T.; Yao, L.; Demanelis, K.; Eloustaz, M.; Yancy, W.S., Jr.; Kelly, T.N.; He, J.; Bazzano, L.A. Effects of low-carbohydrate diets versus low-fat diets on metabolic risk factors: A meta-analysis of randomized controlled clinical trials. *Am. J. Epidemiol.* **2012**, *176* (Suppl. 7), S44–S54. [CrossRef] [PubMed]

62. Nordmann, A.J.; Nordmann, A.; Briel, M.; Keller, U.; Yancy, W.S., Jr.; Brehm, B.J.; Bucher, H.C. Effects of low-carbohydrate vs. low-fat diets on weight loss and cardiovascular risk factors: A meta-analysis of randomized controlled trials. *Arch. Intern. Med.* **2006**, *166*, 285–293. [CrossRef] [PubMed]

63. Vlachos, D.; Ganatopoulou, A.; Stathi, C.; Koutsovasilis, A.; Diakoumopoulou, E.; Doulgerakis, D.; Tentolouris, N.; Melidonis, A.; Katsilambros, N. A low-carbohydrate protein sparing modified diet compared with a low glycaemic index reduced calorie diet in obese type 2 diabetic patients. 47th Annual Meeting of the European Association for the Study of Diabetes, Lisbon, 2011. *Diabetologia* **2011**, *54* (Suppl. 1), S355.

64. Due, A.; Toubro, S.; Skov, A.R.; Astrup, A. Effect of normal-fat diets, either medium or high in protein, on body weight in overweight subjects: A randomised 1-year trial. *Int. J. Obes. Relat. Metab. Disord.* **2004**, *28*, 1283–1290. [CrossRef] [PubMed]

65. Paddon-Jones, D.; Westman, E.; Mattes, R.D.; Wolfe, R.R.; Astrup, A.; Westerterp-Plantenga, M. Protein, weight management, and satiety. *Am. J. Clin. Nutr.* **2008**, *87*, 1558S–1561S. [CrossRef] [PubMed]

66. Halton, T.L.; Hu, F.B. The effects of high protein diets on thermogenesis, satiety and weight loss: A critical review. *J. Am. Coll. Nutr.* **2004**, *23*, 373–385. [CrossRef] [PubMed]

67. Skov, A.R.; Toubro, S.; Ronn, B.; Holm, L.; Astrup, A. Randomized trial on protein vs carbohydrate in ad libitum fat reduced diet for the treatment of obesity. *Int. J. Obes. Relat. Metab. Disord.* **1999**, *23*, 528–536. [CrossRef] [PubMed]

68. Noakes, M.; Keogh, J.B.; Foster, P.R.; Clifton, P.M. Effect of an energy-restricted, high-protein, low-fat diet relative to a conventional high-carbohydrate, low-fat diet on weight loss, body composition, nutritional status, and markers of cardiovascular health in obese women. *Am. J. Clin. Nutr.* **2005**, *81*, 1298–1306. [CrossRef] [PubMed]

69. Layman, D.K.; Boileau, R.A.; Erickson, D.J.; Painter, J.E.; Shiue, H.; Sather, C.; Christou, D.D. A reduced ratio of dietary carbohydrate to protein improves body composition and blood lipid profiles during weight loss in adult women. *J. Nutr.* **2003**, *133*, 411–417. [CrossRef] [PubMed]

70. Layman, D.K.; Shiue, H.; Sather, C.; Erickson, D.J.; Baum, J. Increased dietary protein modifies glucose and insulin homeostasis in adult women during weight loss. *J. Nutr.* **2003**, *133*, 405–410. [CrossRef] [PubMed]

71. Baba, N.H.; Sawaya, S.; Torbay, N.; Habbal, Z.; Azar, S.; Hashim, S.A. High protein vs high carbohydrate hypoenergetic diet for the treatment of obese hyperinsulinemic subjects. *Int. J. Obes. Relat. Metab. Disord.* **1999**, *23*, 1202–1206. [CrossRef] [PubMed]

72. Piatti, P.M.; Monti, F.; Fermo, I.; Baruffaldi, L.; Nasser, R.; Santambrogio, G.; Librenti, M.C.; Galli-Kienle, M.; Pontiroli, A.E.; Pozza, G. Hypocaloric high-protein diet improves glucose oxidation and spares lean body mass: Comparison to hypocaloric high-carbohydrate diet. *Metabolism* **1994**, *43*, 1481–1487. [CrossRef]

73. Vazquez, J.A.; Kazi, U.; Madani, N. Protein metabolism during weight reduction with very-low-energy diets: Evaluation of the independent effects of protein and carbohydrate on protein sparing. *Am. J. Clin. Nutr.* **1995**, *62*, 93–103. [PubMed]

74. Parker, B.; Noakes, M.; Luscombe, N.; Clifton, P. Effect of a high-protein, high-monounsaturated fat weight loss diet on glycemic control and lipid levels in type 2 diabetes. *Diabetes Care* **2002**, *25*, 425–430. [CrossRef] [PubMed]

75. Farnsworth, E.; Luscombe, N.D.; Noakes, M.; Wittert, G.; Argyiou, E.; Clifton, P.M. Effect of a high-protein, energy-restricted diet on body composition, glycemic control, and lipid concentrations in overweight and obese hyperinsulinemic men and women. *Am. J. Clin. Nutr.* **2003**, *78*, 31–39. [CrossRef] [PubMed]

76. Hu, F.B.; Stampfer, M.J.; Manson, J.E.; Rimm, E.; Colditz, G.A.; Speizer, F.E.; Hennekens, C.H.; Willett, W.C. Dietary protein and risk of ischemic heart disease in women. *Am. J. Clin. Nutr.* **1999**, *70*, 221–227. [CrossRef] [PubMed]

77. Skov, A.R.; Toubro, S.; Bulow, J.; Krabbe, K.; Parving, H.H.; Astrup, A. Changes in renal function during weight loss induced by high vs. low-protein low-fat diets in overweight subjects. *Int. J. Obes. Relat. Metab. Disord.* **1999**, *23*, 1170–1177. [CrossRef] [PubMed]

78. Leeds, A.R. Formula food-reducing diets: A new evidence-based addition to the weight management tool box. *Nutr. Bull.* **2014**, *39*, 238–246. [CrossRef] [PubMed]

79. Johansson, K.; Hemmingsson, E.; Neovius, M. Effects of anti-obesity drugs, diet, and exercise on weight-loss maintenance after a very-low-calorie diet or low-calorie diet: A systematic review and meta-analysis of randomized controlled trials. *Am. J. Clin. Nutr.* **2013**, *99*, 14–23. [CrossRef] [PubMed]

80. Sumithran, P.; Prendergast, L.A.; Delbridge, E.; Purcell, K.; Shulkes, A.; Kriketos, A.; Proietto, J. Ketosis and appetite-mediating nutrients and hormones after weight loss. *Eur. J. Clin. Nutr.* **2013**, *67*, 759–764. [CrossRef] [PubMed]

81. Christensen, P.; Bliddal, H.; Riecke, B.F.; Leeds, A.R.; Astrup, A.; Christensen, R. Comparison of a low-energy diet and a very low-energy diet in sedentary obese individuals: A pragmatic randomised controlled trial. *Clin. Obes.* **2011**, *1*, 31–40. [CrossRef] [PubMed]

82. Snel, M.; Gastaldelli, A.; Ouwens, D.M.; Hesselink, M.K.; Schaart, G.; Buzzigoli, E.; Frölich, M.; Romijn, J.A.; Pijl, H.; Meinders, A.E.; et al. Effects of adding exercise to a 16-week very low-calorie diet in obese, insulindependent type 2 diabetes mellitus patients. *J. Clin. Endocrinol. Metab.* **2012**, *97*, 2512–2520. [CrossRef] [PubMed]

83. Christensen, P.; Bliddal, H.; Bartels, E.M.; Leeds, A.; Astrup, A.; Christensen, R. Long-term intervention with weight loss in patients with concomitant obesity and knee osteoarthritis: The LIGHT study—A randomised clinical trial. *Obes. Rev.* **2014**, *15* (Suppl. 2), 152.

84. Johansson, K.; Neovius, M.; Lagerros, Y.T.; Harlid, R.; Rössner, S.; Granath, F.; Hemmingsson, E. Effect of a very-low-energy diet on moderate and severe obstructive sleep apnoea in obese men: A randomised controlled trial. *Br. Med. J.* **2009**, *339*, b4609. [CrossRef] [PubMed]

85.   Geiker, N.R.W.; Jensen, P.; Zachariae, C.; Christensen, R.; Schaadt, B.K.; Stender, S.; Hansen, P.R.; Astrup, A.; Skov, L. Effect of weight loss on the severity of psoriasis: One year follow-up. *Obes. Rev.* **2014**, *15* (Suppl. 2), 170–171.

86.   Colles, S.L.; Dixon, J.B.; Marks, P.; Strauss, B.J.; O'Brien, P.E. Preoperative weight loss with a very low-energy diet: Quantitation of changes in liver and abdominal fat by serial imaging. *Am. J. Clin. Nutr.* **2016**, *84*, 304–311. [CrossRef]

87.   Shai, I.; Schwarzfuchs, D.; Henkin, Y.; Shahar, D.R.; Witkow, S.; Greenberg, I.; Golan, R.; Fraser, D.; Bolotin, A.; Vardi, H.; et al. Dietary Intervention Randomized Controlled Trial (DIRECT) Group. Weight loss with a low-carbohydrate, Mediterranean, or low-fat diet. *N. Engl. J. Med.* **2008**, *359*, 229–241. [CrossRef] [PubMed]

88.   Schwarzfuchs, D.; Golan, R.; Shai, I. Four-year follow-up after two-year dietary interventions. *N. Engl. J. Med.* **2012**, *367*, 1373–1374. [CrossRef] [PubMed]

89.   Trichopoulou, A.; Costacou, T.; Bamia, C.; Trichopoulos, D. Adherence to a Mediterranean diet and survival in a Greek population. *N. Engl. J. Med.* **2003**, *348*, 2599–2608. [CrossRef] [PubMed]

90.   Estruch, R.; Ros, E.; Salas-Salvadó, J.; Covas, M.I.; Corella, D.; Arós, F.; Gómez-Gracia, E.; Ruiz-Gutiérrez, V.; Fiol, M.; Lapetra, J.; et al. PREDIMED (PREvención con DIeta MEDiterránea) Investigators. Primary prevention of cardiovascular disease with a mediterranean diet supplemented with extra-virgin olive oil or nuts. *N. Engl. J. Med.* **2018**, *378*, e34. [CrossRef] [PubMed]

91.   Corella, D.; Carrasco, P.; Sorlí, J.V.; Estruch, R.; Rico-Sanz, J.; Martínez-González, M.Á.; Salas-Salvadó, J.; Covas, M.I.; Coltell, O.; Arós, F.; et al. Mediterranean diet reduces the adverse effect of the TCF7L2-rs7903146 polymorphism on cardiovascular risk factors and stroke incidence: A randomized controlled trial in a high-cardiovascular-risk population. *Diabetes Care* **2013**, *36*, 3803–3811. [CrossRef] [PubMed]

92.   Brinia, M.E.; Spinos, T.; Spinou, M.; Mitsopoulou, D.; Koliaki, C.; Katsilambros, N. The effects of intermittent energy restriction on metabolic and cardiovascular function and overall health. *Arch. Hell. Med.* **2018**, *35*, 1–17.

93.   Chaix, A.; Zarrinpar, A.; Miu, P.; Panda, S. Time-restricted feeding is a preventative and therapeutic intervention against diverse nutritional challenges. *Cell Metab.* **2014**, *20*, 991–1005. [CrossRef] [PubMed]

94.   Harvie, M.; Howell, A. Potential benefits and harms of intermittent energy restriction and intermittent fasting amongst obese, overweight and normal weight subjects—A narrative review of human and animal evidence. *Behav. Sci. (Basel)* **2017**, *7*, 4. [CrossRef] [PubMed]

95.   Catenacci, V.A.; Pan, Z.; Ostendorf, D.; Brannon, S.; Gozansky, W.S.; Mattson, M.P.; Martin, B.; MacLean, P.S.; Melanson, E.L.; Troy Donahoo, W. A randomized pilot study comparing zero-calorie alternate-day fasting to daily caloric restriction in adults with obesity. *Obesity (Silver Spring)* **2016**, *24*, 1874–1883. [CrossRef] [PubMed]

96.   Varady, K.A.; Bhutani, S.; Klempel, M.C.; Kroeger, C.M.; Trepanowski, J.F.; Haus, J.M.; Hoddy, K.K.; Calvo, Y. Alternate day fasting for weight loss in normal weight and overweight subjects: A randomized controlled trial. *Nutr. J.* **2013**, *12*, 146. [CrossRef] [PubMed]

97.   Harvie, M.N.; Pegington, M.; Mattson, M.P.; Frystyk, J.; Dillon, B.; Evans, G.; Cuzick, J.; Jebb, S.A.; Martin, B.; Cutler, R.G.; et al. The effects of intermittent or continuous energy restriction on weight loss and metabolic disease risk markers: A randomized trial in young overweight women. *Int. J. Obes. (Lond.)* **2011**, *35*, 714–727. [CrossRef] [PubMed]

98.   Varady, K.A.; Hudak, C.S.; Hellerstein, M.K. Modified alternate-day fasting and cardioprotection: Relation to adipose tissue dynamics and dietary fat intake. *Metabolism* **2009**, *58*, 803–811. [CrossRef] [PubMed]

99.   Cerqueira, F.M.; da Cunha, F.M.; Caldeira da Silva, C.C.; Chausse, B.; Romano, R.L.; Garcia, C.C.; Garcia, C.C.; Colepicolo, P.; Medeiros, M.H.; Kowaltowski, A.J. Long-term intermittent feeding, but not caloric restriction, leads to redox imbalance, insulin receptor nitration, and glucose intolerance. *Free Radic. Biol. Med.* **2011**, *51*, 1454–1460. [CrossRef] [PubMed]

## 8

Impact of Standardized Prenatal Clinical Training for Traditional Birth Attendants in Rural Guatemala

Sasha Hernandez [1],*, Jessica Oliveira [1], Leah Jones [1], Juan Chumil [2] and Taraneh Shirazian [1]

[1] Saving Mothers, New York, NY 10022, USA; joliveira@savingmothers.org (J.O.);
ljones@savingmothers.org (L.J.); tshirazian@savingmothers.org (T.S.)

[2] Ministerio de Salud Pública y Asistencia Social, Santiago Atitlán, Sololá 07019, Guatemala;
jchumilcuc@hotmail.com

* Correspondence: shernandez@savingmothers.org

Abstract: In low-and-middle-income countries (LMICs), traditional birth attendant (TBA) training programs are increasing, yet reports are limited on how those programs affect the prenatal clinical abilities of trained TBAs. This study aims to assess the impact of clinical training on TBAs before and after a maternal health-training program. A prospective observational study was conducted in rural Guatemala from March to December 2017. Thirteen participants conducted 116 prenatal home visits. Data acquisition occurred before any prenatal clinical training had occurred, at the completion of the 14-week training program, and at six months post program completion. The paired *t*-test and McNemar's test was used and statistical analyses were performed with R Version 3.3.1. There was a statistically significant improvement in prenatal clinical skills before and after the completion of the training program. The mean percentage of prenatal skills done correctly before any training occurred was 25.8%, 62.3% at the completion of the training program (*p*-value = 0.0001), and 71.0% after six months of continued training (*p*-value = 0.034). This study highlights the feasibility of prenatal skill improvement through a standardized and continuous clinical training program for TBAs. The improvement of TBA prenatal clinical skills could benefit indigenous women in rural Guatemala and other LMICs.

Keywords: birth attendant; prenatal care; clinical skills; education; maternal mortality; indigenous health; rural; Guatemala

1. Introduction

Significant worldwide progress has been made towards lowering rates of maternal mortality in the last two decades [1]. Yet maternal mortality ratios (MMR) in the developing world, especially in rural regions and within indigenous populations, continue to be unacceptably high [2]. This holds true in Guatemala where the national average of 88 maternal deaths per 100,000 births [1] does not reflect the major disparities that exist between the MMR for indigenous women which is twice that of their counterparts (163 per 100,000 compared to 78 per 100,000) [3]. In recent years, the Guatemalan government has aimed to decrease this discrepancy by promoting institutional births [4], however, up to 70% of indigenous women living in rural Guatemala continue to deliver at home without receiving adequate prenatal care [5]. This continued preference of home care during pregnancy and delivery is due both due to limited access to essential obstetric care [6] and a non-wavering cultural preference for traditional birth attendants (TBAs) to attend to women at home [7].

TBAs are important to both the local community and national health infrastructure as their training and integration in the current healthcare system can help improve maternal and neonatal outcomes [8–11]. Despite the significant role TBAs hold, there are limitations, as few sustainable training programs exist that properly train TBAs in how to provide basic prenatal care, detect early complications, or refer high-risk pregnancies in a standardized way. TBA participants themselves report that they are not always given sufficient training during these programs [12]. Even for successful programs, challenges exist in measuring Prenatal Clinical Skills (PCS) and reporting trends over time. While some studies have attempted to evaluate PCS, they have focused on simulated sessions [13] and cross-sectional views [14]. Such studies do not provide a direct look at how a training program affects the PCS of their trainees before and after training and how those skills develop after continued training.

The School of POWHER, which stands for Providing Outreach in Women's Health and Educational Resources, is a yearly TBA training program that has been successfully implemented in the rural communities of the department of Sololá, Guatemala over the last four years and supported by both community infrastructure and the regional branch of the Guatemalan Ministry of Health. The School of POWHER training program is an immersive program, delivered in both Spanish and Tz'tujil (a local Mayan language), based on a two-pronged approach. There is a 28-module lecture series (which runs over 14 weeks, with two four-hour lectures given per week) emphasizing signs of referrals for the mom and baby, prenatal care, and initial management of post-partum complications (Figure S1, see Supplementary Materials). A separate 12-month clinical constituent emphasizes basic prenatal home care and appropriate referral. The clinical arm of the school ensures that TBAs refine their traditional midwifery abilities while learning new skills under the supervision of a preceptor. During bi-monthly home visits in the students' communities over twelve months, the TBAs will practice items, including but not limited to, counseling the mother about vaccines, measuring blood pressure, using a fetal Doppler, and correctly estimating delivery date. The School of POWHER respects cultural Mayan practices and its content is in line with current WHO and Guatemalan healthcare guidelines for TBAs [15,16]. Each woman that completes the School of POWHER training program receives a stethoscope, blood pressure equipment, a fetal Doppler, prenatal vitamins, and safe birthing kits. In total, the training program, now a one hundred percent sustainable program as current School of POWHER staff are TBAs who are past graduates of our program, has trained 60 TBAs in southwest Guatemala in focused maternal healthcare with appropriate obstetric referrals as the key to decreasing maternal death and complications in the region [17].

The main objective of the present study was to assess the effect of the School of POWHER's clinical training on its participants after (1) completion of the program and (2) after six months of continued clinical training. The time of notable improvement of PCS, as well as level of adherence over time, was also studied.

2. Materials and Methods

A community-based, prospective observational study was conducted in six rural communities throughout the department of Sololá, Guatemala from March through December 2017 to assess direct PCS acquisition and retention from the School of POWHER training program during prenatal home visits.

All TBAs recruited and then enrolled in the School of POWHER training program during the time of this study were included. TBA demographics are described in Table 1.

Table 1. Traditional birth attendant participant demographics.

Characteristic	Average	Range
Age	40	22–54
Level of Education	2nd grade	No formal education-8th grade (one outlier with one participant pursuing a technical degree in nutrition)
Marital Status	Married	1 single, 1 widowed, 11 married
Years of Experience	9	0–27
Dominant Language	Spanish, Tz'tujil, Kaqcuichel	

Data collection was scheduled at three different time points from March through December 2017 with the goal of capturing PCS during home visits prior to and after School of POWHER clinical training. Home visits were arranged with each TBA student in their respective communities with their existing patients. If a TBA student did not have current pregnant patients and/or a visit could not be scheduled with her patient, the Ministry of Health provided a list of pregnant women in each community to visit. Each time point and the corresponding amount of clinical training are defined in Table 2. The goal was to observe 1–5 prenatal home visits by each TBA student in their own community during each of the three time points. Two weeks were allotted after each time point to collect all observational data from the 13 TBA participants. During each two-week data collection time point, no additional clinical instruction occurred to ensure that each participant had received the same amount of clinical training.

Table 2. The data collection characteristics.

Study Time Point	Dates of Data Collection	Total Weeks of Clinical Training	Total Weeks of Knowledge-Based Learning
Time Point A [1]	March 22–April 7, 2017	0	0
Time Point B [2]	June 30–August 16, 2017	14	14
Time Point C [3]	November 7–December 12, 2017	38	14

[1] Time point A occurred before any clinical instruction had begun; [2] Time point B occurred at the completion of 14-weeks of formalized POWHER curriculum; [3] Time point C occurred after six months of continuous clinical training from completion of the formalized POWHER curriculum.

During each time point of the study period, prenatal home visits were observed with a WHO-adapted prenatal care checklist tested in our prior pilot study [18]. This WHO-adapted checklist covered three broad categories of medical history, clinical skills, and counseling (Figure S2, see Supplementary Materials). The medical history information included age, number of previous pregnancies, complications with previous pregnancies, other significant medical history, current medications, current weeks of gestation, and estimated date of delivery. The clinical skills evaluated included measuring the maternal blood pressure, fundal height, fetal heart rate, and fetal position. Counseling included reviewing signs and symptoms of danger during pregnancy and what course of action to take if danger symptoms presented. A review of the emergency birth plan, the importance of tetanus vaccination, and prenatal vitamins were also evaluated. All study variables and appropriate reasons for referrals are defined in Table 3.

Table 3. The variables included in the prenatal clinical skills observation checklist.

Variable	Definition	Reason for Referral
History		
Accurately calculates EDD	Using Naegele's rule or pregnancy wheel.	If LMP unknown, referral for dating US.
Accurately calculates GA	Only if the mother knows LMP.	If LMP unknown, referral for dating US.
Age	Asks mother for an identification card if age is not known.	Referral recommended if AMA or less than 16 years old.
# of previous pregnancies	All pregnancies, including miscarriages.	
# of living children	All children; follows up if there is a discrepancy between total pregnancies and living children.	
Problems with previous pregnancies	Asks about prolonged labor, hemorrhage, problems with blood pressure, severe headache, fever during or after labor, infection during or after labor, prior C-sections.	Referral recommended if mother reports any prior problem. If C-section less than two years from current pregnancy recommends hospital birth.
Past medical history	Assesses any health conditions outside of pregnancy.	
Current medications	Assesses both OTC medications and street supplements.	

Table 3. *Cont.*

Variable	Definition	Reason for Referral
Documents history	Variables of importance are name, age, EDD, and prior issues of importance in order to report to the MOH. Not applicable for illiterate TBA.	
Clinical skills		
Washes hands	Uses soap and water or antiseptic solution.	
Measures blood pressure	Mother seated or supine, arm below the heart, places cuff 1–2 finger breadths above the elbow, places stethoscope in the area of the brachial artery under the cuff.	Refers if blood pressure greater than 140/90, or in "red zone" if illiterate TBA.
Measures heart rate	Locates radial pulse and measures for 60 s.	
Measures fundal height	Can use a measuring tape or hand measurements if TBA is illiterate.	Refers if there is a difference greater than 4 cm from fundal height compared to GA.
Listens to fetal heart rate	Can find fetal heart rate and distinguish from maternal heart rate and placental vessels.	Refers if fetal distress (FHR > 160 bpm, <100 bpm) persists throughout the visit.
Finds the position of fetus	Uses Leopold's maneuvers.	If the fetal position is oblique, transverse, or breech, in late pregnancy, discusses with mother the dangers of home birth.
Documents all findings	Variables of importance are blood pressure findings to track trends over pregnancy, not applicable if illiterate.	
Counseling		
Discusses severe headaches	Explains to mom the risk of a severe headache and associated changes in vision.	Discusses with mother to report to the health post, local hospital, or private clinic.
Discusses severe abdominal pains	Demonstrates pain in the epigastric region.	Discusses with mother to report to the health post, local hospital, or private clinic.
Discusses vaginal bleeding	Explains the risk of spotting or bleeding at any point during the pregnancy.	Discusses with mother to report to the health post, local hospital, or private clinic.
Discusses fever	Explains chills and night sweats as symptoms of a fever.	Discusses with mother to report to the health post, local hospital, or private clinic.
Discusses location of birth	Discusses with mother and partner (if present) about the risks and benefits of both a home birth and a hospital birth).	
Discusses emergency plan	Discusses with mother and partner (if present) where to report and how to get there if an emergency arises during labor and delivery.	
Distributes prenatal vitamins	Hands a 30 day supply to mother.	
Counsels on the importance of prenatal vitamins	Explains the maternal and fetal benefit of prenatal vitamins to mother.	
Counsels on Td vaccine	Explains the vaccine schedule (1st shot, 2nd shot 2 months later, 3rd shot months later) to mother and the importance of vaccination especially if a home birth is planned.	Refers to either health post or local hospital to received Td vaccine.

Abbreviations: EDD = estimated delivery date; GA = gestational age; LMP = last menstrual period; AMA = advanced maternal age; OTC = over the counter.

On arrival at each home, the evaluator observed the prenatal home visit after patient verbal consent was obtained from the TBA conducting the visit. During the data collection process, one of two evaluators observed all prenatal home visits. These two evaluators were trained on the POWHER curriculum and observation checklist before the commencement of the study. Evaluator A, a senior medical student, was in charge of data collection during the pilot study period to Time Point A. Evaluator B, a medical volunteer with public health experience, observed the prenatal home visits from Time Point B to Time Point C. A translator assisted the evaluator for visits that occurred in native languages (Tz'utujil and Kaqchikel). After the completion of the observed visit, the evaluator had an opportunity to intervene if maternal or fetal referral was indicated, but missed by the TBA during the observation. This referral was not included as part of this study. No personal patient identifiers were collected to maintain the confidentiality of the women.

Data analysis was carried out using standard statistical methods. The paired *t*-test and McNemar's test was used and statistical analyses were performed with R, Version 3.3.1 (R Core Team, Vienna, Austria).

3. Results

A total of 116 prenatal home visits by 13 TBAs were observed. Each TBA participant was evaluated at each of the three time points as no participants were lost to follow-up. A total of 59 visits occurred at Time Point A, 39 visits occurred at Time Point B, and 18 visits occurred at Time Point C. For TBAs with multiple observed home visits during each time point, their results were averaged over their visits (Figure 1).

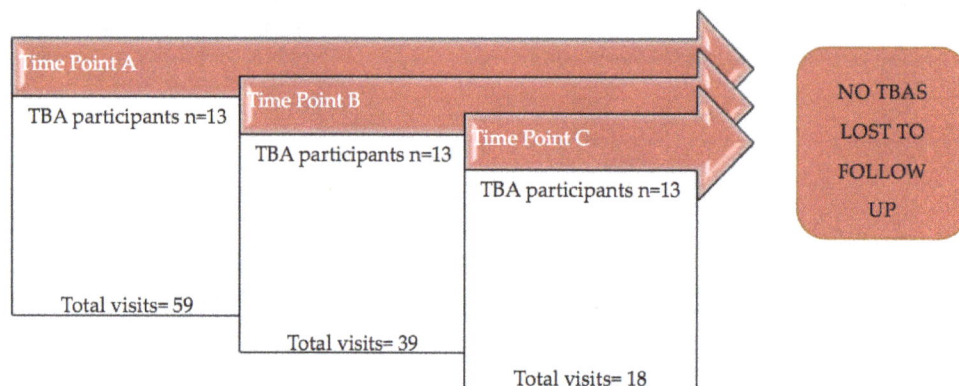

Figure 1. The total participants and observed visits over the study period.

No study participants were lost to follow up from March to December of 2017. Total observed visits differed from each of the three time points due to the difficulty in reaching each rural community due to nationwide transportation strikes. The median number of home visits per TBA during time point A was 3 with a range of 1–9, 2 home visits per TBA during time point B with a range of 1–8, and 1 home visit per TBA during time point C with a range of 1–3.

The overall improvement in prenatal clinical skills is shown in Table 4. The mean percentage correct on the checklist before any training occurred was 25.8% (Time Point A). The mean percentage correct on the checklist after the completion of the School was 62.3% (Time Point B). There was also a statistically significant improvement between the completion of the School of POWHER (Time Point B), a mean of 62.3%, and continued clinical training for 6 months following completion of the School of POWHER with a mean of 71.0% (Time Point C). The largest amount of overall checklist improvement was seen before any clinical training occurred (Time Point A) when compared to completion of the School of POWHER (Time Point B).

Specific improvement in each of the three prenatal skills categories was also statistically significant as seen in Table 5. In the category of history, taking the mean percentage correct on the checklist before any training occurred (Time Point A) was 26.3% compared to 58.8% at the completion of the School of POWHER (*p*-value = 0.005) (Time Point B). After six months of continued clinical training from the completion of the School of POWHER (Time Point C), the percent correct on the checklist improved to 87.1% (*p*-value < 0.0001). In the category of clinical skills, the mean percentage correct on the checklist before any training occurred (Time Point A) was 9.7% compared to 92.4% at the completion of the School of POWHER (*p*-value < 0.0001) (Time Point B). After six months of continued clinical training from the completion of the School of POWHER, the percent correct on the checklist was 81.4% (Time

Point C). This decrease in overall percentage correct was not statistically significant (p-value = 0.19). In the category of counseling, the mean percentage correct on the checklist before any training occurred (Time Point A) was 27.7% compared to 86.2% at the completion of the School of POWHER (p-value < 0.0001) (Time Point B). After six months of continued clinical training from the completion of the School of POWHER (Time Point C), the percent correct in counseling on the checklist was 72.0%. This decrease in overall percentage correct was also not statistically significant (p-value = 0.09).

Table 4. The overall improvements in prenatal clinical skills.[1]

	Time Point A [2]	Time Point B [3]	Time Point C [4]	p-value [5]
Percentage of correctly performed prenatal clinical skills	25.8 (19.6)	62.3 (16.3)	71 (12.5)	Between A and B, 0.0001 Between B and C, 0.034

[1] Values entered as mean percentages (standard deviation); [2] Time point A occurred before any clinical instruction had begun; [3] Time point B occurred at the completion of 14-weeks of formalized POWHER curriculum; [4] Time point C occurred after six months of continuous clinical training from completion of the formalized POWHER curriculum; [5] Paired t-test.

Table 5. The specific checklist improvements per category [1].

Prenatal Skills	Time Point A [2]	Time Point B [3]	Time Point C [4]	p-value [5]
History (overall)	26.3%	58.8%	87.1%	Between A and B, 0.005 Between B and C, <0.0001
Accurately calculates EDD	52.0%	82.0%	90.0%	-
Accurately calculates GA	7.5%	68.0%	90.0%	-
Age	36.0%	64.0%	92.0%	-
# of previous pregnancies	43.5%	64.0%	100.0%	-
# of living children	37.0%	64.0%	100.0%	-
Problems with previous pregnancies	35.5%	50.0%	100.0%	-
Past medical history	10.0%	52.0%	70.0%	-
Current medications	17.5%	44.0%	78.5%	-
Documents history	8.5%	100.0%	100.0%	-
Clinical skills (overall)	9.7%	92.4%	81.4%	Between A and B, ≤0.0001 Between B and C, 0.19
Washes hands	0.0%	78.0%	45.0%	-
Measures blood pressure	0.0%	100.0%	93.0%	-
Measures heart rate	0.0%	94.0%	100.0%	-
Measures fundal height	0.0%	88.0%	93.0%	-
Listens to fetal heart rate	0.0%	100.0%	100.0%	-
Finds position of fetus	64.5%	94.0%	100.0%	-
Documents all findings	0%	100.0%	87.0%	-
Counseling (overall)	27.7%	86.2%	72.0%	Between A and B, ≤0.0001 Between B and C, 0.09
Discusses severe headache	40.5%	89.0%	94.0%	-
Discusses severe abdominal pain	28.0%	89.0%	94.0%	-
Discusses vaginal bleeding	34.0%	89.0%	89.0%	-
Discusses fever	35.0%	89.0%	83.0%	-
Discusses location of birth	41.0%	86.0%	83.0%	-
Discusses emergency plan	43.5%	86.0%	84.0%	-
Distributes prenatal vitamins	0.0%	89.0%	78.0%	-
Counsels on importance of prenatal vitamins	0.0%	85.0%	65.0%	-
Counsels on Td vaccine	29.5%	89.0%	50.0%	-

[1] Values entered as mean percentages; [2] Time point A occurred before any clinical instruction had begun; [3] Time point B occurred at the completion of 14-weeks of formalized POWHER curriculum; [4] Time point C occurred after six months of continuous clinical training from completion of the formalized POWHER curriculum; [5] Paired t-test.

The number of referrals increased over the study period although statistically insignificant. Before any clinical training occurred (Time Point A), only 17.8% of women were referred correctly. At the completion of the School of POWHER (Time Point B), appropriate referrals increased to 52.0% ($p = 0.32$). After six months of continued clinical training from the completion of the School of POWHER (Time Point C), appropriate referrals from the clinical checklist was 27.7%. The largest increase in referrals was seen in the category of clinical skills most commonly referred for the malposition of the fetus during late pregnancy.

4. Discussion

When TBA training is successfully implemented in rural communities, TBAs increase their basic obstetric knowledge, are equipped for safe home deliveries, and are able to identify problems requiring a referral; factors which markedly improve obstetrical outcomes [19]. Recent systematic reviews have identified that successful programs are those that can be integrated into an existing healthcare system, continue skill development (monthly or bi-monthly) of its participants for an extended period of time, and provides them access to birth kits and resuscitation equipment [9,10,12,20].

Our study, in line with these systematic reviews, suggests that standardized and continuous clinical training improves the PCS of TBAs during home visits. Overall, our TBAs were more likely to provide more complete prenatal home visits after the completion of School of POWHER training. An improvement was seen consistently in each broad category (history, clinical skills, and counseling) of basic prenatal care. Continued improvement was seen after six months of post School of POWHER clinical training (10-months of overall clinical training). The finding of this present study are generally encouraging as other studies, including our own previous pilot study, have demonstrated that a lack of continuous training leads to a decrease in PCS [18]. This point is of utmost importance as many TBA programs in low-and-middle-income countries fail to provide follow-up training after the completion of their training program. We have demonstrated how PCS continue to improve, and the average amount of improvement expected to be seen within each broad category of prenatal care, when clinical training is structured and continuous.

One of the biggest challenges that TBA training programs face is successfully measuring and reporting the outcomes of their didactic and clinical curriculum. We have previously published on the details of our 14-week School of POWHER training program [17]. With this present study, we focus on the standardization of our clinical curriculum and measuring its impact on PCS of our participant with a prenatal skills checklist. Our choice of standardization of clinical skills through a checklist was influenced by the success of other checklists in maternal healthcare [21–23]. The initial development of our prenatal skills checklist occurred from November 2016 through March 2017. Our own School of POWHER curriculum [17], WHO healthcare practices for birth attendants [15], and current guidelines for TBAs from the Guatemalan Ministry of Health [16] were consulted. By using this checklist to both standardize our clinical curriculum and measure PCS over time, we were able to report on a promising improvement of PCS during home visits. We believe our checklist had this effect via two ways: (1) our educators who trained the TBAs had an easy instrument that highlighted the key aspects of prenatal care from the clinical curriculum, (2) our TBAs had a simple and systematic approach during their prenatal home visits that reflected the curriculum learned during their training. Ultimately, the prenatal checklist standardized the clinical curriculum and successfully measured PCS improvement of each participant.

Additionally, the results of our study demonstrated the referral capacities of our TBAs throughout their training. Our study participants saw a significant increase in appropriate referrals after the completion of the School of POWHER training program (Time Point B). Referrals decreased after six months of continuous, focused PCS training (Time Point C) but remained higher than referral capacities when TBAs had no training at all (Time Point A). It is likely that there was a decrease in referrals from Time Point B to Time Point C due to the strong emphasis on standardized PCS training during this six month time period. During this period, there was focused exposure and training on PCS where referral teaching by the clinical educators was not as structured. Furthermore, study observers reported that during time Point C, study participants verbalized that they were more comfortable waiting on certain referral points until the mother was more advanced in her pregnancy (for example maternal age or past medical history), thus, the study tool would not pick up this later referral as it was not captured during the observed visit. Despite this, even at Time Point B, when the most referrals were occurring by study participants, only 52% of women were accurately referred. Our study suggests that a major focus on PCS during continued training does not indicate an equivalent increase in referrals. Our results on referral capacities also demonstrate the need to have a structured teaching approach for referrals taught parallel to standardized PCS.

This latter point is key as referrals must be timely and appropriate, which will only occur with access to properly trained birth attendants. Despite the push towards institutionalized births, the WHO has recognized that quality care during labor and delivery does not necessarily occur once a birth occurs in a hospital [24]. Specifically in Guatemala where there has been a push to birth in hospitals [4], untimely referrals during pregnancy by untrained healthcare personnel has inundated hospital waiting rooms leading to a minimal decrease in MMR. A possible solution to this problem lies in a new model of Birthing Homes (Casa Maternas) which have helped to reduce inappropriate referrals to the national hospitals in Guatemala [25]. This effective hybrid model between a home and institutional birth relies on the referral capacities of trained birth attendants that run the birthing homes. We propose that effective clinical training of TBAs not only affects the healthcare of women in rural settings but also has a larger impact on the burden of institutional births.

Findings from our study should be interpreted within its limitations. Our sample size of 13 TBA participants was small. Nonetheless, our study was able to capture each participant before and after exposure to the School of POWHER training program and follow PCS outcomes over a considerable amount of time as the last data collection point was at eight and a half months of total clinical training. The small sample size potentially affected our statistical analysis of referrals performed by our TBA study participants, as the analytic sample at Time Point C is approximately 1/3 of the analytical sample at Time Point B and C. This difference in an already small sample size could mean that it is possible that there is not a sufficient sample size to detect subtle improvements in accurate referrals. Convenience sampling may introduce study bias but was unavoidable in the current study as it was extremely difficult to recruit and observe TBAs that were not participating in the School of POWHER training program. Additionally, participants knew that they were being observed and this could have unintentionally influenced their behavior during prenatal home visits. Participants might have been driven to practice the PCS they learned during the training program when the observer was present but this does not indicate that TBA participants were routinely implementing PCS during routine unobserved home visits.

Despite these limitations, the strength and originality of our study counteracts many of the biases put forth. Our standardization of prenatal clinical care and subsequent measurement of PCS prior to and after our training program via observation allows for a direct method to collect data that is superior to self-reporting.

5. Conclusions

This study highlights the feasibility of PCS improvement through a standardized and continuous clinical training program for TBAs. The prenatal checklist assessment tool also serves as an objective means to quantify TBA skills in order to evaluate and maintain their skills in low resource settings. The improvement of TBA prenatal clinical skills could benefit indigenous women in rural Guatemala, and other low-and middle-income countries that prefer and/or have no other option except home care during pregnancy and birth.

Author Contributions: S.H. helped with the implementation of the training program and clinical study, acquired and analyzed study data, drafted, and revised the manuscript. J.O. contributed to the conception, initial development, and implementation of the training program and the initial development of the clinical study. J.C. helped with the implementation of the training program and clinical study and recruitment of study participants. L.J. helped with the implementation of the clinical study, and acquired and analyzed study data. T.S. contributed to the initial conception and development of the training program, the design and implementation of the clinical study, and revised the manuscript. All authors approve the manuscript.

Acknowledgments: Financial support was provided by a Global Health Education Grant from the Consortium of Universities for Global Health.

References

1. Alkema, L.; Chou, D.; Hogan, D.; Zhang, S.; Moller, A.B.; Gemmill, A.; Fat, D.M.; Boerma, T.; Temmerman, M.; Mathers, C.; et al. Global, regional, and national levels and trends in maternal mortality between 1990 and 2015, with scenario-based projections to 2030: A systematic analysis by the UN Maternal Mortality Estimation Inter-Agency Group. *Lancet* **2016**, *387*, 462–474. [CrossRef]

2. Zureick-Brown, S.; Newby, H.; Chou, D.; Mizoguchi, N.; Say, L.; Suzuki, E.; Wilmoth, J. Understanding Global Trends in Maternal Mortality. *Int. Perspect. Sex Reprod. Health* **2013**, *39*, 32–41. [CrossRef] [PubMed]

3. MSPAS. Estudio Nacional de Mortalidad Materna 2011. Guatemala City. 2011. Available online: http://www.mspas.gob.gt/index.php/component/jdownloads/send/94-muerte-materna/805-estudio-nacional-de-mortalidad-materna-2011?option=com_jdownloads (accessed on 28 September 2016).

4. Walton, A.; Kestler, E.; Dettinger, J.C.; Zelek, S.; Holme, F.; Walker, D. Impact of a low-technology simulation-based obstetric and newborn care training scheme on non-emergency delivery practices in Guatemala. *Int. J. Gynaecol. Obstet.* **2016**, *132*, 359–364. [CrossRef] [PubMed]

5. Ministerio de Salud Publica y Asistencia Social. *Encuesta Nacional de Salud Materno Infantil: Informe Interno Priliminario*; Ministerio de Salud Publica y Asistencia Social: Guatemala City, Guatemala, 2017.

6. Bailey, P.E.; Szaszdi, J.A.; Glover, L. Obstetric complications: Does training traditional birth attendants make a difference. *Rev. Panam. Salud Publica* **2002**, *11*, 15–23. [CrossRef] [PubMed]

7. Walsh, L. Beliefs and rituals in traditional birth attendant practice in Guatemala. *J. Transcult. Nurs.* **2006**, *17*, 148–152. [CrossRef] [PubMed]

8. Mahler, H. The safe motherhood initiative: A call to action. *Lancet* **1987**, *1*, 668–670. [CrossRef]

9. Byrne, A.; Morgan, A. How the integration of traditional birth attendants with formal health systems can increase skilled birth attendance. *Int. J. Gynaecol. Obstet.* **2011**, *115*, 127–134. [CrossRef] [PubMed]

10. Wilson, A.; Gallos, I.D.; Plana, N.; Lissauer, D.; Khan, K.S.; Zamora, J.; MacArthur, C.; Coomarasamy, A. Effectiveness of strategies incorporating training and support of traditional birth attendants on perinatal and maternal mortality: Meta-analysis. *BMJ* **2011**, *343*. [CrossRef] [PubMed]

11. Sakala, C.; Newburn, M. Meeting needs of childbearing women and newborn infants through strengthened midwifery. *Lancet* **2014**, *384*, e39–e40. [CrossRef]

12. Munabi-Babigumira, S.; Glenton, C.; Lewin, S.; Fretheim, A.; Nabudere, H. Factors that influence the provision of intrapartum and postnatal care by skilled birth attendants in low- and middle-income countries: A qualitative evidence synthesis. *Cochrane Database Syst. Rev.* **2017**, *11*, Cd011558. [CrossRef] [PubMed]

13. Carlough, M.; McCall, M. Skilled birth attendance: What does it mean and how can it be measured? A clinical skills assessment of maternal and child health workers in Nepal. *Int. J. Gynaecol. Obstet.* **2005**, *89*, 200–208. [CrossRef] [PubMed]

14. Ayiasi, R.M.; Criel, B.; Orach, C.G.; Nabiwemba, E.; Kolsteren, P. Primary healthcare worker knowledge related to prenatal and immediate newborn care: A cross sectional study in Masindi, Uganda. *BMC Health Serv. Res.* **2014**, *14*, 65. [CrossRef] [PubMed]

15. WHO; ICM; FIGO. *Making Pregnancy Safer: The Critical Role of the Skilled Birth Attendant Geneva*; World Health Organization: New York, NY, USA, 2004.

16. Ministry of Health and Public Assistance. *Training Manual for Traditional Birth Attendants in Neonatal Maternal Care*; Program, N.R.H., Ed.; Ministry of Health and Public Assistance: Guatemala City, Guatemala, 2016.

17. Hernandez, S.; Oliveira, J.B.; Shirazian, T. How a training program is transforming the role of traditional birth attendants from cultural practitioners to unique health-care providers: A community case study in rural Guatemala. *Front. Public Health* **2017**, *5*. [CrossRef] [PubMed]

18. Hernandez, S.; Oliveira, J.; Cuc, J.C.; Shirazian, T. *Prenatal Skills Pilot Study of Graduates from a Traditional Birth Attendant Training Program in Rural Guatemala*; American College of Obstetrics and Gynecology: Austin, TX, USA, 2018.

19. McCord, C.; Premkumar, R.; Arole, S.; Arole, R. Efficient and effective emergency obstetric care in a rural Indian community where most deliveries are at home. *Int. J. Gynaecol. Obstet.* **2001**, *75*, 297–307. [CrossRef]

20. Jokhio, A.H.; Winter, H.R.; Cheng, K.K. An Intervention involving traditional birth attendants and perinatal and maternal mortality in Pakistan. *N. Engl. J. Med.* **2005**, *352*, 2091–2099. [CrossRef] [PubMed]

21. Spector, J.M.; Agrawal, P.; Kodkany, B.; Lipsitz, S.; Lashoher, A.; Dziekan, G.; Bahl, R.; Merialdi, M.; Mathai, M.; Lemer, C.; et al. Improving quality of care for maternal and newborn health: Prospective pilot study of the WHO safe childbirth checklist program. *PLoS ONE* **2012**, *7*, e35151. [CrossRef] [PubMed]

22. Patabendige, M.; Senanayake, H. Implementation of the WHO safe childbirth checklist program at a tertiary care setting in Sri Lanka: A developing country experience. *BMC Pregnancy Childbirth* **2015**, *15*, 12. [CrossRef] [PubMed]

23. True, B.A.; Cochrane, C.C.; Sleutel, M.R.; Newcomb, P.; Tullar, P.E.; Sammons, J.H., Jr. Developing and Testing a Vaginal Delivery Safety Checklist. *J. Obstet. Gynecol. Neonatal. Nurs.* **2016**, *45*, 239–249. [CrossRef] [PubMed]

24. Individualized, Supportive Care Key to Positive Childbirth Experience, Says WHO: World Health Organization 2018. Available online: http://www.who.int/mediacentre/news/releases/2018/positive-childbirth-experience/en/ (accessed on 16 February 2018).

25. Stollak, I.; Valdez, M.; Rivas, K.; Perry, H. Casas Maternas in the rural highlands of Guatemala: A Mixed-methods case study of the introduction and utilization of birthing facilities by an indigenous population. *Glob. Health Sci. Pract.* **2016**, *4*, 114–131. [CrossRef] [PubMed]

## 9

Developing a Case-Based Blended Learning Ecosystem to Optimize Precision Medicine: Reducing Overdiagnosis and Overtreatment

Vivek Podder [1] (ORCID), Binod Dhakal [2], Gousia Ummae Salma Shaik [3], Kaushik Sundar [4], Madhava Sai Sivapuram [5], Vijay Kumar Chattu [6] (ORCID) and Rakesh Biswas [3,*]

[1] Department of Internal Medicine, Tairunnessa Memorial Medical College, Gazipur 1704, Bangladesh; drvivekpodder@gmail.com

[2] Division of Hematology/Oncology, Medical College of Wisconsin, Milwaukee, WI 53226, USA; bdhakal@mcw.edu

[3] Department of Internal Medicine, Kamineni Institute of Medical Sciences, Narketpally 508254, India; drshaiksalma@gmail.com

[4] Department of Neurology, Rajagiri Hospital, Chunanangamvely, Aluva 683112, India; skaushik85@gmail.com

[5] Department of Internal Medicine, Dr. Pinnamaneni Siddhartha Institute of Medical Sciences and Research Foundation, Chinaoutapalli 521101, India; madhavasai2011@gmail.com

[6] Department of Paraclinical Sciences, Faculty of Medical Sciences, The University of the West Indies, St. Augustine 0000, Trinidad and Tobago; vijay.chattu@sta.uwi.edu

* Correspondence: rakesh7biswas@gmail.com

Abstract: Introduction: Precision medicine aims to focus on meeting patient requirements accurately, optimizing patient outcomes, and reducing under-/overdiagnosis and therapy. We aim to offer a fresh perspective on accuracy driven "age-old precision medicine" and illustrate how newer case-based blended learning ecosystems (CBBLE) can strengthen the bridge between age-old precision approaches with modern technology and omics-driven approaches. Methodology: We present a series of cases and examine the role of precision medicine within a "case-based blended learning ecosystem" (CBBLE) as a practicable tool to reduce overdiagnosis and overtreatment. We illustrated the workflow of our CBBLE through case-based narratives from global students of CBBLE in high and low resource settings as is reflected in global health. Results: Four micro-narratives based on collective past experiences were generated to explain concepts of age-old patient-centered scientific accuracy and precision and four macro-narratives were collected from individual learners in our CBBLE. Insights gathered from a critical appraisal and thematic analysis of the narratives were discussed. Discussion and conclusion: Case-based narratives from the individual learners in our CBBLE amply illustrate their journeys beginning with "age-old precision thinking" in low-resource settings and progressing to "omics-driven" high-resource precision medicine setups to demonstrate how the approaches, used judiciously, might reduce the current pandemic of over-/underdiagnosis and over-/undertreatment.

Keywords: overdiagnosis; overtreatment; CBBLE (case-based blended learning ecosystem); case studies; precision medicine; omics driven; low resource setting; high resource setting

1. Introduction

The term "Precision Medicine" was first coined by Clayton Christensen in his book the "Innovator's Prescription", published in 2009 [1]. According to the early definition given by the Institute of Precision Medicine, "Precision medicine is targeted, individualized care that is tailored to each patient based on his or her specific genetic profile and medical history" [2].

While the above definitions allow us to assume that precision medicine is focused on meeting patients' requirements accurately, we need to review the scientific nature of accuracy, precision and their relationship with each other to put things in perspective. This is essential toward optimizing patient requirements and outcomes, minimizing damage to the healthcare ecosystem by reducing under-overdiagnosis and therapy. To quote from Thomas (2014), "The healthcare 'system' is now better understood as an 'ecosystem' of interconnected stakeholders, each one charged with a mission to improve the quality of care while lowering its cost. To ensure patient safety and quality care while realizing savings, these stakeholders are building new relationships—often outside the four walls of the hospital" [3].

We illustrate current concepts borrowed from existing scientific literature around accuracy and precision with Figures 1 and 2. We have modified the figure in reference to paper [4] to offer a fresh perspective on accuracy-driven "precision medicine", which is an age-old tool for physicians, currently augmented by technology.

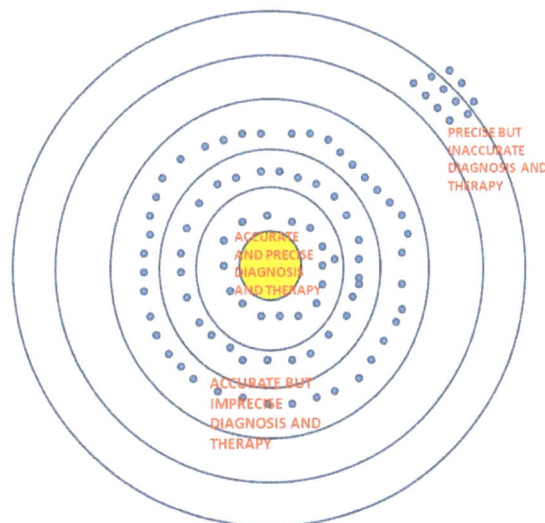

Figure 1. Mapping 'Precision' and 'Accuracy' in Medicine (Accuracy—achieving patients' requirement of best outcome, and Precision—the narrowest path to achieve it).

1.1. Precision versus Accuracy

We illustrate the above concepts with micro case studies below:

"An elderly patient from a country endemic with tuberculosis presented with a chronic cough and weight loss. A lung pathology was detected on imaging that was not amenable to further biopsy efforts as a result of unavailable resources. He was started on empirical treatment for tuberculosis after sending a sputum for acid-fast bacillus (AFB) and culture."

In tuberculosis endemic countries, physicians often treat empirically for tuberculosis in suspicious lung pathologies, although lung malignancy is a close differential in such situations. In the above patient's context, physicians were being obviously imprecise in starting treatment for tuberculosis empirically even when the tuberculosis bacilli was undetectable. This is an acceptable standard practice with established protocols for treating sputum-negative tuberculosis utilized globally by many countries that are endemic for tuberculosis.

Now to illustrate the concepts further, the above case may have the following mentioned outcomes:

(a)   The elderly patient's sputum comes out to be positive and once he is begun on antitubercular therapy, he recovers. His cough subsides and weight improves and his sputum culture report that comes after 6 weeks also turns out to be positive for tuberculosis. This is an example of precise and accurate diagnosis and treatment.

(b)   The elderly patient's sputum turns out to be negative and yet once he is begun on antitubercular therapy, he recovers. His cough subsides and weight improves and his sputum culture report that comes after 6 weeks turns out to be positive for tuberculosis although his initial sputum smear was negative. This would be an example of initially imprecise, but finally accurate outcomes.

(c)   The elderly patient's sputum turns out to be negative and a cartridge-based nucleic acid amplification assay test (CBNAAT) sent at the same time also turns out to be negative for tuberculosis and once he is begun on antitubercular therapy, he does not appear to recover at all. His cough worsens along with his appetite and his weight loss increases. A bronchoscopy with bronchoalveolar lavage is performed and sent again for malignant cytology, AFB, CBNAAT, and culture. His sputum culture report that comes after 6 weeks turns out to be positive for drug-resistant tuberculosis. Although, he receives second-line therapy for his drug-resistant tuberculosis, his condition worsens, and he dies.

The above is an example of a precise approach that still leads to inaccurate patient outcomes. We can be inaccurate in spite of being precise because of the current limitation of information and knowledge that does not always allow us to be accurate. The role of research and learning is to address this limitation and push the boundaries of current knowledge. Precision medicine develops and positively evolves with better research and learning.

(d)   The elderly patient's sputum turns out to be negative for tuberculosis and no further tests are done due to lack of resources. He is put on empirical antitubercular therapy, but he does not appear to recover at all. His cough worsens along with his appetite and his weight loss increases. One day he has a sudden shortness of breath and dies. An autopsy reveals bronchogenic carcinoma and pulmonary embolism.

The above is an example of imprecise and inaccurate outcomes. Here again, the obvious precipitants are low resources that prevent further probing toward a precise diagnosis, leading one to resort to imprecise treatment.

Out of the descriptions of a–d above, let's focus on (b), which illustrates imprecise approaches to arrive at accuracy. This is also known as the trial and error method in common parlance. Over the past centuries, medicine has often relied on this imprecise trial and error method, particularly on individual patients before it was replaced by the population-based randomized controlled trial approach to collect generalizable average evidence that is often applied on individual patients. The problem with this current approach is that the requirements of the individual at hand may not always match the average requirements.

Nevertheless, modern-day, evidence-based precision demands that the individual is first viewed through the 'average evidence' lens. Once the individual's response to the 'average' evidence-based available therapy is suboptimal or the therapy itself is unavailable, a therapeutic trial on the individual can be undertaken as a single subject 'n of 1' study design.

Coming back to (b), which is about a situation where empirical therapy is provided to an individual who may have a substantial chance of having an alternative diagnosis, and in (b) that individual turns out to be lucky to have that very diagnosis that was targeted. This imprecise approach may often be overdone in low-resource settings, where one often comes across prescriptions listing out 9–10 medications where the strategy is to target all possible differentials with whatever medicine appears to have the slightest evidence of success. While this form of irrational overuse of medication is a global problem, it appears to be more pronounced in low-resource settings [5]. This problem, a lack of system to make practitioners aware of their follies, is more common in low-resource settings also because of arcane medical education strategies that do not train students in critical appraisal, neither in terms of recognizing nor applying current best evidence. This deficit often stems from the education system's overreliance on rote memorization based on a curriculum that discourages students to ask questions [6]. One solution to the current curricular conundrum is to create more CBBLEs in every medical college, where patient-centered, evidence-based, self-directed learning is the prime emphasis [7].

Behnke LM et al. has defined overutilization as *"use of unnecessary care when alternatives may produce similar outcomes, results in a higher cost without increased value"* [8]. Overuse has a huge burden on low- and middle-income countries, where much healthcare is provided by ill-regulated, private providers and with fee-for-service. As a result, healthcare costs significantly increase and potentially harm patients through inappropriate interventions.

While our above description of overuse is true for multiple medication overuse in single patients, some single interventions can be scaled rapidly in larger populations. Current global concerns are mounting over inappropriate interventions such as percutaneous coronary intervention (PCI) for patients who are unlikely to benefit.

Brownlee S et al. reported that in an Indian second opinion setting, 55% of recommended PCIs were ill-advised [9]. A study in a tertiary care center in India showed that ST-elevation myocardial infarction (STEMI) patients constituted 55% of all inappropriate elective PCIs. These PCI procedures were performed on totally occluded infarct-related vessels after 12 h of symptom onset. The same study also showed that patients with stable angina with single or double vessel disease, low-risk group and sub-optimal medical therapy constituted 45% of all inappropriate elective PCIs [10]. It has been reported that the prevalence of inappropriate PCI procedures is 3.7% in Korea; 12% in the USA; 14% in Germany; 16% in Italy; 22% in Israel and 20% in Spain [9].

Over the last decade, we have adopted an evidence-based precision medicine approach that enables utilizing the best available evidence toward optimizing care for individual patients. Our individual patient requirements have led us to adopt a blended learning platform to enable an informational support for our patients. It also helps medical students to have a platform to help patients locally while learning from global experts in an online ecosystem [11]. Our online learning ecosystem is a community of computer and mobile users comprised of medical students, their physician teachers, other health professionals and patients and their relatives, each one of whom provide inputs (in terms of case-based information) to this ecosystem through devices. They receive learning feedback on the same cases such that their learning outcomes can be potentially translated into patient outcomes. This system, labeled "user-driven healthcare" (UDHC), is not restricted to our CBBLE, but represents an evolving global "phenomenon". Here "improved healthcare is achieved through concerted collaborative learning between multiple users and stakeholders, primarily patients, health professionals and other actors in the caregiving collaborative network across a web interface". This has been described in detail elsewhere [12–18].

1.2. Case-based Blended Learning Ecosystem (CBBLE): Current Case Studies and Implications for Precision Medicine

"The idea of sharing and learning around patients has been alive since the beginning of medicine, when physicians would present their cases to a large audience to primarily learn from the inputs of other physicians." With the invention of the printing press, instead of restricting themselves to verbal face-to-face case presentations, many physicians published their cases in journals and slowly the medical fraternity started naming those published diseases after their first authors. "In this way, case reporting became a gainful activity not only in terms of scientific advancement towards patient benefits, but also as an important instrument of physician fame." We have utilized this case reporting model to help our patients and to train our medical students about disease and patient experience [18,19].

By reporting cases, this model allows more engagement both from patients and medical students to reach a precise and accurate diagnosis, and also helps as an educational tool.

Our healthcare learning ecosystem is currently based offline in the Kamineni Institute of Medical Sciences, and this offline base keeps shifting with the various university locations in India where our corresponding authors are based for varying numbers of years. The online component of this blended learning ecosystem began on email groups, and then shifted to social media groups such as "Tabula Rasa" [14]. It currently exists in WhatsApp groups with a global audience of medical students and physicians. Gauging by the mentions in our past publications that have flowered through offline inputs processed further online, the students and faculty driving our online discussions range from universities in the US; India; Oxford, UK; Ontario, Canada; Montpellier, France; and Monash, Australia; as well as in the Maldives, Nepal, and Bangladesh.

What follows is a series of case narratives by the physicians in our case-based learning ecosystem and our critical appraisal of them through the "precision lens". We have previously published detailed patient narratives of online patient users of our ecosystem [18], and this article focuses on the physician narratives to provide a qualitative perspective of our workflow.

2. Materials and Methods

These case studies were taken from our "case-based blended learning ecosystem" (CBBLE) and were narrated by the physicians, students, and their senior teachers. We illustrated current concepts of scientific accuracy and precision using two analogies. The first was an age-old analogy of "scientific precision" and the second was a creative analogy comparing the medical endeavor of our CBBLE to a game of cricket where health professional bowlers and fielders try to get the batting disease team out in time to win the match. While this is not far from established analogies of "battling" disease, the cricket stadium offers a detailed perspective of our CBBLE framework. A group of our CBBLE online students visited Kamineni Institute of Medical Sciences (KIMS), Narketpally, where its offline component is currently ongoing. They worked with the team of students, physically managing the patients and developing insights into the nature of precision that enabled further analysis of the narratives obtained from our CBBLE students past and present.

This was done to attain our objective of illustrating the role of accuracy-driven "age-old precision medicine" in the framework of our current CBBLE, parallel to current "OMICS-driven" precision medicine narratives, and how we may create a bridge between the two systems.

3. Results

3.1. Precision Medicine through a Physician Resident's Narrative Lens (in Relatively Low-Resource Settings)

SS is a postgraduate resident physician managing critically ill patients, as well as chronic patients in the outpatient department (OPD) as part of her formal residency program in medicine. She also works part of the time on a thesis that involves clinical decision making around management of thyroid disorders.

What follows is her own narrative of experiences with one recent critically ill patient that she managed onsite, offline along with her other resident colleague as well as other first-year postgraduate colleagues, also known as interns. This was observed in real time by the online members of our CBBLE, who supported with their input once SS shared the patient's deidentified online record on a blog. This was preceded by a snippet of the patient's computed tomography (CT) images, as well as a very brief history of her problem. The online record blog link is accessible in [20].

After dinner on my night duty, I rushed to casualty as a patient was brought who needed immediate attention. On going to casualty, I saw that a 60-year-old lady was struggling to breathe and appeared tachypneic. Her % oxygen saturation was only 86% at room air. We had to provide her immediate oxygen support which improved her saturation but she was still tachypneic, and opening her mouth to take in the air, basically struggling to take the air in.

After making sure that her saturation was well maintaining I had called the attenders to take a detailed history. Her complaints were not of recent onset. She had complaints since the past 4 months. The lady had been having complaints of burning micturition since 4 months. She had been visiting the hospital often for the above complaints. This time, she had the same complaints of burning micturition, fever, abdominal pain and decreased urine output.

On asking further the attenders related that she hadn't passed urine since 3–4 days. So I had immediately asked for a Foley's catheterization. The moment we had inserted the Foley's the urine was milky white for the initial few minutes. By this time we had got a few of their old prescriptions which showed a urology op card and the urologist made a diagnosis based upon the history of "thin stream of urine" as stricture urethra. Now everything was falling into place. Her persistent complaints from the past few months, her burning micturition, fever.

We got the necessary investigations done, firstly sent a blood and urine culture as I could sense that she may deteriorate. Sent immediately blood for an arterial blood gas (ABG) analysis which showed a metabolic acidosis thus ruling out any lung pathology leading to shortness of breath. She needed dialysis. Blood counts showed elevated leukocytes. Her urine routine microscopy showed plenty of pus cells. Her ultrasonogram (USG)of the abdomen revealed pyonephrosis with dilated ureters.

Had got her dialysis done the next day. In her Foley's interestingly we noted some debris. We had a discussion around it as what it could be. But post dialysis though her acidosis resolved she went into hypotension. We had to start her on inotropic support. Had to monitor her blood pressure (BP) closely to tailor the dose accordingly. We were eagerly waiting for her culture reports as the leucocyte count showed an increasing trend. By this time we had got all her previous outpatient cards which not only revealed her past history and procedures done but were also a representation of the case-based workflow of multiple departments in our rural tertiary medical college hospital.

Her previous outpatient cards revealed that her first visit was in December last year. She had first gone to a gynecologist with complaints of burning micturition, whitish discharge per vaginum and fever. Probably the gynecologist had asked her to void and come as they wanted to examine her per vaginally. But this is where we lost track of the information in her outpatient card progress notes. She then landed up in urology OPD where her op card revealed that she had a thin stream of urine. The diagnosis of stricture urethra was made solely based on this and a dilatation procedure was done, she was catheterized with Foley's and urine culture sensitivity was sent. She was started on antibiotic and asked to turn up after 3 days which she did. She got her Foley's removed and was prescribed the 1st line antibiotic for urinary tract infection (UTI). The urine culture report was, unseen by the care provider, and unasked by the patients. She was prescribed the same 1st line antibiotic as in the first visit. She was then asymptomatic for the next 2 months. When she developed her current symptoms she turned up in the casualty this time.

The organism was the same since the first report, but sadly the culture reports being unseen she was getting the antibiotic for which the organism was never sensitive. The organism had been evolving since then into a more virulent one.

3.1.1. Analogy-Driven Analysis: Retrospective Notes from the Dugout

We draw below an analogy of our blended ecosystem with a cricket match (Figure 2), where the bowler is the treating physician, along with the rest of the fielders as a part of the treating team. The dugout is the online team sending inputs to the bowler, also known as, the offline treating physician team for taking the wicket of that batsman, also known as, the disease.

The main aim of the entire offline and the online team is to take an accurate wicket using a precise strategy that minimizes overuse and overtreatment and successfully banishes the disease to the pavilion and accurately meets patient requirements. Precision medicine ensures the narrowest path toward accuracy.

The healthcare professional team, as bowlers and fielders, rushed to the casualty (field) to battle the disease of this patient and win the match to meet the patient requirements within a narrowest path possible to attain precision and accuracy without overdiagnosis and overtreatment (Figure 2).

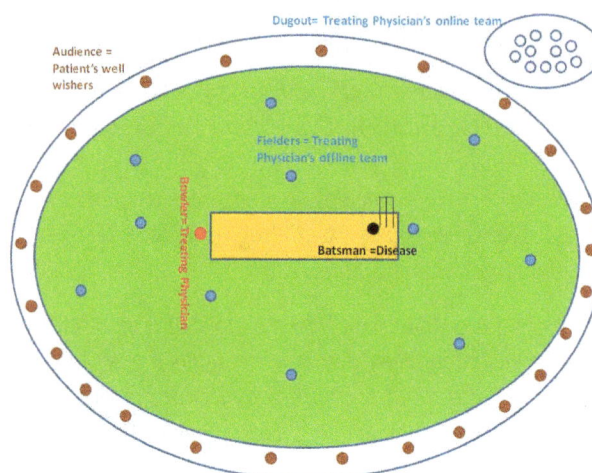

Figure 2. Illustrates the analogy of healthcare ecosystem functioning in the form of a cricket match.

The postmenopausal woman was prescribed first-line antibiotics for UTI without following the urine c/s reports that precisely pointed toward the sensitivity. This permitted the E. coli to strengthen, as the antibiotic in use was a poor match. Moreover, an estrogen ointment was prescribed for local use, although evidence of efficacy for this intervention for UTI prevention or treatment is inconclusive [21]. Lacking adequate diagnosis and follow-up, she returned to casualty with life-threatening symptoms.

The above is an example of an initial accurate diagnosis managed with an imprecise approach leading to inaccuracy.

Physician resident's narrative, continued

We got a CT abdomen done for her as the USG abdomen revealed pyonephrosis. We had something very unusual and unexpected in store for us in the CT. She had air pockets in the kidney, in the erector spinae muscle and spinal canal. We decided to change the antibiotic. We were still waiting for the culture report and had started her on a higher antibiotic. But to our dismay, our microbiology department didn't have the sensitivity checking disc for the antibiotic which we had started her on.

3.1.2. Online Work flow in Parallel with the Offline Component of Our CBBLE

At this point, the patient data was shared online in our CBBLE and the online team (analogous to the stadium dugout) swung into action (Figures 3 and 4). This enriched the decision-making capacities of the bowling and fielding team by sharing current evidence-based inputs gathered through search engines. This considerably helped the offline treating team (the bowlers and fielders) to intensify their strategy to finally get all the batsmen out. This patient's course was such that one batsman after another tried to score as much as possible, as once she appeared to have recovered from the sepsis, she developed a myocardial infarction. Once that was out, she developed recurrent seizures, which were possibly a result of her uremic encephalopathy. She finally recovered, with all the wickets taken. A graphical representation of the entire hospital course of her illness is shared (Figure 5), here.

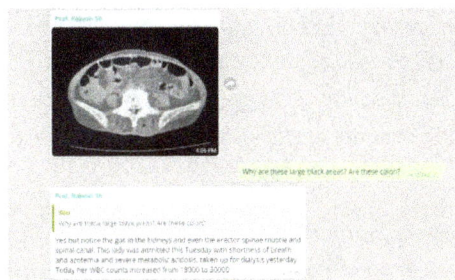

Figure 3. Illustrating the patient data shared online into our CBBLE online network.

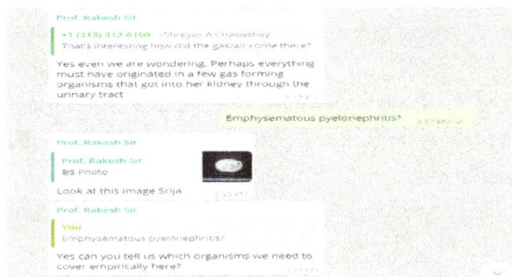

Figure 4. Illustrating the patient data shared online into our CBBLE online network.

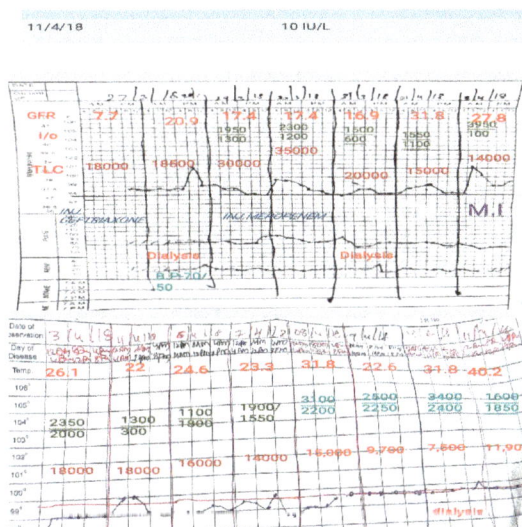

Figure 5. Illustrates the graphical representation of her illness during her stay in the hospital.

3.2. Precision Medicine through a Neurologist's Narrative Lens (in Relatively High-Resource Settings)

KS has been a member of our CBBLE since 2006, when RB, his offline teacher in his medical college in Bangalore migrated on a teaching assignment to Malaysia and he chose to keep in touch online. Since then, he has completed his postgraduate residency in medicine and fellowship in neurology. He currently practices interventional neurology in a high-resource setting in India, where he often works in the neuro cath lab performing angiography and stenting of cerebral blood vessels. What follows is a case-based narrative in his voice.

A 29-year-old male, presented to our Neurology Clinic with his first known episode of generalized tonic-clonic seizures. He denies drug or alcohol usage and his growth and developmental history was normal. Prior to this hospital visit, he had not attended any medical consultation. He was not on any medications for any other ailment. His neurological examination was normal. He was then subjected to an electroencephalography (EEG) and magnetic resonance (MR)imaging of the brain. EEG was normal. However, MR imaging (with contrast) revealed a single ring-enhancing lesion in the left temporal lobe with a visible scolex. A diagnosis of Neurocysticercosis was made. The patient was prescribed Albendazole and steroids for the acute problem and then prescribed T. Levetiracetam 500 mg twice a day for the seizures.

Two weeks into treatment he was brought to the emergency room (ER) in an unresponsive state. His parents found him unresponsive and noticed that he had inadvertently passed urine in his clothes. On examination, his vitals were stable. He had a gaze preference to the left, with paucity of movements on the right side. The possibility of an unwitnessed seizure, Todd's palsy, and postictal confusion were suspected. A repeat MR imaging revealed acute infarct in the left middle cerebral artery (MCA) and left anterior cerebral artery (ACA) territories. MR angiogram revealed a left carotid occlusion. His older MR images were reviewed and showed no evidence of carotid or intracranial vascular disease. He was transferred to the angiography suite and a diagnostic cerebral angiogram was performed. Digital subtraction angiography (DSA) revealed a left carotid T occlusion. A mechanical thrombectomy was successfully performed. However, there was also evidence of left MCA occlusion. Mechanical thrombectomy was repeated, with partial recanalization. Repeat brain imaging revealed significant. Left hemispheric infarct with evidence of evolving cerebral edema. A decompressive craniectomy was done 3 days after the surgery, repeat imaging revealed persistent cerebral edema and hence he was referred for re-exploration. He underwent left frontal and temporal lobectomy. The patient is slowly recovering with occupational and rehabilitative therapies.

A young stroke workup was considered. Routine blood investigations were normal. Autoimmune markers including antinuclear antibody (ANA) and antineutrophil cytoplasmic antibodies (ANCA) were normal. He had normal homocysteine levels and a normal echocardiogram. Holter monitoring was normal. We screened him for genetic thrombophilic conditions. He was found to have a homozygous MTHFR C677T gene mutation. MTHFR mutation has been previously linked to ischemic strokes.

Two hit hypothesis is well discussed in the field of oncology where a reactive genetic mutation can be triggered by an epigenetic event such as an infection. However, if we are to apply the same principle in this case scenario, our patient had a 'first hit' with a homozygous MTHFR C677T mutation. The 'second hit' may have been the neurocysticercosis infection, followed by the interventions or the resultant systemic distress and functional recovery.

Analogy-Driven Analysis: Retrospective Notes from the Dugout

In the above game, the bowling and fielding team of KS played with the best possible strategy (precision), but was unable to get the disease out (accuracy), and the game appeared to be drawn, if not lost.

3.3. Precision Medicine (in Relatively Low-Resource Settings) through the Lens of a Medical Student's Online Interaction with Our CBBLE

VP is a medical student from Tairunnessa Memorial Medical College, Gazipur, Bangladesh and an active member of our CBBLE who has attended the offline component of our CBBLE, which is also organized in collaboration with BMJ case reports [22]. After finishing his offline elective stint a year back in our host Institute, he has subsequently remained active online and regularly collates patient data shared by different members of our CBBLE into deidentified online patient records and ensures that all the signed informed consents from these patients are maintained and preserved in secure locations. The physicians in our CBBLE share their patient data in the hope of obtaining online feedback through conversational engagement with peers along with current best evidence support which VP provides through extensive searches of online and offline electronic resources. The patient narrative below was posted on our WhatsApp discussion forum by a CBBLE member and collated by VP.

A 52 year old woman, who was visiting us from North Bengal said she was watching TV in her apartment one day in the summer of 2015 and suddenly noticed that the TV was swinging followed by swinging walls and even the stairs of her apartment when she quickly started running down to safety and amidst all this commotion she noticed a buzz of people shouting earthquake! Earthquake!! She remembers that is the first time she had experienced severe palpitations since then which she complains of repeatedly experiencing over the years. However, she didn't notice the swelling in front of her neck that we noticed. We didn't notice any protruding eyes or tremors etc. USG neck showed nodules in the thyroid that was sent for fine-needle aspiration cytology (FNAC) and her T4 was double the normal value and TSH was very low.

Toxic adenoma is a toxic thyroid nodule which produces excessive thyroid hormones. They are managed either by prolonged thionamide therapy, surgery or radioiodine ablation. In this non-diabetic patient, a non-velvety, hyperpigmented area involving skin folds was noticed at the back of the neck that was very atypical of acanthosis nigricans. In view of thyroid nodule and hyperpigmentation in the neck, paraneoplastic acanthosis nigricans was brought into consideration. Later, FNAC report was available which showed features of benign thyroid lesion with foci of mild atypia.

Once the above narrative was posted by one of our CBBLE users feedback started pouring in, in the form of queries and clarifications sought (Figure 6).

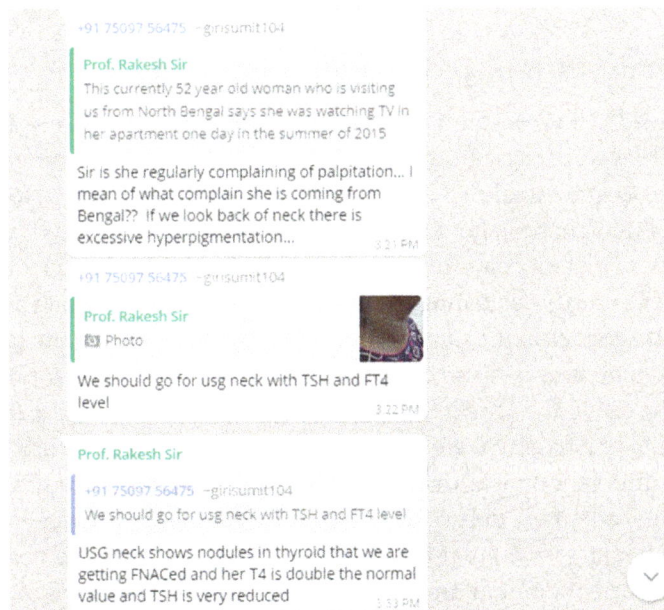

Figure 6. Illustrates the feedback and the queries posted from the CBBLE online network.

3.3.1. After the Discussion, the Following Questions about the Patient Were Raised

If FNAC is positive, we would know what to do next, but what are the chances of false negativity after FNAC? What is the frequency of having to obtain excision/incision biopsies in such situations? What if we miss an underlying malignancy and go for radioiodine? Based on FNAC findings, how would you decide between surgery and medical management in this patient?

These were answered by VP after searching online and offline resources and illustrated by him below along with interactions with the initial CBBLE user who had posted the patient data.

3.3.2. If FNAC Is Positive, We Would Know What to Do Next, But What Are the Chances of False Negativity after FNAC?

This made us look up specificity and sensitivity of FNAC in detecting thyroid malignancy. A study showed FNAC is more specific (98%) than sensitive (80%) in detecting malignancy [23]. Here if FNAC is more specific than sensitive so what should we do if the FNAC is negative? There is still 20% chance of its being malignant.

3.3.3. What Is the Frequency of Having to Obtain Excision/Incision Biopsies in Such Situations?

The decision to go for excision biopsy primarily for histopathological examination (HPE) to rule out malignancy is often a judgement call. In this context from a precision medicine perspective would a liquid biopsy be feasible or help? A feasibility study was conducted by detecting BRAF(V600E) circulating tumour DNA (ctDNA) in the plasma of patients with thyroid nodules to distinguish between benign and malignant nodules. Results showed that BRAF(V600E) ctDNA could distinguish between the two [24].

3.3.4. Based on FNAC Findings, How Would You Decide between Surgery and Medical Management in This Patient?

The problem with both radioiodine and surgery is that the patient would become hypothyroid eventually and end up in a lifelong dose of maintenance thyroxine. The problem with carbimazole is that we may not be sure of the response.

Eventually, the patient was started on carbimazole after shared decision making with her and her relatives.

3.3.5. Analogy-Driven Analysis: Retrospective Notes from the Dugout

This game involved a fair amount of precision even in a relatively low-resource setting. It appears to have achieved a fair amount of accuracy, although the game is going to be long, as thyroid-suppressive treatment takes a long time to maintain remission in toxic adenomas. There is always a chance of a malignancy showing up sometime later. This patient was actually referred to our CBBLE from a very distant community, nearly 2000 km away from our tertiary care teaching hospital. VP and RB were already evaluating the patient's inputs posted by one our CBBLE community health workers, who also resides in the same community 2000 km away, in the patient's village/town. A tentative plan for evaluation was made online, following which the patient was further evaluated in the hospital after she made the long journey. The revised inputs on the patient after evaluation by the hospital residents and faculty were again posted to the online network on WhatsApp, and a final plan of available intervention was drawn. There was a question raised by the team evaluating the patient in the hospital about the uncertainty of future malignancy prediction in this patient when an online CBBLE member suggested that this could become feasible in the near future using BRAF (V600E) ctDNA. At the current point in time, this is out of reach from a rural Indian tertiary teaching hospital perspective, but it is possible that resources and research could make this available even in less than a decade, in the coming years. Until then, we may have to live with the uncertainty posed.

3.4. Precision Medicine through a Hematoncologists Narrative Lens (in Relatively High-Resource Settings)

Author BD is one of the earliest students of our CBBLE from the purely email era, when he published some of his cases even as a graduate student in Manipal College of Medical Sciences, Pokhara, Nepal, way back in 2002. He is currently working at the cutting edge of precision medicine in a high-resource setting at the Medical College of Wisconsin, as a hemat-oncologist focused on multiple myeloma and other plasma cell disorders.

In a frigid Wisconsin morning last December, I received a phone call from my friend, whose brother was in the battle for his life against Multiple Myeloma. This patient's disease had progressed after multiple lines of chemotherapy including two stem cell transplants in the span of 4 years. My friend was desperate for a ray of hope to help his brother. He had exhausted all available options, and enrollment in a clinical trial was the only potential solution for his disease. As a myeloma focussed physician, I was aware of a clinical trial that was exploring an experimental agent for the subtype of myeloma he had; myeloma with chromosomal translocation 11 and 14; t(11:14). With ample caution, I routed them towards relevant myeloma clinical trials in their area. Fast forward a few months, my friend called me again, but this time excitement was palpable through the phone. His brother was enrolled in a clinical trial using bcl 2-inhibitor (venetoclax)—a drug active against a particular subtype of multiple myeloma with t(11:14) [25]. This result, a remission, was shared by others and this would open a new era of precision medicine in the therapeutic armamentarium of multiple myeloma.

Analogy-Driven Analysis: Retrospective Notes from the Dugout

The patient's disease was difficult to drive out in spite of the best possible efforts by the fielding team over 4 years, and a chemical that targeted a precise molecular pathway in the pathogenesis of the disease offered promise of finally making a dent in the disease.

4. Discussion

4.1. Current Narratives in Precision Oncogenomics

In 1927, a brilliant physicist from Germany, Werner Heisenberg, introduced a principle, well known as "The Heisenberg Uncertainty Principle", which would become pivotal for the development of quantum mechanics. The principle asserts the fundamental limit to the precision with which certain pairs of physical properties of a particle can be known. Modern medicine, particularly within the field of oncology, is rapidly moving towards a precision approach, as the molecular underpinnings of disease evolution are made known. As one of the major goals of cancer research is the gaining of understanding of the genetic changes responsible for the establishment of the "cancer clone" and the "key pathways", they could be targeted therapeutically. New insights into human cancers are emerging from basic research, and this has the potential to augment disease diagnostics, therapeutics, and clinical decision-making.

"Precision Medicine"—an abundant term in medical literature—refers to the tailoring of medical treatment guided by genomic or molecular features of the disease and not by the clinicopathological features [26]. Since cancer is a disease of the genome, the field has been the perfect choice to enhance the impact of precision medicine [27]. Because every single cancer patient exhibits a different genetic profile, and that profile can change over time, "tailored" treatment, rather than a "one-size-fits-all" approach, is likely to benefit patients, and hence is an attractive concept. Whether it is a mere concept or realistically assures a better future in oncology continues to remain a debate. The precision medicine approach has transformed the outlook for some deadly cancers. One of the most notable examples is the discovery of bcr-abl gene fusion and the development of imatinib for Chronic Myelogenous Leukemia (CML). CML treated by imatinib resulted in unprecedented results, with a 5-year survival of 90% and some patients even inching towards cure [28]. Other examples include the human epidermal growth factor receptor-2 (HER-2) and development of agents like trastuzumab. Compared to conventional chemotherapy, the addition of this agent has resulted in significant improvement in progression-free survival and reduction of death by 20% [29]. These examples illustrate how the identification of key molecular pathways targeted therapeutically could alter the disease course and result in the desired outcomes. What about other cancers? Has precision medicine delivered its promise in other cancers, as well, and is it a time to celebrate? Or has our approach for more "precision" resulted in more "uncertainty", as described by Heisenberg?

In this context, the design and the results of the SHIVA trial are worth a discussion. It is a phase 2, randomized multicenter trial, which assessed the efficacy of several molecularly targeted therapies based on molecular profiling compared to conventional therapies in patients with advanced cancers [30]. The results showed no improvement in progression-free survival (the primary end-point) with the use of molecularly targeted agents compared to physician's choice of chemotherapy. However, it is important to realize that the majority of the patients in the trial received a hormone modulator or mTOR inhibitor, and thus the justification of the failure of the precision approach based on this limited data is not reasonable. The other was that the study was powered to determine whether the use of an algorithm-based approach to treatment allocation can improve patient outcomes—regardless of the nature of such allocated treatments [30]. In the trial, each patient served as his or her own control in terms of primary end-point assessment. This calls for novel methods of designing the trials, with clinically meaningful endpoints using precision medicine. One of the other concerns has been the possible lack of valid biomarkers. We are experiencing another revolution in personalized treatment, with the introduction of various immune-based approaches. Cancer immunotherapy used to have limited applications, mainly for selected cancers like melanoma and renal cancers and involved the use of interleukin 2 (IL-2). With the dramatic progress in the last few years, this approach has moved into the mainstream in several cancers. Currently, immune-based approaches represent the most exciting area for diseases like melanoma, non-small lung cell cancer, and hematological cancers including multiple myeloma. The immune approach includes both active and passive immunotherapies: monoclonal antibodies, checkpoint inhibitors, and cellular immunotherapy. Recently, Rosenberg et al. demonstrated a new approach to immunotherapy, in which "adoptive transfer of mutant-protein-specific tumour-infiltrating lymphocytes (TILs) in conjunction with interleukin (IL)-2 and checkpoint blockade mediated the complete durable regression of metastatic breast cancer, which is now ongoing for >22 months" [31]. However, not all patients respond to immunotherapy, and there is a variability in response. One of the reasons for the variability in patient response with immunotherapy is the lack of predictive biomarkers. Identifying predictive biomarkers is a challenge in immunotherapy, and the other challenges include cost, toxicity and tumor heterogeneity, which impede the efficacy of immune-based therapy. For checkpoint inhibition, PDL1 has been proposed as a putative biomarker, as pembrolizumab (anti-PD 1) is approved in non-small-cell lung carcinoma (NSCLC) only in patients whose tumor PD-L1 levels are $\geq$50% [32]. Unfortunately, with the different temporal, spatial and methodological heterogeneity, it remains an unreliable biomarker [27]. The other unreliable biomarker includes the ERCC1 for NSCLC to platinum therapy [33].

Despite the challenges, precision medicine holds a lot of potential in cancer therapy. While we need to conduct well-designed randomized trials to assess broader efficacy of personalized medicine and validate the bio-markers, we can also enjoy the tremendous success of KIT mutations in gastrointestinal stromal tumor (GIST), BRAF (V600E) in melanoma, EGFR, ALK, and ROS1 alterations in NSCLC [34–36]. In a study in which my friend's brother participated, venetoclax monotherapy resulted in unprecedented response rates of 40% in heavily pre-treated patients with multiple myeloma [25]. Biomarker analysis confirmed that response to venetoclax correlated with higher BCL2:BCL2L1 and BCL2:MCL1 mRNA expression ratios, which are predominantly seen in patients with t (11:14). These outcomes show potential in results, for the first time, that pave the way for precision medicine in multiple myeloma with a significant potential to change practice in specific subgroups of patients and the hope is that knowledge in the field will increase to include other subgroups.

Clinical trials are evolving to investigate tumor heterogeneity from patient to patient in their design. The Molecular Analysis for Therapy Choice (NCI-MATCH) is a clinical trial selecting treatments based on genetic features of patients, not traditional tumor histology [32]. Thusfar, 2500 patients in the USA have been enrolled in one of the 24 arms of this trial, representing one half of the recruitment goals [37]. The Molecular Profiling-based Assignment of Cancer Therapy (NCI-MPACT) is another innovative clinical trial to test the hypothesis that targeting an oncogenic driver mutation is more efficacious than not targeting it. NCI-MPACT will recruit advanced cancer patients who have been unresponsive to standard therapeutic options and possess mutations in one of three genetic pathways that include DNA repair, PI3K/mTOR (phosphoinositide-3 kinase/mammalian target of rapamycin), and Ras/Raf/MEK (mitogen-activated protein kinase). The efficacy of diagnosis and therapies using precision medicine could be significantly enhanced, should results deliver the outcomes investigated in these trials.

With the development of novel technologies, it is hoped that understanding of tumor complexity and the immune system will be increased. These will be critical in designing future tailored combination therapies. The recent advances in the development of sequencing technologies have enhanced the ability to sequence cancers at both population and single-cell levels. Diverse mechanisms that lead to disease evolution, disease response, and refractoriness are slowly being understood. These advancements, we hope, will translate to more targeted therapies with better outcomes in patients with cancers in future.

The above discussion by author BD perhaps reflects and echoes the thoughts of many of his peers, who are working to make the dream of precision medicine a reality; while at the same time, this is an evolving area, where there are unseen threats (for patients) and opportunities (for pharma) in terms of aggravating the pandemic of overdiagnosis and overtreatment [38–40].

4.2. Age-Old Precision Medicine

The patient of KS presented to a relatively high-resource set-up in India, where the practitioner worked in a highly specialized and narrow domain of precision medicine (interventional neurology) and made the best precise efforts to address the problem in this critically ill patient, but the results were far from accurate. We are not sure of the outcomes that may have been achieved if the same patient had visited a low-resource setting; would the approach have been imprecise but the outcomes serendipitously better? Currently, what are the available strategies for predicting patient outcomes in response to highly specialized precision intervention? Randomized controlled trials have looked at catheter-based interventions in cerebral vessels, and available data supports the use of mechanical thrombectomy from 6 to 24 h for patients with occlusion of the intracranial carotid or proximal middle cerebral artery who present to a stroke center with expertise in both mechanical thrombectomy and automated infarct volume determination using MR imaging or perfusion CT [41]. While the data continues to evolve, there shall remain a grey zone where the push of newer innovations in terms of pharmacological and non-pharmacological devices will encourage overdiagnosis and overtreatment. This appears directly reactionary to combat pre-existing underdiagnosis and undertreatment, particularly in parts of the globe that are plagued by it.

The two patient narratives from relatively low-resource settings naturally reflect the danger of underdiagnosis and undertreatment. This is apparent beginning with the very first narrative, where the urinary tract infection was undertreated due to underdiagnosis. This was again a result of informational discontinuity. This is another malady that our CBBLE is striving to address by tracking each patient record online and encouraging physicians to communicate around their online patient records, which can be accessed through our CBBLE. The solution to this lies in concerted team communication. Ideally, if this patient had first approached our CBBLE, we could have utilized our online network, connected to microbiologists, to collect her results. While this is easier in patients admitted to our hospital, the same may not be true with outpatients. For such situations, we have in the past tried to train community health workers to follow up with our outpatients even after they return to their homes. We have tried to integrate this with rudimentary home health care programs, but we must admit that we have not been able to scale this approach beyond just one or two towns in rural India [42].

Identification, elucidation and correlation of external life event pathways through traditional history taking and internal cellular and molecular event pathways through current precision medicine approaches could serve as a superior predictor of outcomes than the binary preference-bound "patient-related outcome". It can begin with recording and documentation of individual case-based experiences of the external and internal pathways that are otherwise routinely lost to science, and all this data can be harnessed using case-based reasoning (CBR) techniques. Many labels, such as case-based informatics and evidence farming, have been applied to these currently fledgling endeavors [43–46]. Our elective students have begun the process through their case records in their online learning portfolios [47], and in the next few months to years, once the number of cases in our database improves, we shall be able to utilize algorithms for "experiential evidence farming" to demonstrate improved patient outcomes with recording, sharing, reusing and recycling steps in the CBR evidence farming cycle.

5. Conclusions

The above paper was written to illustrate how CBBLE can strengthen the bridge between age-old precision approaches with modern omics-driven approaches to deliver precision healthcare and reduce overdiagnosis and overtreatment. The narratives from our CBBLE found that physicians naturally aim for precision and accuracy, although accuracy may remain elusive in spite of our best focused precise approaches. One can considerably increase one's chances of obtaining accuracy if one is regularly supported by a CBBLE that not only offers evidence-based decision tools, but also a regular connection with peers that can go a long way toward improved documentation, transparency and newer learning insights.

We hope to scale the CBBLE approach in the near future to not only reduce overdiagnosis and overtreatment, but also promote transparency, accountability, and innovation toward optimizing solutions for individual patients, integrating age-old as well as technology-driven precision medicine approaches.

Author Contributions: Conceptualization: R.B., V.P. and M.S.S.; Writing Original Draft Preparation: R.B., V.P., B.D., K.S., G.U.S.S., M.S.S., V.K.C.; Writing-Review& Editing: R.B.; Images: M.S.S. and V.P.

Funding: This research received no external funding.

Acknowledgments: For case 1, we would like to acknowledge faculty and students of Kamineni Institute of Medical Sciences, which was presented by Akhil Sugandhi and Salma to the Department of Microbiology, Gynecology, Hospital Administration, Urology and Emergency Medicine before being finally presented to everyone in the Thursday morning CME for their inputs; Venkat Kishan, Department of Radiodiagnosis for identifying the gas in the kidneys, spinal canal, and erector spinae. We also acknowledge the online members of our CBBLE namely Abhishek Choudary, Monika Pathania, Avinash Kumar Gupta, Srija Katta, Shreyas Chawathey, Ashwini Ronghe, Deepak Badhani, Yogesh Sharma, Kuldeep Gupta, Aadipta Ghosh and all other students in our current offline location for our CBBLE, Kamineni Institute of Medical Sciences (KIMS), Narketpally. We also acknowledge Amy Price, Namrata Dass, Michele Meltzer, Bhavik Shah, Boudhayan Das Munshi, Rajib Sengupta, Amit Taneja, Nidhi Sehgal, Sujoy Dasgupta, Able Lawrence, Rajendra Takhar, Debasish Acharjee, Karthik Balachandran, Binidra Banerjee, Leelavati Thakur, Pradip Kar and other active online members of our CBBLE.

References

1. Christensen, C.M.; Grossman, J.H.; Hwang, J. The innovator's prescription. In *Soundview Executive Book Summaries*; McGraw-Hill: New York, NY, USA, 2009.

2. Institute for Precision Medicine. Available online: http://ipm.weill.cornell.edu/about/definition(2015) (accessed on 14 May 2018).

3. Thomas, B.; UST Global Health Group. The New Healthcare Ecosystem: 5 Emerging Relationships. Available online: https://www.beckershospitalreview.com/hospital-management-administration/the-new-healthcare-ecosystem-5-emerging-relationships.html (accessed on 28 January 2018).

4. Peter, A. How Does Accuracy Differ from Precision in Scientific Measurements? Socratic Questions. Available online: https://socratic.org/questions/how-does-accuracy-differ-from-precision-in-scientific-measurements (accessed on 1 March 2018).

5. Nagashree, B.; Manchukonda, R.S. Prescription audit for evaluation of present prescribing trends in a rural tertiary care hospital in South India: An observational study. *Int. J. Basic Clin. Pharmacol.* **2016**, *5*, 2094–2097.

6. Krishna, P. Medical education. *Health Millions* **1992**, *18*, 42–44.

7. Shankar, P.R.; Chandrasekhar, T.S.; Mishra, P.; Subish, P. Initiating and strengthening medical student research: Time to take up the gauntlet. *Kathmandu Univ. Med. J.* **2006**, *4*, 135–138.

8. Behnke, L.M.; Solis, A.; Shulman, S.A.; Skoufalos, A. A targeted approach to reducing overutilization: Use of percutaneous coronary intervention in stable coronary artery disease. *Popul. Health Manag.* **2013**, *16*, 164–168. [CrossRef] [PubMed]

9. Brownlee, S.; Chalkidou, K.; Doust, J.; Elshaug, A.G.; Glasziou, P.; Heath, I.; Nagpal, S.; Saini, V.; Srivastava, D.; Chalmers, K.; et al. Evidence for overuse of medical services around the world. *Lancet* **2017**, *390*, 156–168. [CrossRef]

10. Patil, D.; Lanjewar, C.; Vaggar, G.; Bhargava, J.; Sabnis, G.; Pahwa, J.; Phatarpekar, A.; Shah, H.; Kerkar, P. Appropriateness of elective percutaneous coronary intervention and impact of government health insurance scheme—A tertiary centre experience from Western India. *Indian Heart J.* **2017**, *69*, 600–606. [CrossRef] [PubMed]

11. Podder, V. A Large Force of Health System—The Medical Students: Have They Been Utilized Adequately? Available online: https://blogs.bmj.com/case-reports/2017/12/12/a-large-force-of-health-system-the-medical-students-have-they-been-utilized-adequately/ (accessed on 27 January 2018).

12. Price, A.; Chandra, S.; Bera, K.; Biswas, T.; Chatterjee, P.; Wittenberg, R.; Mehta, N.; Biswas, R. Understanding clinical complexity through conversational learning in medical social networks: Implementing user-driven health care. In *Handbook of Systems and Complexity in Health*; Springer: New York, NY, USA, 2013; pp. 767–793.

13. Biswas, R.; Sturmberg, J.P.; Martin, C.M. The User Driven Learning Environment. In *User-Driven Healthcare and Narrative Medicine: Utilizing Collaborative Social Networks and Technologies*; IGI Global: Hershey, PA, USA, 2011; pp. 229–241.

14. Purkayastha, S.; Price, A.; Biswas, R.; Ganesh, A.J.; Otero, P. From Dyadic Ties to Information Infrastructures: Care-Coordination between Patients, Providers, Students and Researchers: Contribution of the Health Informatics Education Working Group. *Yearb. Med. Inform.* **2015**, *10*, 68. [CrossRef] [PubMed]

15. Biswas, R. Clinical audit and lifelong reflective practice as game changers to integrate medical education and practice. *J. Fam. Med. Prim. Care* **2015**, *4*, 476. [CrossRef] [PubMed]

16. Price, A.I.; Djulbegovic, B.; Biswas, R.; Chatterjee, P. Evidence-based medicine meets person-centred care: A collaborative perspective on the relationship. *J. Eval. Clin. Pract.* **2015**, *21*, 1047–1051. [CrossRef] [PubMed]

17. Price, A.; Chatterjee, P.; Biswas, R. Comparative effectiveness research collaboration and precision medicine. *Ann. Neurosci.* **2015**, *22*, 127. [CrossRef] [PubMed]

18. Arora, N.; Tamrakar, N.; Price, A.; Biswas, R. Medical Students Meet User Driven Health Care for Patient Centered Learning in Clinical Medicine. *Int. J. User Driven Healthc. (IJUDH)* **2014**, *4*, 7–17. [CrossRef]

19. Price, A.; Biswas, T.; Biswas, R. Person-centered healthcare in the information age: Experiences from a user driven healthcare network. *Eur. J. Pers. Cent. Healthc.* **2013**, *1*, 385–393. [CrossRef]

20. Case Based Blended Learning Ecosystem Narratives. Available online: http://cbblenarratives.blogspot.com/2018/05/cbble-narratives.html (accessed on 30 March 2018).

21. Raz, R. Urinary tract infection in postmenopausal women. *Korean J. Urol.* **2011**, *52*, 801–808. [CrossRef] [PubMed]

22. BMJ Case Report Student Electives. Available online: https://promotions.bmj.com/jnl/bmj-case-reports-student-electives-2/ (accessed on 30 March 2018).

23. Basharat, R.; Bukhari, M.H.; Saeed, S.; Hamid, T. Comparison of fine needle aspiration cytology and thyroid scan in solitary thyroid nodule. *Pathol. Res. Int.* **2011**, *2011*, 754041. [CrossRef] [PubMed]

24. Patel, K.B. *Detection of Circulating Thyroid Tumor DNA in Patients with Thyroid Nodules*; Electronic Thesis and Dissertation Repository: London, ON, Canada, 2015.

25. Kumar, S.; Kaufman, J.L.; Gasparetto, C.; Mikhael, J.; Vij, R.; Pegourie, B.; Benboubker, L.; Facon, T.; Amiot, M.; Moreau, P.; et al. Efficacy of venetoclax as targeted therapy for relapsed/refractory t (11; 14) multiple myeloma. *Blood* **2017**, *130*, 2401–2409. [CrossRef] [PubMed]

26. Hunter, D.J. Uncertainty in the era of precision medicine. *N. Engl.J. Med.* **2016**, *375*, 711–713. [CrossRef] [PubMed]

27. Collins, F.S.; Varmus, H. A new initiative on precision medicine. *N. Engl. J. Med.* **2015**, *372*, 793–795. [CrossRef] [PubMed]

28. Saußele, S.; Krauß, M.-P.; Hehlmann, R.; Lauseker, M.; Proetel, U.; Kalmanti, L.; Hanfstein, B.; Fabarius, A.; Kraemer, D.; Berdel, W.E.; et al. Impact of comorbidities on overall survival in patients with chronic myeloid leukemia: Results of the randomized CML Study IV. *Blood* **2015**, *126*, 42–49. [CrossRef] [PubMed]

29. Slamon, D.J.; Leyland-Jones, B.; Shak, S.; Fuchs, H.; Paton, V.; Bajamonde, A.; Fleming, T.; Eiermann, W.; Wolter, J.; Pegram, M.; et al. Use of chemotherapy plus a monoclonal antibody against HER2 for metastatic breast cancer that overexpresses HER2. *N. Engl. J. Med.* **2001**, *344*, 783–792. [CrossRef] [PubMed]

30. Le Tourneau, C.; Delord, J.-P.; Gonçalves, A.; Gavoille, C.; Dubot, C.; Isambert, N.; Campone, M.; Trédan, O.; Massiani, M.-A.; Mauborgne, C.; et al. Molecularly targeted therapy based on tumour molecular profiling versus conventional therapy for advanced cancer (SHIVA): A multicentre, open-label, proof-of-concept, randomised, controlled phase 2 trial. *Lancet Oncol.* **2015**, *16*, 1324–1334. [CrossRef]

31. Zacharakis, N.; Chinnasamy, H.; Black, M.; Xu, H.; Lu, Y.C.; Zheng, Z.; Pasetto, A.; Langhan, M.; Shelton, T.; Prickett, T.; et al. Immune recognition of somatic mutations leading to complete durable regression in metastatic breast cancer. *Nat. Med.* **2018**, *24*, 724–730. [CrossRef] [PubMed]

32. McLaughlin, J.; Han, G.; Schalper, K.A.; Carvajal-Hausdorf, D.; Pelekanou, V.; Rehman, J.; Velcheti, V.; Herbst, R.; LoRusso, P.; Rimm, D.L. Quantitative assessment of the heterogeneity of PD-L1 expression in non–small-cell lung cancer. *JAMA Oncol.* **2016**, *2*, 46–54. [CrossRef] [PubMed]

33. Lee, S.M.; Falzon, M.; Blackhall, F.; Spicer, J.; Nicolson, M.; Chaudhuri, A.; Middleton, G.; Ahmed, S.; Hicks, J.; Crosse, B.; et al. Randomized prospective biomarker trial of ERCC1 for comparing platinum and nonplatinum therapy in advanced non-small-cell lung cancer: ERCC1 trial (ET). *J. Clin. Oncol.* **2016**, *35*, 402–411. [CrossRef] [PubMed]

34. Demetri, G.D.; Von Mehren, M.; Blanke, C.D.; Van den Abbeele, A.D.; Eisenberg, B.; Roberts, P.J.; Heinrich, M.C.; Tuveson, D.A.; Singer, S.; Janicek, M.; et al. Efficacy and safety of imatinib mesylate in advanced gastrointestinal stromal tumors. *N. Engl. J. Med.* **2002**, *347*, 472–480. [CrossRef] [PubMed]

35. Ascierto, P.A.; Kirkwood, J.M.; Grob, J.-J.; Simeone, E.; Grimaldi, A.M.; Maio, M.; Palmieri, G.; Testori, A.; Marincola, F.M.; Mozzillo, N.; et al. The role of BRAF V600 mutation in melanoma. *J. Transl. Med.* **2012**, *10*, 85. [CrossRef] [PubMed]

36. Desai, A.; Menon, S.P.; Dy, G.K. Alterations in genes other than EGFR/ALK/ROS1 in non-small cell lung cancer: Trials and treatment options. *Cancer Biol. Med.* **2016**, *13*, 77. [CrossRef] [PubMed]

37. Do, K.; O'Sullivan Coyne, G.; Chen, A.P. An overview of the NCI precision medicine trials—NCI MATCH and MPACT. *Chin. Clin. Oncol.* **2015**, *4*. [CrossRef]

38. Bhatt, J.R.; Klotz, L. *Overtreatment in Cancer–Is It a Problem?* Taylor &Francis: Didcot, UK, 2016.

39. Klotz, L. Cancer overdiagnosis and overtreatment. *Curr. Opin. Urol.* **2012**, *22*, 203–209. [CrossRef] [PubMed]

40. Esserman, L.J.; Thompson, I.M.; Reid, B.; Nelson, P.; Ransohoff, D.F.; Welch, H.G.; Hwang, S.; Berry, D.A.; Kinzler, K.W.; Black, W.C.; et al. Addressing overdiagnosis and overtreatment in cancer: A prescription for change. *Lancet Oncol.* **2014**, *15*, e234–e242. [CrossRef]

41. Nogueira, R.G.; Jadhav, A.P.; Haussen, D.C.; Bonafe, A.; Budzik, R.F.; Bhuva, P.; Yavagal, D.R.; Ribo, M.; Cognard, C.; Hanel, R.A.; et al. Thrombectomy 6 to 24 hours after stroke with a mismatch between deficit and infarct. *N. Engl. J. Med.* **2018**, *378*, 11–21. [CrossRef] [PubMed]

42. Biswas, R. User Driven Health Care. Available online: http://userdrivenhealthcare.blogspot.com/2016/08/role-of-patient-information.html?m=0 (accessed on 27 January 2018).

43. Andritsos, P.; Jurisica, I.; Glasgow, J.I. Case-Based Reasoning for Biomedical Informatics and Medicine. In *Springer Handbook of Bio-/Neuroinformatics*; Springer: New York, NY, USA, 2014; pp. 207–221.

44. Pantazi, S.V.; Arocha, J.F.; Moehr, J.R. Case-based medical informatics. *BMC Med. Inform. Decis. Mak.* **2004**, *4*, 19. [CrossRef] [PubMed]

45. Hay, M.C.; Weisner, T.S.; Subramanian, S.; Duan, N.; Niedzinski, E.J.; Kravitz, R.L. Harnessing experience: Exploring the gap between evidence-based medicine and clinical practice. *J. Eval. Clin. Pract.* **2008**, *14*, 707–713. [CrossRef] [PubMed]

46. Dussart, C.; Pommier, P.; Siranyan, V.; Grelaud, G.; Dussart, S. Optimizing clinical practice with case-based reasoning approach. *J. Eval. Clin. Prac.* **2008**, *14*, 718–720. [CrossRef] [PubMed]

47. BMJ Elective Case Log. Available online: http://bmjcaselogvivek.blogspot.com/ (accessed on 30 May 2018).

High Income Protects Whites but Not African Americans against Risk of Depression

Shervin Assari [1,2] (iD)

[1] Center for Research on Ethnicity, Culture, and Health (CRECH), School of Public Health,
University of Michigan, Ann Arbor, MI 48104, USA; assari@umich.edu
[2] Department of Psychiatry, University of Michigan, 4250 Plymouth Rd., Ann Arbor, MI 48109-2700, USA

Abstract: *Background:* Built on the Blacks' diminished return theory, defined as smaller effects of socioeconomic status (SES) on a wide range of health outcomes for African Americans compared to Whites, the current study compared African Americans and Whites for the association between household income and risk of lifetime, 12-month, and 30-day major depressive disorder (MDD). *Methods:* For the current cross-sectional study, we used data from the Collaborative Psychiatric Epidemiology Surveys (CPES), 2001–2003. With a nationally representative sampling, CPES included 4746 non-Hispanic African Americans and 7587 non-Hispanic Whites. The dependent variables were lifetime, 12-month, and 30-day MDD, measured using Composite International Diagnostic Interview (CIDI). The independent variable was household income. Age, gender, education, chronic medical conditions, and obesity were covariates. Race was the focal moderator. Logistic regression models were used to test the protective effects of household income against MDD in the overall sample and also by race. *Results:* In the overall sample, household income was inversely associated with the risk of 12-month and 30-day MDD. We found a significant interaction between race and household income on 12-month and 30-day MDD, suggesting a smaller protective effect of household income against MDD for African Americans compared to Whites. *Conclusion:* In line with the Blacks' diminished return theory, household income better protects Whites than African Americans against MDD. The contribution of diminished return of SES as an underlying mechanism behind racial disparities in health in the United States is often overlooked. Additional research is needed on why and how SES resources generate smaller health gain among minority groups.

Keywords: socioeconomic status; depression; major depressive disorder; ethnic health disparities; race; African Americans

1. Introduction

Longitudinal and cross-sectional studies have strongly established the protective effects of socioeconomic status (SES) on population health [1–6]. SES indicators such education [7], employment [8,9], and income [1,4,5] protect individuals against morbidity [10] and mortality [11–13]. Income has protective effects against risk of depression [14].

However, population sub-groups do not similarly gain health from their SES indicators [15–17]. Some of the sociodemographic factors that alter the effects of SES include age [18], gender [3,19–22], race [19–21], and their intersections [22]. This is in line with the Blacks' "diminished return" theory, suggesting that the protective effect of SES on health of populations is systemically smaller for African Americans in comparison to Whites [15,16,21]. Education [20], employment [23], and income [24] better reduce mortality and morbidity of the socially privileged than the socially disadvantaged group.

Research that shows SES effects are conditional by race [25,26] suggest that it is race and SES not race or SES that cause racial disparities [15,16]. If it is race and SES not race or SES, then SES does not fully explain the effects of race, and for the elimination of racial disparities in health, more needs to be done than merely eliminating racial disparities in SES [15,16]. That is, the elimination of SES disparities will not fully eliminate the racial disparities in health.

Regarding the effects of high SES on major depressive disorder (MDD), a meta-analysis showed that the prevalence, incidence, and persistence of MDD is lower in high-SES individuals compared to low-SES individuals [27]. However, individual studies have shown mixed results regarding the protective effects of SES indicators against risk of MDD [19,22,28,29]. Studies have suggested that the protective effects of SES indicators such as education and income against MDD and depressive symptoms may be larger for Whites than non-Whites [19,22]. In line with this literature, some research has documented an increase in the risk of depression in high-SES African Americans [22,28].

Aims

The current study compared African Americans and Whites for the association between household income and lifetime, 12-month, and 30-day MDD.

2. Methods

2.1. Design and Setting

With a cross-sectional design, the current study used data from the Collaborative Psychiatric Epidemiology Surveys (CPES), 2001–2003. The CPES was conducted by the University of Michigan (UM, Ann Arbor, MI, USA). Although the CPES methods have been described in detail elsewhere [29], we briefly summarize the study methodology here.

CPES is composed of three national surveys: (1) the National Comorbidity Survey- Replication (NCS-R) [30], (2) the National Latino and Asian American Study (NLAAS) [31], and (3) the National Study of American Life (NSAL) [29]. The CPES data were collected by the University of Michigan (UM) Institute for Social Research (ISR), Ann Arbor.

2.2. Sampling

White and African American participants were recruited using the CPES core sampling. Core sampling of the CPES was a multistage stratified area probability sample that recruited a nationally representative household sample. All participants were adults (18 years of age and older). Participants were recruited from households in the coterminous 48 states. The sample was limited to individuals who were able to conduct an interview in English. This study did not include any institutionalized individuals. Thus, being in prisons, jails, nursing homes, and medical facilities were exclusion criteria [29]. African Americans and Whites in the CPES were selected from large cities, other urban areas, or rural areas [29]. The analysis for the current study included a total of 4746 non-Hispanic African Americans and 7587 non-Hispanic Whites.

2.3. Ethics

The CPES study protocol was approved by the University of Michigan (UM) Institutional Review Board (IRB # B03-00004038-R1). Informed written consent was received from all participants. Data were kept anonymous. Participants were financially compensated for their time. Publicly available CPES data were downloaded from Interuniversity Consortium for Political and Social Research (ICPSR https://www.icpsr.umich.edu), located at the University of Michigan Institute for Social Research.

2.4. Data Collection

CPES collected data using structured interviews (survey questionnaires). Most of the data were collected using computer-assisted face-to-face interviews. Telephone interviews were only used for the remaining data collection. Interviews lasted between two hours on average. The overall response rate of the CPES is 69%.

2.5. Measures

2.5.1. Independent Variable

Household income was self-reported. Income was treated as a continuous measure in this study. To increase interpretability of the income coefficients, we divided income by USD 10,000. So, our income coefficients reflect the effect of a USD 10,000 increase in income on odds of MDD.

2.5.2. Dependent Variable

Major Depressive Disorder (MDD). The presence of MDD (lifetime, 12-month, and 30-day) was evaluated using the World Mental Health (WMH) Composite International Diagnostic Interview (CIDI). The CIDI can be administered by trained interviewers who are not clinicians. Participants were assessed for meeting the DSM criteria for MDD. CIDI is frequently used for African Americans and Whites [32–36].

2.5.3. Covariates

Covariates in this study included demographic characteristics (age and gender), health (chronic medical conditions and obesity), and socioeconomic status (education). Age was operationalized as a continuous variable. Gender was conceptualized as a dichotomous variable (male 1 vs. female 0). The socioeconomic covariate included education, which was measured as an ordinal variable with the following four categories: (1) less than 11 years, (2) 12 years, (3) between 13 and 15 years, and (4) 16 years or more. Education was operationalized as a categorical variable [37]. Chronic medical conditions and obesity were health covariates. Participants indicated whether or not they were ever told by a doctor or health professional that they had chronic medical conditions, including heart diseases, hypertension, chronic lung disease, asthma, diabetes, peptic ulcer, epilepsy, and cancer. Chronic medical conditions were defined as the number of chronic medical conditions, with a potential range from 0 to 8 [38–40]. Obesity was defined as having a body mass index (BMI) equal to or larger than 30. BMI was calculated using participants' self-reported height and weight. The use of self-reported height and weight in the calculation of BMI has been validated [41,42].

2.5.4. Moderator

Race. Race was self-identified in the CPSE [43–46]. African-Americans were defined as Blacks without any ancestral ties to the Caribbean. Race was treated as a dichotomous variable, with Whites being the reference category. (African Americans = 1 vs. Whites = 0). All African Americans and Whites entered in this analysis were non-Hispanic.

2.6. Statistical Analysis

2.6.1. Weights

To accommodate the CPES's sampling weight, which was due to the multi-stage sampling design of the NCS-R, NSAL, and NLAAS, Stata 13.0 (Stata Corp., College Station, TX, USA) was applied for all our data analysis. This approach will consider applying the CPES sampling weights. We used Taylor series linearization to re-estimate our standard errors. To perform our subsample analyses, we applied sub-pop survey commands in Stata.

2.6.2. Analytical Plan

For descriptive purposes, we used mean (SE) and proportions (relative frequency). Bivariate analyses included independent sample t-test, Pearson Chi square, and Spearman correlation tests in the pooled sample and by race. For multivariable analysis, we used four logistic regression models. From independent sample *t*-test and Pearson Chi square tests, we only reported *p*-values. From Spearman correlation tests, we reported *rho* values. Adjusted odds ratios (OR), 95% confidence intervals (CIs), and *p*-values were reported. In our logistic regression models, we used household income as the independent variable, MDD (lifetime, 12-month, and 30-day) as the dependent variable, and socio-demographics as covariates. Race was the focal moderator. The first two logistic regression models were estimated in the pooled sample composed of both African Americans and Whites. *Model 1* did not include race by household income interaction. *Model 2* included the race by household income interaction term. Subsequently, we estimated race-specific logistic regression models. *Model 3* was estimated for Whites and *Model 4* was calculated for African Americans.

3. Results

3.1. Descriptive Statistics

Table 1 provides a summary of the descriptive statistics in the overall sample and by race. African Americans had lower education and household income in comparison to Whites. African Americans had lower odds of MDD than Whites (Table 1).

Table 1. Summary of descriptive statistics in the overall sample and by race.

Characteristics	All		Whites		African Americans	
	%	95% CI	%	95% CI	%	95% CI
Gender						
Men	52.00	50.72–53.28	51.59	50.09–53.10	54.68	53.34–56.02
Women	48.00	46.72–49.28	48.41	46.90–49.91	45.32	43.98–46.66
Education (≥12 years) *,a						
0–11 years	14.58	13.25–16.02	13.18	11.57–14.98	23.76	21.92–25.70
12 years	32.01	29.66–34.45	31.30	28.57–34.15	36.66	35.11–38.23
13–15 years	27.76	26.30–29.27	28.16	26.44–29.95	25.14	23.55–26.80
16 years+	25.65	23.33–28.12	27.36	24.63–30.28	14.44	12.74–16.33
Obesity *,a						
No	75.35	74.09–76.58	76.86	75.34–78.31	65.52	64.03–66.97
Yes	24.65	23.42–25.91	23.14	21.69–24.66	34.48	33.03–35.97
Lifetime Major Depressive Disorder *,a						
No	82.98	81.95–83.96	81.98	80.85–83.06	89.51	88.55–90.40
Yes	17.02	16.04–18.05	18.02	16.94–19.15	10.49	9.60–11.45
12-Month Major Depressive Disorder *,a						
No	93.14	92.59–93.66	92.93	92.31–93.51	94.52	93.74–95.21
Yes	6.86	6.34–7.41	7.07	6.49–7.69	5.48	4.79–6.26
30-Day Major Depressive Disorder *,a						
No	97.42	97.04–97.75	97.33	96.90–97.70	98.01	97.50–98.42
Yes	2.58	2.25–2.96	2.67	2.30–3.10	1.99	1.58–2.50
	Mean	95% CI	Mean	95% CI	Mean	95% CI
Age (years) *	43.09	42.37–43.82	44.65	43.64–45.65	40.78	38.66–42.90
Chronic medical conditions (CMC) *,b	0.68	0.65–0.71	0.73	0.70–0.77	0.83	0.73–0.93
Household Income (USD 10,000) *,b	5.99	5.69–6.28	6.34	5.92–6.76	4.40	3.78–5.02

* *p* < 0.05 for comparisons of Whites and African Americans. [a] Pearson Chi square. [b] Independent samples *t* test. CI: confidence interval.

3.2. Bivariate Correlations

Table 2 presents the results of bivariate correlations in the pooled sample and by race. Household income showed negative correlation with 12-month and 30-day MDD in the pooled sample and White, but not African Americans (Table 2).

Table 2. Spearman correlations in the pooled sample and by race.

Characteristics	1	2	3	4	5	6	7	8	9	10
All										
1 Race (African Americans)	1.00									
2 Gender (Women)	−0.05	1.00								
3 Age	−0.08	−0.04	1.00							
4 Chronic Medical Conditions	0.05	−0.01	0.37 *	1.00						
5 Obesity	0.09	−0.02	0.05	0.17 *	1.00					
6 Education (≥12 years)	−0.11 *	−0.02	−0.09	−0.12 *	−0.06	1.00				
7 Household Income (USD 10,000)	−0.14 *	0.12 *	−0.05	−0.12 *	−0.06	0.31 *	1.00			
8 Lifetime Major Depressive Disorder (MDD)	−0.07	−0.11 *	−0.03	0.01	0.03	0.05	0.01	1.00		
9 12-Month Major Depressive Disorder (MDD)	−0.02	−0.08	−0.08	0.03	0.01	0.00	−0.06	0.58 *	1.00	
10 30-Day Major Depressive Disorder (MDD)	−0.01	−0.05	−0.03	0.02	0.00	−0.02	−0.05	0.34 *	0.58 *	1.00
Whites										
2 Gender (Women)	1.00									
3 Age	−0.05	1.00								
4 Chronic Medical Conditions	−0.01	0.37 *	1.00							
5 Obesity	0.00	0.05	0.18 *	1.00						
6 Education (≥12 years)	−0.02	−0.10	−0.12 *	−0.06	1.00					
7 Household Income (USD 10,000)	0.12 *	−0.06	−0.12 *	−0.05	0.29 *	1.00				
8 Lifetime Major Depressive Disorder (MDD)	−0.12 *	−0.03	0.02	0.05	0.04	0.00	1.00			
9 12-Month Major Depressive Disorder (MDD)	−0.09	−0.08	0.03	0.02	−0.01	−0.07	0.57 *	1.00		
10 30-Day Major Depressive Disorder (MDD)	−0.05	−0.04	0.01	0.01	−0.02	−0.06	0.33 *	0.57 *	1.00	
African Americans										
2 Gender (Women)	1.00									
3 Age	−0.01	1.00								
4 Chronic Medical Conditions	−0.02	0.36	1.00							
5 Obesity	−0.10 *	0.04	0.13 *	1.00						
6 Education (≥12 years)	−0.06	−0.09	−0.07	−0.03	1.00					
7 Household Income (USD 10,000)	0.12 *	−0.02	−0.13 *	−0.08	0.37 *	1.00				
8 Lifetime Major Depressive Disorder (MDD)	−0.06	−0.09	−0.03	0.00	0.04	−0.01	1.00			
9 12-Month Major Depressive Disorder (MDD)	−0.06	−0.09	0.02	−0.02	0.05	0.00	0.65 *	1.00		
10 30-Day Major Depressive Disorder (MDD)	−0.04	−0.02	0.02	−0.07	0.01	0.02	0.39 *	0.60 *	1.00	

$* p < 0.05.$

3.3. Logistic Regressions in the Overall Sample

Table 3 presents the results of three sets of logistic regression models in the pooled sample. Both models have household income as the independent variable, and lifetime, 12-month, and 30-day MDD as the dependent variables. *Model 1* only included the main effects. *Model 2* also included the race by household income interaction term. *Model 1* showed that high household income was associated with lower odds of MDD above and beyond the covariates. *Model 2* also showed an interaction between race and household income, suggesting that the protective effects of household income against 12-month and 30-day MDD are smaller for African Americans relative to Whites (Table 3).

Table 3. Summary of logistic regressions between household income and major depressive disorder (MDD) in the pooled sample.

Characteristics	Model 1 Main Effects		Model 2 Model 1 + Interactions	
	B	95% CI	B	95% CI
Lifetime MDD				
Race (African Americans)	0.57 ***	0.43–0.74	0.55 ***	0.40–0.74
Gender (Women)	0.60 ***	0.53–0.69	0.60 ***	0.53–0.69
Age	0.99 *	0.99–1.00	0.99 *	0.99–1.00
Chronic Medical Conditions	1.08 #	0.99–1.16	1.08 #	0.99–1.16
Obesity	1.28 ***	1.12–1.45	1.28 ***	1.12–1.45
Education (≥12 years)				
0–11 years				
12 years	1.03	0.77–1.39	1.03	0.77–1.39
13–15 years	1.15	0.94–1.40	1.15	0.94–1.40
16 years+	1.24 #	0.97–1.57	1.24 #	0.97–1.57
Household Income (USD 10,000)	1.00	0.99–1.02	1.00	0.99–1.02
Household Income (USD 10,000) × Race	-	-	1.01	0.97–1.05
Intercept	0.52 ***	0.39–0.69	0.52 ***	0.39–0.69

Table 3. *Cont.*

Characteristics	Model 1 Main Effects		Model 2 Model 1 + Interactions	
	B	95% CI	B	95% CI
12-Month MDD				
Race (African Americans)	0.65 *	0.47–0.91	0.49 ***	0.34–0.73
Gender (Women)	0.56 ***	0.47–0.66	0.56 ***	0.47–0.66
Age	0.98 ***	0.97–0.98	0.98 ***	0.97–0.98
Chronic Medical Conditions	1.26 ***	1.10–1.44	1.26 ***	1.10–1.44
Obesity	1.14	0.92–1.41	1.14	0.92–1.41
Education (≥12 years)				
0–11 years				
12 years	0.72	0.49–1.07	0.72	0.49–1.07
13–15 years	0.81	0.62–1.04	0.80 #	0.62–1.04
16 years+	0.92	0.67–1.26	0.91	0.67–1.26
Household Income (USD 10,000)	0.96 **	0.93–0.99	0.96 **	0.93–0.99
Household Income (USD 10,000) × Race	-	-	1.07 *	1.00–1.14
Intercept	0.54 ***	0.39–0.75	0.55 ***	0.39–0.76
30-Day MDD				
Race (African Americans)	0.69	0.43–1.10	0.43	0.23–0.79
Gender (Women)	0.56 ***	0.41–0.77	0.56	0.41–0.77
Age	0.98 **	0.98–0.99	0.98	0.98–0.99
Chronic Medical Conditions	1.09	0.94–1.26	1.09	0.94–1.26
Obesity	1.42	0.78–2.62	1.43	0.78–2.62
Education (≥12 years)				
0–11 years				
12 years	0.55 *	0.31–0.97	0.55	0.31–0.97
13–15 years	0.55 *	0.33–0.92	0.55	0.33–0.92
16 years+	0.82	0.45–1.47	0.81	0.45–1.46
Household Income (USD 10,000)	0.94 *	0.89–0.99	0.94	0.89–0.99
Household Income (USD 10,000) × Race	-	-	1.12	1.00–1.26
Intercept	0.18 ***	0.10–0.34	0.19	0.10–0.35

# $p < 0.1$, * $p < 0.05$, ** $p < 0.01$, *** $p < 0.001$.

3.4. Logistic Regressions by Race

Table 4 provides a summary of the results of two logistic regression models specific to Whites and African Americans. *Model 3* showed that in Whites, high household income was associated with lower odds of 12-month and 30-day MDD. *Model 4* showed that in African Americans, household income was not associated with odds of 12-month or 30-day MDD (Table 4).

Table 4. Summary of logistic regressions between household income and major depressive disorder (MDD) in Whites and African Americans.

Characteristics	Model 1 Whites		Model 2 African Americans	
	B	95% CI	B	95% CI
Lifetime MDD				
Gender (Women)	0.60 ***	0.52–0.69	0.69 #	0.46–1.05
Age	0.99 *	0.99–1.00	0.99 #	0.98–1.00
Chronic Medical Conditions	1.08 #	0.99–1.17	1.03	0.82–1.30
Obesity	1.30 ***	1.14–1.47	0.84	0.55–1.27
Education (≥12 years)				
0–11 years				
12 years	1.02	0.75–1.38	1.48	0.70–3.13
13–15 years	1.13	0.92–1.39	1.56	0.73–3.33
16 years+	1.23 #	0.96–1.58	1.32	0.64–2.75
Household Income (USD 10,000)	1.00	0.99–1.02	1.00	0.96–1.04
Intercept	0.52 ***	0.38–0.69	0.30 ***	0.13–0.71

Table 4. *Cont.*

Characteristics	Model 1 Whites		Model 2 African Americans	
	B	95% CI	B	95% CI
12-Month MDD				
Gender (Women)	0.51 *	0.28–0.92	0.56 ***	0.47–0.67
Age	0.98 *	0.96–0.99	0.98 ***	0.97–0.98
Chronic Medical Conditions	1.31	0.91–1.87	1.26 **	1.09–1.45
Obesity	0.76	0.43–1.34	1.16	0.93–1.44
Education (≥12 years)				
0–11 years				
12 years	1.55	0.61–3.95	0.70 #	0.47–1.06
13–15 years	1.57	0.59–4.20	0.78 #	0.60–1.03
16 years+	2.03	0.68–6.10	0.89	0.65–1.23
Household Income (USD 10,000)	1.01	0.93–1.09	0.96 **	0.93–0.99
Intercept	0.19 ***	0.06–0.56	0.55 ***	0.39–0.78
30-Day MDD				
Gender (Women)	0.56	0.41–0.78	0.40 *	0.18–0.93
Age	0.98	0.98–0.99	0.99	0.97–1.02
Chronic Medical Conditions	1.08	0.93–1.26	1.20	0.76–1.90
Obesity	1.49	0.81–2.76	0.31 *	0.11–0.87
Education (≥12 years)				
0–11 years				
12 years	0.54	0.30–0.97	0.92	0.31–2.77
13–15 years	0.52	0.31–0.89	1.83	0.52–6.43
16 years+	0.81	0.44–1.48	0.74	0.11–5.17
Household Income (USD 10,000)	0.94	0.89–0.99	1.03	0.93–1.14
Intercept	0.19	0.10–0.35	0.06 **	0.01–0.31

# $p < 0.1$, * $p < 0.05$, ** $p < 0.01$, *** $p < 0.001$.

4. Discussion

Built on the Blacks' diminished return theory [15,16], the current study aimed to explore racial variation in the association between household income and 12-month and 30-day MDD. Our findings showed that while higher household income is associated with lower risk of 12-month and 30-day MDD overall, this health gain is disproportionate and unequal for Whites and African Americans.

By documenting the diminished mental health returns of household income for African Americans compared to Whites, our results support the Blacks' diminished return theory [15,16]. Previously, smaller health effects of education, employment, and income were shown for physical health outcomes such as chronic disease and mortality in African Americans relative to Whites [20,21,23]. For instance, a recent study showed smaller protective effects of income on chronic medical conditions for African Americans compared to Whites [24]. The life expectancy gain that is expected to follow employment is smaller for African Americans compared to Whites [23]. Similar differential effects of education on health behaviors such as drinking between Whites and African Americans are shown [21]. In addition to economic resources, psychological assets such as affect, coping, sleep, self-rated health, and self-efficacy better serve the health of Whites than African Americans [47–57].

Blacks' diminished return theory has attributed the diminished return of African Americans to the discrimination and structural racism that are embedded in the fabric of American society. American society functions in a way that constantly maximizes the benefits of Whites, with the unintended consequence of minimum health return for non-Whites including African Americans, Latinos, and Native Americans [15,16,23].

The results do not suggest that African Americans have a tendency to mismanage their economic resources such as income, or that Whites more effectively use their resources. Instead, we argue that the American social structure is failing the African American families, even high SES African American families who have successfully climbed the social ladder and earn high income. Regardless of their ambitions, the U.S. society makes them pay extra psychological costs for their social mobility. This is particularly shown in the studies showing poor mental health of high SES African Americans [19,58].

One major contribution of this study is to the theoretical models that are commonly used for health disparities research. In line with the Blacks' diminished return theory, at least some of the disparities are not due to differential exposures, but differential effects of the very same exposures [15,16]. Unfortunately, differential effects of socioeconomic factors between African Americans and Whites is traditionally overlooked [20,21]. We believe that without an assumption that the protective effects of SES indicators are universal, researchers should systemically explore interactions between race and resources on health [15,16]. Another theoretical contribution of this study is that it may not be African Americans but Whites whose health declines more rapidly due to low SES. Several existing theories such as Double Jeopardy [28,59], Triple Jeopardy [60], Multiple Jeopardy [61], and Multiple Disadvantage [62] conceptualize minority status as a vulnerable status, meaning that minority populations' health is more strongly dependent upon the presence or absence of very same risk or protective factor [61].

This is not the first study to show that race alters the health effects of SES indicators; however, most of this literature has focused on physical health outcomes such as mortality [63–67]. Relative to physical health outcomes [63–67], less is known about differential gains that follow SES indicators such as income on depression.

Similar to our findings, there is some research [19,21,63,64,68] showing that SES does not explain the effect of race on health, but interacts with race on health [39]. In this view, race limits how much individuals and groups can benefit from the very same SES resource [15,16]. These patterns will result in high levels of racial disparities in high levels of SES [39,60].

A greater differential effect of education is shown than the differential effects of income. This is partially because given the racism in the labor market and segregation, education is more likely than income to generate different outcomes [69–72]. Racial inequity in pay causes differential health gains of education and employment by race [60,71]. The current study shows that the same racial gap exists between Whites and African Americans in how they can use their income to gain mental health. The low mental health gain of high-SES African Americans may be because high-SES African Americans are commonly more discriminated against than low-SES African Americans [72].

4.1. Implications

Our findings have policy and public health implications. Policies and programs should also aim to reduce the diminished returns of African Americans as a strategy to eliminate health disparities [15,16]. Addressing health disparities should go beyond merely equalizing access to the SES resources or reducing extra risk factors in the lives of minorities [15,16].

The diminished health return of very same SES resources should be regarded as a major contributor of racial health disparities in the USA [73–76]. Policies that merely focus on a universal increase of all populations to SES indicators may widen the existing health disparities. Policy makers and program planners who are interested in eliminating the persisting racial health disparities in the USA should think beyond equalizing access to resources across populations. Tailored programs may be needed to ensure that all social groups equally benefit from the very same resources, regardless of their race and color. Policy and program evaluations should also consider the evaluation of the same policy or program by race, in order to understand how the very same policy is affecting population sub-groups, and whether our interventions are widening the existing gaps or not.

4.2. Limitations

Our study had its own limitations. Due to the cross-sectional design, the current study does not allow the establishment of causal associations between household income and CMC. Not only SES impacts mental health; poor mental health may interfere with productivity and income generation. Future research should also consider the risk of reverse causality between MDD and household.

Another potential limitation of the current study is omitted confounders. We did not include several factors such as insurance, health care use, and history of encounters with the mental health care system. Similarly, this study was limited to individual characteristics. Future research should include higher-level SES indicators that reflect policy and communities for Whites and African Americans. Similar to other studies that compare racial groups for the effects of the same variable, differential validity may be a threat. MDD may be of different severity in Whites and African Americans [77].

5. Conclusions

To conclude, race was found to alter the magnitude of the association between household income and 12-month and 30-day MDD in the U.S. The effect of race is not just on the amount of SES indicators such as income, but also on how SES indicators impact the health of individuals. This may be because race is a very important social construct in the United States and shapes treatment by society and access to the opportunity structure.

Acknowledgments: Shervin Assari is partially supported by the Heinz C. Prechter Bipolar Research Fund and the Richard Tam Foundation at the University of Michigan Depression Center. This research is supported by National Institute of Mental Health Research Grants MH06220, MH62207, MH62209, HD049142 and RWJ DA18715 with generous support from SAMHSA and OBSSR. The National Survey of American Life (NSAL) was supported by the National Institute of Mental Health (U01-MH57716) with supplemental support from the National Institutes of Health Office of Behavioral and Social Science Research; National Institute on Aging (5R01 AG02020282) with supplemental support from the National Institute on Drug Abuse; and the University of Michigan. Preparation of this article was also aided by grants from the National Institute of Mental Health (1P01 MH58565, 1T32 MH67555, and 5TMH16806). This publication was also made possible by Grant Number 1KL2RR025015-01 from the National Center for Research Resources (NCRR), a component of the National Institutes of Health (NIH) and NIH Roadmap for Medical Research.

References

1. Dowd, J.B.; Albright, J.; Raghunathan, T.E.; Schoeni, R.F.; Leclere, F.; Kaplan, G.A. Deeper and wider: Income and mortality in the USA over three decades. *Int. J. Epidemiol.* **2011**, *40*, 183–188. [CrossRef] [PubMed]
2. Marmot, M.G.; Shipley, M.J. Do socioeconomic differences in mortality persist after retirement? 25 year follow up of civil servants from the first Whitehall study. *Br. Med. J.* **1996**, *313*, 1170–1180. [CrossRef]
3. Morris, J.K.; Cook, D.G.; Shaper, A.G. Loss of employment and mortality. *Br. Med. J.* **1994**, *308*, 1135–1139. [CrossRef]
4. Van Groenou, M.I.B.; Deeg, D.J.; Penninx, B.W. Income differentials in functional disability in old age: Relative risks of onset, recovery, decline, attrition and mortality. *Aging Clin. Exp. Res.* **2003**, *15*, 174–183. [CrossRef]
5. Berkman, C.S.; Gurland, B.J. The relationship among income, other socioeconomic indicators, and functional level in older persons. *J. Aging Health* **1998**, *10*, 81–98. [CrossRef] [PubMed]
6. Burgard, S.A.; Elliott, M.R.; Zivin, K.; House, J.S. Working conditions and depressive symptoms: A prospective study of US adults. *J. Occup. Environ. Med.* **2013**, *55*, 1007–1014. [CrossRef] [PubMed]
7. Baker, D.P.; Leon, J.; Smith Greenaway, E.G.; Collins, J.; Movit, M. The education effect on population health: A reassessment. *Popul. Dev. Rev.* **2011**, *37*, 307–332. [CrossRef] [PubMed]
8. Eliason, M. Alcohol-related morbidity and mortality following involuntary job loss: Evidence from Swedish register data. *J. Stud. Alcohol Drugs* **2014**, *75*, 35–46. [CrossRef] [PubMed]
9. Noelke, C.; Beckfield, J. Recessions, job loss, and mortality among older US adults. *Am. J. Public Health* **2014**, *104*, e126–e134. [CrossRef] [PubMed]
10. Herd, P.; Goesling, B.; House, J.S. Socioeconomic position and health: The differential effects of education versus income on the onset versus progression of health problems. *J. Health Soc. Behav.* **2007**, *48*, 223–238. [CrossRef] [PubMed]
11. Hummer, R.A.; Lariscy, J.T. Educational attainment and adult mortality. In *International Handbook of Adult Mortality*; Springer: Dordrecht, The Netherlands, 2011; pp. 241–261.
12. Masters, R.K.; Hummer, R.A.; Powers, D.A. Educational differences in US adult mortality a cohort perspective. *Am. Soc. Rev.* **2012**, *77*, 548–572. [CrossRef] [PubMed]

13. Brown, D.C.; Hayward, M.D.; Montez, J.K.; Hummer, R.A.; Chiu, C.T.; Hidajat, M.M. The significance of education for mortality compression in the United States. *Demography* **2012**, *49*, 819–840. [CrossRef] [PubMed]

14. Lorant, V.; Deliege, D.; Eaton, W.; Robert, A.; Philippot, P.; Ansseau, M. Socioeconomic inequalities in depression: A meta-analysis. *Am. J. Epidemiol.* **2003**, *157*, 98–112. [CrossRef] [PubMed]

15. Assari, S. Health Disparities Due to Diminished Return among Black Americans: Public Policy Solutions. *Soc. Issues Policy Rev.* **2018**, *12*, 112–145. [CrossRef]

16. Assari, S. Unequal gain of equal resources across racial groups. *Int. J. Health Policy Manag.* **2017**, *6*, 1–6. [CrossRef] [PubMed]

17. Assari, S.; Thomas, A.; Caldwell, C.H.; Mincy, R.B. Blacks' Diminished Health Return of Family Structure and Socioeconomic Status; 15 Years of Follow-up of a National Urban Sample of Youth. *J. Urban Health* **2017**. [CrossRef] [PubMed]

18. Roelfs, D.J.; Shor, E.; Davidson, K.W.; Schwartz, J.E. Losing life and livelihood: A systematic review and meta-analysis of unemployment and all-cause mortality. *Soc. Sci. Med.* **2011**, *72*, 840–854. [CrossRef] [PubMed]

19. Assari, S. Combined racial and gender differences in the long-term predictive role of education on depressive symptoms and chronic medical conditions. *J. Racial Ethn. Health Disparit.* **2016**, *4*, 385–396. [CrossRef] [PubMed]

20. Assari, S.; Lankarani, M.M. Race and urbanity alter the protective effect of education but not income on mortality. *Front. Public Health* **2016**, *4*. [CrossRef] [PubMed]

21. Assari, S.; Lankarani, M.M. Education and alcohol consumption among older Americans. Black-White Differences. *Front. Public Health* **2016**, *4*. [CrossRef] [PubMed]

22. Assari, S. Social Determinants of Depression: The Intersections of Race, Gender, and Socioeconomic Status. *Brain Sci.* **2017**, *7*, 156. [CrossRef] [PubMed]

23. Assari, S. Life expectancy gain due to employment status depends on race, gender, education, and their intersections. *J. Racial Ethn. Health Disparit.* **2017**. [CrossRef] [PubMed]

24. Assari, S. The Benefits of Higher Income in Protecting against Chronic Medical Conditions Are Smaller for African Americans than Whites. *Healthcare* **2018**, *6*, 2. [CrossRef] [PubMed]

25. Steenland, K.; Henley, J.; Thun, M. All-cause and cause-specific death rates by educational status for two million people in two American Cancer Society cohorts, 1959–1996. *Am. J. Epidemiol.* **2002**, *156*, 11–21. [CrossRef] [PubMed]

26. Montez, J.K.; Hayward, M.D.; Brown, D.C.; Hummer, R.A. Why is the educational gradient of mortality steeper for men? *J. Gerontol. Ser. B Psychol. Sci. Soc. Sci.* **2009**, *64*, 625–634. [CrossRef] [PubMed]

27. Lorant, V.; Deliège, D.; Eaton, W.; Robert, A.; Philippot, P.; Ansseau, M. Socioeconomic inequalities in depression: A meta-analysis. *Am. J. Epidemiol.* **2003**, *157*, 98–112. [CrossRef] [PubMed]

28. Assari, S.; Caldwell, C.H. High Risk of Depression in High-Income African American Boys. *J. Racial Ethn. Health Disparit.* **2017**, 1–12. [CrossRef] [PubMed]

29. Heeringa, S.; Wagner, J.; Torres, M.; Duan, N.H.; Adams, T.; Berglund, P. Sample designs and sampling methods for the collaborative psychiatric epidemiology studies (CPES). *Int. J. Methods Psychiatr. Res.* **2004**, *13*, 221–240. [CrossRef] [PubMed]

30. Kessler, R.C.; Merikangas, K.R. The National Comorbidity Survey Replication (NCS-R): Background and aims. *Int. J. Methods Psychiatr. Res.* **2004**, *13*, 60–68. [CrossRef] [PubMed]

31. Alegria, M.; Takeuchi, D.; Canino, G.; Duan, N.; Shrout, P.; Meng, X.; Vega, W.; Zane, N.; Vila, D.; Woo, M.; et al. Considering context, place and culture: The National Latino and Asian American Study. *Int. J. Methods Psychiatr. Res.* **2004**, *13*, 208–220. [CrossRef] [PubMed]

32. Kessler, R.C.; Calabrese, J.R.; Farley, P.A.; Gruber, M.J.; Jewell, M.A.; Katon, W.; Keck, P.E.; Nierenberg, A.A.; Sampson, N.A.; Shear, M.K.; et al. Composite International Diagnostic Interview screening scales for DSM-IV anxiety and mood disorders. *Psychol. Med.* **2013**, *43*, 1625–1637. [CrossRef] [PubMed]

33. Kessler, R.C.; Wittchen, H.-U.; Abelson, J.M.; McGonagle, K.; Schwarz, N.; Kendler, K.S.; Knäuper, B.; Zhao, S. Methodological studies of the Composite International Diagnostic Interview (CIDI) in the US National Comorbidity Survey. *Int. J. Methods Psychiatr. Res.* **1998**, *7*, 33–55. [CrossRef]

34. Robins, L.N.; Wing, J.; Wittchen, H.U.; Helzer, J.E.; Babor, T.F.; Burke, J.; Farmer, A.; Jablenski, A.; Pickens, R.; Regier, D.A.; et al. The Composite International Diagnostic Interview. An epidemiologic instrument suitable for use in conjunction with different diagnostic systems and in different cultures. *Arch. Gen. Psychiatry* **1988**, *45*, 1069–1077. [CrossRef] [PubMed]

35. Williams, D.R.; González, H.M.; Neighbors, H.; Nesse, R.; Abelson, J.M.; Sweetman, J.; Jackson, J.S. Prevalence and distribution of major depressive disorder in African Americans, Caribbean blacks, and nonHispanic whites: Results from the National Survey of American Life. *Arch. Gen. Psychiatry* **2007**, *64*, 305–315. [CrossRef] [PubMed]

36. Hu, W. Reliability and validity studies of the WHO-Composite International Diagnostic Interview (CIDI): A critical review. *J. Psychiatr. Res.* **1994**, *200*, 57–84.

37. Kessler, R.C.; Neighbors, H.W. A new perspective on the relationships among race, social class, and psychological distress. *J. Health Soc. Behav.* **1986**, *27*, 107–115. [CrossRef] [PubMed]

38. Assari, S. Chronic Medical Conditions and Major Depressive Disorder: Differential Role of Positive Religious Coping among African Americans, Caribbean Blacks and Non-Hispanic Whites. *Int. J. Prev. Med.* **2014**, *5*, 405–413. [PubMed]

39. Assari, S. Number of Chronic Medical Conditions Fully Mediates the Effects of Race on Mortality; 25-Year Follow-Up of a Nationally Representative Sample of Americans. *J. Racial Ethn. Health Disparit.* **2017**, *4*, 623–631. [CrossRef] [PubMed]

40. Assari, S.; Lankarani, M.M. Chronic Medical Conditions and Negative Affect; Racial Variation in Reciprocal Associations over Time. *Front. Psychiatry* **2016**, *7*, 140. [CrossRef] [PubMed]

41. Spencer, E.A.; Appleby, P.N.; Davey, G.K.; Key, T.J. Validity of self-reported height and weight in 4808 EPIC-Oxford participants. *Public Health Nutr.* **2002**, *5*, 561–565. [CrossRef] [PubMed]

42. Stewart, A.L. The reliability and validity of self-reported weight and height. *J. Chronic Dis.* **1982**, *35*, 295–309. [CrossRef]

43. Chou, T.; Asnaani, A.; Hofmann, S.G. Perception of racial discrimination and psychopathology across three U.S. ethnic minority groups. *Cult. Divers. Ethn. Minor. Psychol.* **2012**, *18*, 74–81. [CrossRef] [PubMed]

44. Asnaani, A.; Richey, J.A.; Dimaite, R.; Hinton, D.E.; Hofmann, S.G. A cross-ethnic comparison of lifetime prevalence rates of anxiety disorders. *J. Nerv. Ment. Dis.* **2010**, *198*, 551–555. [CrossRef] [PubMed]

45. Asnaani, A.; Gutner, C.A.; Hinton, D.E.; Hofmann, S.G. Panic disorder, panic attacks and panic attack symptoms across race-ethnic groups: Results of the collaborative psychiatric epidemiology studies. *CNS Neurosci. Ther.* **2009**, *15*, 249–254. [CrossRef] [PubMed]

46. Gavin, A.R.; Walton, E.; Chae, D.H.; Alegria, M.; Jackson, J.S.; Takeuchi, D. The associations between socio-economic status and major depressive disorder among Blacks, Latinos, Asians and non-Hispanic Whites: Findings from the Collaborative Psychiatric Epidemiology Studies. *Psychol. Med.* **2010**, *40*, 51–61. [CrossRef] [PubMed]

47. Lampe, F.C.; Walker, M.; Lennon, L.T.; Whincup, P.H.; Ebrahim, S. Validity of a self-reported history of doctor-diagnosed angina. *J. Clin. Epidemiol.* **1999**, *52*, 73–81. [CrossRef]

48. Assari, S.; Lankarani, M.M.; Burgard, S. Black-white difference in long-term predictive power of self-rated health on all-cause mortality in United States. *Ann. Epidemiol.* **2016**, *26*, 106–114. [CrossRef] [PubMed]

49. Assari, S.; Burgard, S.; Zivin, K. Long-term reciprocal associations between depressive symptoms and number of chronic medical conditions: Longitudinal support for black-white health paradox. *J. Racial Ethn. Health Disparit.* **2015**, *2*, 589–597. [CrossRef] [PubMed]

50. Assari, S.; Moazen-Zadeh, E.; Lankarani, M.M.; Micol-Foster, V. Race, depressive symptoms, and all-cause mortality in the United States. *Front. Public Health* **2016**, *4*, 40. [CrossRef] [PubMed]

51. Assari, S.; Lankarani, M.M. Depressive symptoms are associated with more hopelessness among white than black older adults. *Front. Public Health* **2016**, *4*, 82. [CrossRef] [PubMed]

52. Assari, S.; Burgard, S. Black-White differences in the effect of baseline depressive symptoms on deaths due to renal diseases: 25 year follow up of a nationally representative community sample. *J. Ren. Inj. Prev.* **2015**, *4*, 127–134. [PubMed]

53. Assari, S. Hostility, anger, and cardiovascular mortality among Blacks and Whites. *Res. Cardiovasc. Med.* **2016**. [CrossRef]

54. Assari, S. Race, sense of control over life, and short-term risk of mortality among older adults in the United States. *Arch. Med. Sci.* **2016**. [CrossRef] [PubMed]

55. Assari, S.; Lankarani, M.M. Association between stressful life events and depression; intersection of race and gender. *J. Racial Ethn. Health Disparit.* **2016**, *3*, 349–356. [CrossRef] [PubMed]

56.   Assari, S.; Sonnega, A.; Pepin, R.; Leggett, A. Residual effects of restless sleep over depressive symptoms on chronic medical conditions: Race by gender differences. *J. Racial Ethn. Health Disparit.* **2016**. [CrossRef] [PubMed]

57.   Assari, S. Perceived neighborhood safety better predicts 25-year mortality risk among Whites than Blacks. *J. Racial Ethn. Health Disparit.* **2016**. [CrossRef]

58.   Chen, E.; Martin, A.D.; Matthews, K.A. Understanding health disparities: The role of race and socioeconomic status in children's health. *Am. J. Public Health* **2006**, *96*, 702–708. [CrossRef] [PubMed]

59.   Dowd, J.J.; Bengtson, V.L. Aging in minority populations an examination of the double jeopardy hypothesis. *J. Gerontol.* **1978**, *33*, 427–436. [CrossRef] [PubMed]

60.   Wilson, K.B.; Thorpe, R.J.; LaVeist, T.A. Dollar for dollar: Racial and ethnic inequalities in health and health-related outcomes among persons with very high income. *Prev. Med.* **2017**, *96*, 149–153. [CrossRef] [PubMed]

61.   Bowleg, L.; Huang, J.; Brooks, K.; Black, A.; Burkholder, G. Triple jeopardy and beyond: Multiple minority stress and resilience among Black lesbians. *J. Lesbian Stud.* **2003**, *7*, 87–108. [CrossRef] [PubMed]

62.   King, D.K. Multiple jeopardy, multiple consciousness: The context of a Black feminist ideology. *Signs J. Women Cult. Soc.* **1988**, *14*, 42–72. [CrossRef]

63.   Hayward, M.D.; Hummer, R.A.; Sasson, I. Trends and group differences in the association between educational attainment and U.S. adult mortality: Implications for understanding education's causal influence. *Soc. Sci. Med.* **2015**, *127*, 8–18. [CrossRef] [PubMed]

64.   Backlund, E.; Sorlie, P.D.; Johnson, N.J. A comparison of the relationships of education and income with mortality: The national longitudinal mortality study. *Soc. Sci. Med.* **1999**, *49*, 1373–1384. [CrossRef]

65.   Everett, B.G.; Rehkopf, D.H.; Rogers, R.G. The nonlinear relationship between education and mortality: An examination of cohort, race/ethnic, and gender differences. *Popul. Res. Policy Rev.* **2013**, *32*, 893–917. [CrossRef] [PubMed]

66.   Cutler, D.M.; Lleras-Muney, A. Education and Health: Evaluating Theories and Evidence. National Bureau of Economic Research. Available online: http://www.nber.org/papers/w12352/ (accessed on 9 September 2017).

67.   Holmes, C.J.; Zajacova, A. Education as "the great equalizer": Health benefits for black and white adults. *Soc. Sci. Q.* **2014**, *95*, 1064–1085. [CrossRef]

68.   Assari, S.; Nikahd, A.; Malekahmadi, M.R.; Lankarani, M.M.; Zamanian, H. Race by gender group differences in the protective effects of socioeconomic factors against sustained health problems across five domains. *J. Racial Ethn. Health Disparit.* **2017**, *4*, 884–894. [CrossRef] [PubMed]

69.   Oliver, M.L.; Shapiro, T.M. *Black Wealth, White Wealth: A New Perspective on Racial Inequality*; Taylor & Francis: Abingdon, UK, 2006.

70.   Williams, D.R.; Collins, C. Racial residential segregation: A fundamental cause of racial disparities in health. *Public Health Rep.* **2001**, *116*, 404–416. [CrossRef]

71.   Williams, D.R.; Mohammed, S.A.; Leavell, J.; Collins, C. Race, socioeconomic status, and health: Complexities, ongoing challenges, and research opportunities. *Ann. N. Y. Acad. Sci.* **2010**, *1186*, 69–101. [CrossRef] [PubMed]

72.   Assari, S.; Caldwell, C.H. Social Determinants of Perceived Discrimination among Black Youth: Intersection of Ethnicity and Gender. *Children* **2018**, *5*, 24. [CrossRef] [PubMed]

73.   Navarro, V. Race or class, or race and class. *Int. J. Health Serv.* **1989**, *19*, 311–314. [CrossRef] [PubMed]

74.   Mehta, N.; Preston, S. Are major behavioral and sociodemographic risk factors for mortality additive or multiplicative in their effects? *Soc. Sci. Med.* **2016**, *154*, 93–99. [CrossRef] [PubMed]

75.   Williams, D.R.; Collins, C.U.S. socioeconomic and racial differences in health: Patterns and explanations. *Ann. Rev. Sociol.* **1995**, *21*, 349–386. [CrossRef]

76.   Farmer, M.M.; Ferraro, K.F. Are racial disparities in health conditional on socioeconomic status? *Soc. Sci. Med.* **2005**, *60*, 191–204. [CrossRef] [PubMed]

77.   Assari, S.; Moazen-Zadeh, E. Ethnic Variation in the Cross-sectional Association between Domains of Depressive Symptoms and Clinical Depression. *Front. Psychiatry* **2016**, *7*, 53. [CrossRef] [PubMed]

## 11

A 40-Day Journey to Better Health: Utilizing the DanielFast to Improve Health Outcomes in Urban Church-Based Settings

Nicole A. Vaughn [1,2,3,*], Darryl Brown [4], Beatriz O. Reyes [5], Crystal Wyatt [6], Kimberly T. Arnold [7], Elizabeth Dalianis [8], Paula J. Kalksma [1], Caryn Roth [9], Jason Langheier [9], Maria Pajil-Battle [10] and Meg Grant [11]

[1] Department of Health & Exercise Sciences, School of Health Professions, Rowan University, Glassboro, NJ 08028, USA; kalksma@rowan.edu
[2] Department of Biomedical Sciences, Cooper Medical School of Rowan University, Camden, NJ 08103, USA
[3] Department of Family Medicine, School of Osteopathic Medicine, Rowan University, Stratford, NJ 08084, USA
[4] Department of Health Management & Policy, School of Public Health, Drexel University, Philadelphia, PA 19104, USA; drb48@drexel.edu
[5] Department of Anthropology, Global Health Studies Program, Northwestern University, Evanston, IL 60208, USA; beatriz.reyes@northwestern.edu
[6] Ride & Rebuild, LLC, Philadelphia, PA 19151, USA; cwyatt1119@gmail.com
[7] Department of Health Policy & Management, Bloomberg School of Public Health, Johns Hopkins University, Baltimore, MD 21205, USA; karnol14@jhmi.edu
[8] Community College of Philadelphia, Philadelphia, PA 19130, USA; edalianis@ccp.edu
[9] Zipongo, Inc., San Francisco, CA 94133, USA; carynroth@gmail.com (C.R.); jason.langheier@zipongo.com (J.L.)
[10] AmeriHealth Caritas Partnership, Philadelphia, PA 19113, USA; riarudybattle@aol.com
[11] Keystone First, Philadelphia, PA 19113, USA; mgrant@keystonefirstpa.com
* Correspondence: vaughnn@rowan.edu

Abstract: *Background:* As the costs associated with obesity increase, it is vital to evaluate the effectiveness of chronic disease prevention among underserved groups, particularly in urban settings. This research study evaluated Philadelphia area Keystone First members and church participants enrolled in a group health education program to determine the impact of the Daniel Fast on physical health and the adoption of healthy behaviors. *Methods:* Participants attended six-weekly health education sessions in two participating churches, and were provided with a digital healthy eating platform. *Results:* There was a statistically significant decrease from baseline to post assessment for weight, waist circumference and cholesterol. Participants reported a significant improvement in their overall well-being, social and physical functioning, vitality and mental health. *Conclusion:* Results of this study demonstrate that dietary recommendations and comprehensive group health education delivered in churches and reinforced on a digital platform can improve physical health, knowledge and psychosocial outcomes.

Keywords: African American; community intervention; urban settings; health disparity; technology; weight loss; nutrition education

1. Introduction

Seven of the top 10 leading causes of death in the U.S. are due to chronic diseases. 8.6% of the nation's $2.7 trillion annual health care expenditure goes toward treating these diseases. Approximately 50% of adults (117 million people) have one or more chronic diseases or conditions [1]. Cardiovascular disease (CVD), diabetes and obesity are the most prevalent and costly chronic diseases. The top two leading causes of death, heart disease and cancer, account for 46% of deaths in the U.S. and over 80% of all health care costs [1,2]. Cardiovascular disease claims the lives of approximately 600,000 Americans each year and CVD and stroke, combined, cost an estimated $316.1 billion [3,4]. In 2010, more than one-third of adults were obese [3]. Medical costs related to obesity were estimated to exceed $147 billion. Additionally, diabetes expenditures approached $245 billion and affect over 29 million people in the U.S. [5,6].

Despite the complex etiologies of many chronic diseases, many are preventable through healthy behaviors, such as diet and regular physical activity. Studies have shown that individuals who lose weight, modify their eating behaviors, and increase their physical activity can prevent many chronic conditions (e.g., diabetes, hypertension, and cardiovascular disease) [7]. As the physical, economic and societal cost associated with overweight and obesity increase, it is vital to evaluate the effectiveness of chronic disease prevention interventions among high-risk groups, especially African Americans living in urban settings.

Health disparities do exist for some racial and ethnic groups with particularly large health disparities and inequities among African Americans [8]. Inadequate access to health care, lack of education, poverty, racism, and community conditions lead to health disparities, resulting in poor health outcomes and higher healthcare costs [8]. Among African Americans, one out of every two persons is obese, which increases the risk for developing chronic conditions. According to the Centers for Disease Control and Prevention (CDC), African Americans aged 18–49 years are twice as likely to die from heart disease compared to Caucasians, and African Americans aged 35–64 years are 50% more likely to have high blood pressure than Caucasians [9,10].

Currently, 31.8% of Pennsylvanians are obese. Of this third, approximately 36.4% are African Americans [9]. Among the top 10 most populous cities, Philadelphia experiences the highest prevalence of hypertension (34.5%), type II diabetes (16%), and adult obesity (32%), exceeding the national average by 3.7%, 3.3%, and 4.5% respectively [11]. Stark racial/ethnic health disparities exist for all of these diseases, with African-Americans carrying the heaviest burden of hypertension (47.1%), type II diabetes (20.2%), and obesity (41.8%) compared to non-Hispanic Whites, Hispanic/Latinos, and Asians [11]. In order to reduce adverse health outcomes associated with obesity, especially for African Americans, it is important to design and implement targeted programs to improve health behaviors where people live.

Background

The "40-Day Journey to Better Health (40-Day Journey)" program, designed by AmeriHealth Caritas Partnership, encourages individuals to change their nutrition and physical activity behaviors during the Lenten season (a Christian religious observance that occurs 40 days before Easter and promotes fasting and sacrifice). The program included a group health education curriculum, digital engagement, and the Daniel Fast (Fast), a plant-based diet based on the book of Daniel in the Bible. The Fast promotes eating fruits, vegetables and whole foods, drinking water, and eliminating sweeteners and bread for 40 days [12]. The Fast excludes the consumption of meat, dairy, sweeteners, and bread, consistent with a strict vegan diet [12,13]. AmeriHealth Caritas Partnership and Keystone First worked with Zipongo, a web- and app-based nutrition platform, and a local Philadelphia chef to develop a series of recipes and meal plans based on the diet. Zipongo introduced a digital healthy eating platform to the intervention that included sending recipes, meal plans and text messages to support users in adopting and maintaining the Fast. Also, Healthy Measures, Inc. was contracted to collect biometric data and the university-based research team collected behavioral health data and evaluated the study.

Recently, the Daniel Fast has gained interest and popularity among congregations across the U.S. Many church leaders have presented the plan to their congregants despite a paucity of research on its impact on health and the programming necessary to drive adoption. Although there is limited research, the Fast has been promoted by prominent and influential figures (e.g., Pastor Rick Warren) and some members of the medical community.

Despite the limited research, prior study results have suggested a positive impact on health outcomes. Specifically, Bloomer et al. (2010) found that people who adopted the Fast experienced improvements in many metabolic and cardiovascular disease risk factors and concluded that the Fast is an effective strategy in chronic disease prevention [14]. Compared to baseline, white blood cell count, blood urea nitrogen, protein, total cholesterol, low-density lipoprotein (LDL) cholesterol, high-density lipoprotein (HDL) cholesterol, and blood pressure all significantly lowered after the Fast. Although not statistically significant, there were also clinically meaningful outcomes which included improvements in insulin, homeostatic model assessment of insulin resistance (HOMA-IR), and C-Reactive Protein (CRP) [14]. In another evaluation of the 21-day version of the Fast, participants had improvements in selected biomarkers of antioxidant status and oxidative stress [13]. Furthermore, individuals who had adopted either a traditional or a modified Daniel Fast diet had significant improvements in blood lipids and reduced inflammation [15,16]. A 2010 review concluded that the Daniel Fast can yield improved health outcomes of reduced blood pressure, blood lipids, insulin sensitivity, and oxidative stress [17]. If the traditional or modified diet is sustained over time, individuals may improve blood pressure and blood lipids [14–16].

In addition to diet change, previous randomized control studies have shown similar successes changing health behaviors through text messaging in order to increase support [18]. A weight loss program targeted at obese African American women found that the group receiving daily text messages lost weight while the control group receiving only didactic health education gained weight [19]. The researchers hypothesized that the text messaging helped with daily self-monitoring of diet, which has previously been linked to increased weight loss. Another randomized controlled trial which compared weight loss for participants receiving paper-based health education to those also receiving two-five daily text messages found that the text messaging group lost significantly more weight [20].

The Zipongo digital healthy eating platform was used in this intervention to support participants adopting new healthy eating behaviors. During the maintenance phase (six-week–six-month follow-up), in accordance with the Fast, participants were provided specific recipes and meal plans in print, web, smartphone and text messaging format. Text messaging included dinner recipe recommendations and weekly grocery lists with discounts from each user's preferred grocery stores. Prior programs have assessed text messaging to help people with diabetes improve habits such as fruit and vegetable consumption with some success, but a comprehensive healthy eating program, or one using the Fast with churches, has not been previously explored.

The purpose of this research study was to evaluate the impact of the 40-Day Journey—a faith-based dietary guidance program paired with digital and text messaging platform—on weight change, health knowledge, health behaviors and clinical outcomes in churches located in an urban setting. Participants were advised to adopt the Daniel Fast for their 2013 observation of Lent.

2. Materials and Methods

2.1. Design

Participants attended a six-week intervention to improve eating and exercising behaviors at two predominantly African American churches in Philadelphia, PA, USA. These churches served as the site for the 40-Day Journey. The active phase of this intervention started in February 2013, follow-up occurred at six months, and data analysis occurred in 2014. The Drexel University Institutional Review Board approved this study protocol.

Two predominantly African American churches were selected by AmeriHealth based on established pastoral relationships, interest in health programming, congregation size, space availability and being located in areas with high chronic disease statistics (i.e., overweight, obesity, CVD, etc.).

Participants were then recruited by AmeriHealth Caritas Partnership through flyers. Keystone First identified health plan members with type 2 diabetes in the zip codes surrounding the two churches. They were also provided transportation to the weekly sessions if needed. All participants gave informed consent prior to enrollment. All participants were eligible to participate in weekly raffle drawings as an incentive (e.g., blender, pedometers, cookbooks).

During the intervention, participants attended a two-hour session each week that focused on an overview of the 40-Day Daniel Fast, fitness and exercise, how stress can trigger chronic disease, including diabetes, heart health and stroke prevention, why taking your medication matters, and sharing program experiences. They also attended live cooking and food sampling demonstrations. Meal plans and corresponding recipes for each meal item were provided by the partners (Figure 1). The chef aligned the recommendations for the Fast to create culturally-relevant recipes for African Americans. A weekly grocery list linked to in-store discounts and loyalty card coupons was also provided.

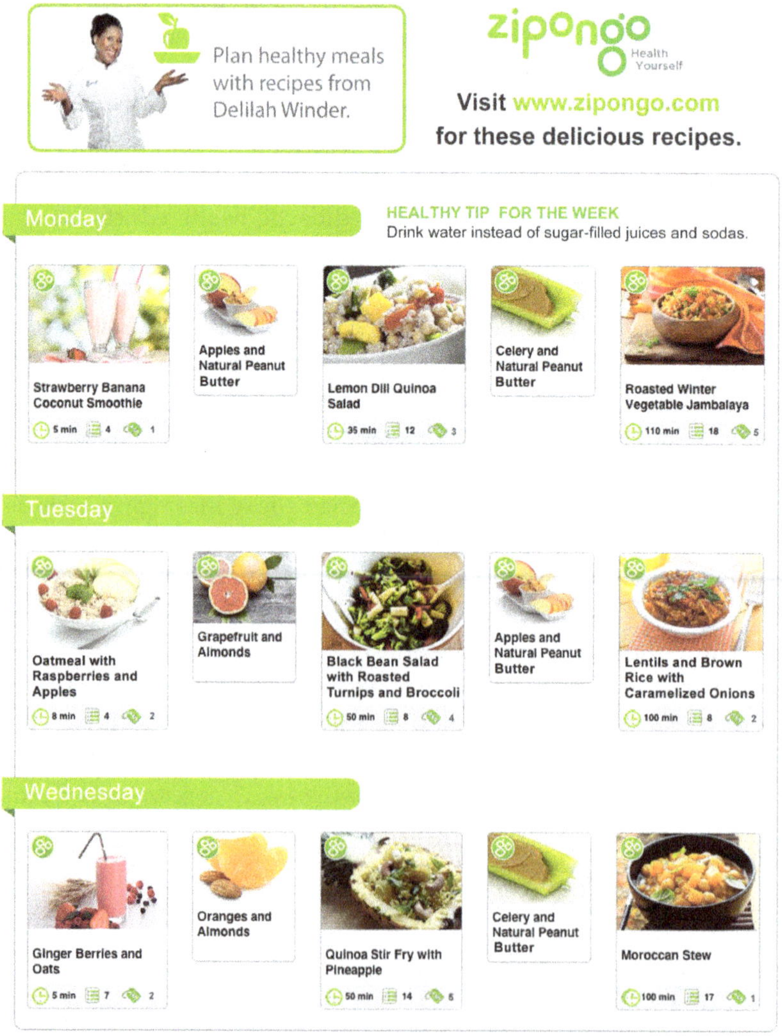

Figure 1. Sample Recommended Meal Plan Provided to Participants (ONLINE MATERIAL).

Daily or bi-weekly texts were sent with healthy eating tips and users could opt-in for additional daily recipe suggestions via text. Zipongo's registered dietitian called participants to discuss personal nutrition and to ensure intervention materials were able to be utilized. At the conclusion of 6 weeks, participants continued to receive healthy eating and recipe tips via text from Zipongo.

2.2. Measures

Baseline, week 6 and 6-month follow-up measures were collected by the Drexel research team, Healthy Measures and Zipongo personnel. The primary study outcomes were changes in biomarkers (i.e., weight, LDL, HDL, waist circumference, body mass index (BMI), glucose, HgA1C). Body weight was collected using a calibrated scale with participants wearing no shoes and light clothes. Pre- and post-Fast measurements of cholesterol, glucose, waist circumference, and body mass index were also collected. HgA1c was assessed with a Unistik lancet from a fingerstick capillary whole-blood sample, collecting 40 microliters of blood using a capillary tube and measured using the A1cNow+. Total cholesterol was also measured from capillary whole blood sample. Blood pressure was assessed with an Omron BP760 automatic BP cuff, while participants were seated, relaxed for three minutes.

Paper-pencil measures were administered and participants completed Sallis' scale to measure social support from family and friends for diet and exercise behaviors [21]. Higher scores indicated more social support was provided by either a family or friend. They also completed the validated Food Choice Questionnaire (FCQ) [22,23].

The FCQ is designed to capture the multidimensional nature of food choice. Participants reported factors they considered important when selecting food items. The nine subscales within the FCQ are health, mood, sensory appeal, price, natural content, convenience, familiarity, ethical concern, and weight control.

Overall, physical and mental health was assessed using the SF-12 Health Survey. The SF-12 assessed eight dimensions of physical and mental health outcomes: Physical functioning, Role Physical, Bodily Pain, General Health, Social Functioning, Role Emotional, Mental Health, and Vitality. A program assessment survey was used to collect participants' feedback on the cooking demonstrations, food samples, web-based grocery deals, fitness information, disease prevention, medication matters, social support, and recipes. The participants used a 5-point Likert Scale (from strongly disagree to strongly agree) to report whether the material was relevant, easy to implement, easy to follow, and if the information helped to change their behaviors.

Finally, self-reported data were collected on whether participants used the digital platform, how they used it, and whether they found it helpful during the 40-Day Journey. User engagement data was also gathered through telephone calls by a dietitian, text messages, and post-intervention paper surveys.

2.3. Statistical Analyses

Respondent data from both churches were combined, a priori, to maximize sample size. Generalized linear models were run to test for statistical heterogeneity to validate the assumption of no difference between churches. For study measures where this assumption was not held, analysis was limited to the respective church. All data were input into SPSS version 20 and analyzed in SAS version 9.3 and STATA version 11.

Chi-square tests and simple means were used to compare descriptive data. Psychosocial and biometric measurements at baseline and the change in these measures at the end of study were examined for all participants with completed pre- and post-Fast measurements. The within-individual change from baseline was evaluated by using paired t tests for data distributed normally and matched-pair Wilcoxon signed rank sum tests for non-normally distributed data.

3. Results

3.1. Participant Demographics

Across both churches, 135 participants were initially enrolled from Church 1 ($n = 47$) and Church 2 ($n = 88$). At the six-week culmination of the "40-Day Journey", 69 participants completed surveys from Church 1 ($n = 27$) and Church 2 ($n = 42$). A majority of the participants were women ($n = 57$). The mean age across churches was 49.2 years (SD = 12.65 years). Participants from Church 1 were older ($m = 51.1$ years, SD = 11.96 years) than participants from Church 2 ($m = 45.8$ years, SD = 13.31 years). This difference in age was statistically significant (t(115) = 2.20, $p = 0.03$).

3.2. Biometric Data

The key outcomes of interest in this study were changes in biomarkers that indicate improvement in health. Table 1 presents these data. Participants experienced a statistically significant weight loss during the 40-Day Journey. They lost an average of 3.9 lbs (t(60) = 2.93, $p = 0.0004$). The decrease in waist circumference was 0.7 inches between pre ($m = 41.50$ in, SD = 6.69 in) and post assessment ($m = 40.80$ in, SD = 6.38 in). Overall, there was no statistically significant change in body mass index (BMI) between pre- and post-Fast. The mean Total Cholesterol (TC) dropped significantly between pre ($m = 171.70$ mg/dL, SD = 12.02 mg/dL) and post testing ($m = 158.80$ mg/dL, SD = 30.60 mg/dL). A Wilcoxon Signed Rank Test for non-normally distributed data indicated a statistically significant difference between the pre and post TC (t(62) = 5.17, $p = 0.0001$).

Table 1. Participants' Biometric Data.

	Pre-Test Mean (SD)	Post-Test Mean (SD)	df	T-Score	p-Value
Weight (lbs)	210.00 (52.00)	206.10 (51.96)	60	2.93	0.005 *
Waist circumference (in)	41.50 (6.69)	40.80 (6.38)	61	1.83	0.07
BMI (kg/m^2)	34.84 (7.32)	34.52 (7.56)	61	1.35	0.18
Total Cholesterol (mg/dL)	171.7 (12.02)	158.8 (30.60)	62	5.17	0.0001 *
Glucose (mg/dL)	126.95 (51.30)	117.60 (35.88)	61	1.81	0.071
Systolic BP (mm/Hg)	134.59 (19.16)	130.92 (19.05)	62	1.64	0.11
Diastolic BP (mm/Hg)	83.03 (10.56)	82.76 (10.51)	62	0.18	0.86

* $p = 0.03$ (Wilcoxon Signed-Rank test).

Zipongo text messaging continued after the completion of the 40-Day Journey (i.e., week six) through six months. Self-report data collected via survey also indicated that participants maintained improvements in mood and weight loss over six months. Overall, 90% of participants that completed the intervention stated that the program made them feel happier ($n = 40$), and 71% of participants reported losing weight, with an average weight loss of nine pounds ($n = 35$).

3.3. Blood Pressure Data by Church

While overall blood pressure did not approach significance for participants (Table 1), systolic blood pressure decreased by 9 mm/Hg between pre ($m = 142$ mm/Hg, SD = 19.9 mm/Hg) and post assessment ($m = 133$ mm/Hg, SD = 20.8 mm/Hg) amongst participants at Church 1. This change was statistically significant (t(22) = 2.46, $p = 0.02$). The decrease in pre ($m = 88$ mm/Hg, SD = 10.30 mm/Hg) and post ($m = 83.90$ mm/Hg, SD = 11.40 mm/Hg) of diastolic blood pressure amongst Church 1 participants approached significance (t(22) = 1.75, $p = 0.09$).

3.4. SF-12 across Church and by Church

Out of the eight scales in the SF-12, three scales were statistically significant across (Table 2) both churches between pre- and post-Fast assessments. Participants reported statistically improved mean scores in social functioning between pre ($m = 72.75$, SD = 28.45) and post ($m = 80.65$, SD = 30.08;

t(23) = 3.00, *p* = 0.01). Mental health scores also improved between pre (*m* = 69.41, SD = 22.94) and post (*m* = 75.81, SD = 23.49); t(23) = 2.65, *p* = 0.01). Additionally, vitality scores improved significantly from pre (*m* = 51.57, SD = 25.55) to post (*m* = 62.58, SD = 25.69; t(23) = 2.33, *p* = 0.02). The breakdown by church show that the statistically significant improvements in mental health (*p* < 0.01) and vitality (*p* < 0.01) were for Church 2 participants and the improvements in social functioning were for Church 1 participants (*p* < 0.05).

Table 2. SF-12 Results for Congregants.

SF-12 Domain	Pre-Test Mean (SD)	Post-Test Mean (SD)	df	T-Score	*p*-Value
Physical functioning	61.46 (37.58)	67.71 (36.47)	23	0.97	0.34
Role physical	72.92 (44.18)	77.08 (38.95)	23	0.46	0.65
Bodily pain	73.95 (30.82)	78.13 (28.85)	23	0.7	0.49
General health	48.95 (20.16)	46.88 (16.99)	23	−0.49	1
Social functioning	69.79 (33.77)	83.33 (27.25)	23	3	0.01 *
Role emotional	68.75 (43.77)	77.08 (36.05)	23	1.16	0.26
Mental health	70.00 (22.26)	79.17 (21.45)	23	2.65	0.01 *
Vitality	52.50 (24.18)	65.00 (23.77)	23	2.33	0.03 *

* *p* < 0.05.

3.5. Food Choice

Subscales that emerged as statistically significant from pre- and post-Fast assessments were natural content, convenience, familiarity, and weight control. Participants reported natural content was an important factor in their food choice at post (*m* = 3.32, SD = 0.62) compared to pre assessment (*m* = 3.04, SD = 0.75; (t(59) = 3.12, *p* = 0.003; Table 3). Also, between pre (*m* = 3.30, SD = 0.68) and post (*m* = 3.17, SD = 0.63), participants reported that convenience became a less important factor in food choice (t(59) = 2.18, *p* = 0.03). Similarly, participants began to eat less familiar foods which indicated that they were trying new foods and not eating their usual foods between pre (*m* = 2.66, SD = 0.91) and post (*m* = 2.44, SD = 0.95; (t(59) = −2.62, *p* = 0.01). Finally, weight control was statistically significant between pre (*m* = 3.25, SD = 0.83) and post (*m* = 3.47), t(58) = 2.02, *p* = 0.048). These all represent positive changes with respect to knowledge and food choice behaviors directly related to participating in the 40-Day Journey.

Table 3. Food Choice Questionnaire (FCQ) Results for Participants.

FCQ Dimension	Pre-Test Mean (SD)	Post-Test Mean (SD)	df	T-Score	*p*-Value
Natural content	3.04 (0.75)	3.32 (0.62)	59	3.12	0.003 *
Convenience	3.30 (0.68)	3.17 (0.63)	59	2.18	0.03 *
Familiarity	2.66 (0.91)	2.44 (0.95)	59	−2.62	0.01 *
Weight control	3.25 (0.83)	3.47 (0.57)	58	2.02	0.048 *
Ethical concern	2.51 (1.05)	2.60 (0.91)	59	0.8	0.43
Price	3.24 (0.74)	3.13 (0.76)	59	−1.3	0.2
Mood	2.95 (0.90)	2.83 (0.95)	59	1.15	0.26
Sensory appeal	3.30 (0.67)	3.26 (0.68)	59	−0.061	0.54
Health	3.27 (0.73)	3.40 (0.62)	59	−1.52	0.13

* *p* < 0.05.

3.6. Zipongo: Digital Engagement for Healthier Eating

Initially, 181 participants consented and enrolled in the Zipongo platform; 57 participants (31%) opted to receive emails, and average open rate was 30%. Additionally, 155 participants (86%) opted to receive text messages. Of these, 66% opted to receive daily text messages and 34% opted to receive bi-weekly text messages. Also, 57% and 19% of those receiving daily and bi-weekly tips, respectively, texted back. Some text participants (n = 48; 31%) also opted to receive additional daily recipe texts. These participants were even more responsive, with 100% texting back at least once throughout the 6 weeks of recipes. These responses showed their interest in and attitudes towards the health tips and recipes and that they were changing eating behaviors and following suggestions from the tips (Table 4).

Table 4. Text Responses from 40-Day Journey Participants.

Healthy Tips and Recipe Responses
"Good information for me to know. Thank you"
"I luv [sic] the daily tips pls [sic] cont [sic] thank you"
"Soup was delicious, great using veg [sic] stock"
"I am enjoying the recipes. They are easy and quick to make. I have a new appreciation for beans. Please keep them coming. I like new dishes. Thanks!"

Responses Indicating Behavior Change
"I made some soup and I ate lots of salad last week. No meat!!!"
"I made ur [sic] wonderful meals. My favorite so far is the black bean chili and lentil/sweet potato"
"eating more healthier, made spagetti [sic] squash and califlower [sic]with parsnips blended together instead of mash potatoes topped with veggie chee[se]" [sic]
"Thank u [sic] for the Healthy meals!!!!! I m [sic] on day 3 eating veggies Just loving it. Thank u [sic]again"

At the conclusion of the text program, participants were also asked to rate their satisfaction with Zipongo through text message and through a follow-up survey during biometric screening. From the written assessments, 72% of participants reported that Zipongo's web-based grocery deals and recipes increased their knowledge about healthy nutrition, and 66% said that these deals helped change eating behaviors. Further when prompted to respond on a 5-point Likert through text message on, "How helpful have our tips have been?", 98% responded with 4 or 5, indicating high satisfaction (n = 49). On a 10-point scale, participants gave an average rating of 9 for whether they would recommend Zipongo to a friend (n = 39). Though assessed on different scales, the combined quantitative and qualitative engagement and satisfaction data suggest that SMS messaging had a greater impact than web and email, for this population.

4. Discussion

4.1. Program Assessment

Overall, participants rated the program highly across all domains. Individuals agreed that the information presented from Cooking Demonstrations and Food Samples were relevant (93%, 96.5%, respectively). It is of note that the food samples provided seemed to be an important component for participants as they were able to taste-test novel foods. This demonstrated how slight modifications for traditional foods could make a potentially positive impact on food choices. Ninety-four percent of participants surveyed stated that this could have an influence as they consider changing their eating behaviors. Finally, the fitness, disease prevention, and medication topics covered were also highly rated as being relevant, easy to follow and influential in increasing knowledge.

This study demonstrates the importance of integrating multiple approaches to improve health, particularly in urban settings. In order to begin to address reducing health disparities, underserved and underrepresented minority groups may require hybrid approaches, such as this project as it fits within community culture, context and religious practices and religious norms. The core interventions of the 40-Day Journey included in-person classes, personalized digital recipe and grocery list recommendations, and biometric data collection in a familiar setting. Each of these components may be critical in this model to engage a hard to reach population at high risk for many chronic conditions. By working with individuals in the context of a trusted setting (i.e., church) we were able to bring traditional health education together with technology. In addition, cooking demonstrations by the chef paired with personalized guidance for specific foods to buy, cook and eat via image-based print materials for web, email and text messaging were critical to the program success. The call from the dietitian helped participants navigate and understand the recipes and meal plans. Research has shown that only prescribing a diet and offering nutrition tracking, or health education alone but lacking a maintenance program can impact the success of adoption of new health knowledge and healthy behaviors [24–26].

4.2. Limitations

This study recruited church members from churches who partnered with the AmeriHealth program. Thus, this was a convenience sample of church members which may limit generalizability to a broader non-church going population. The overall sample included more middle aged women than men which may also limit our understanding of younger populations as well as men in urban settings. Most church-based interventions in African American communities have similar demographics for church attenders with women more likely to regularly attend. Finally, while there was support for individuals in using the nutrition-based application on their phone, individuals who may have had difficulty with technology may not have used all features available to them in the app.

5. Conclusions

To our knowledge, this is the first community research evaluation of the Daniel Fast in conjunction with a digital engagement component in a church-based setting. The 40-Day Journey results are promising given the positive impact on blood pressure, cholesterol, weight outcomes and mental wellness outcomes. This project also demonstrates how multiple partners can come together (university-community-industry) for evaluation projects in the community.

The authors believe that there may be interest in these types of projects to introduce and initiate healthful eating as it is connected to faith beliefs. Understanding the types of programs used in faith settings with an urban African American population may be of value, particularly as the DanielFast continues to gain momentum with churches across the country. Understanding more about the incentives to engage in a healthy lifestyle change in a familiar setting with the support of others in their church community adds to the research literature on strategies to reduce health disparities. Finally, adding a technology component with high touch points between sessions may also be cost effective and nationally scalable across diverse communities. Further studies are needed to evaluate longer-term follow-up at 12 and 18 months, and to understand the relative contributions of different elements of the 40-Day Journey integrated intervention for participants

Acknowledgments: The authors would like to thank AmeriHealth Caritas Partnership for funding this program and the study. The funding sponsors had no role in the collection, analyses, or interpretation of data; in the writing of the manuscript, and in the decision to publish the results. We would also like to extend special thanks to Sandra Ludewig & Zachary Babel at Rowan University in the Department of Health and Exercise Sciences in Glassboro, NJ for their role in preparing this manuscript.

Author Contributions: Nicole A. Vaughn (lead evaluator) along with the research team (Darryl Brown, Beatriz O. Reyes, Crystal Wyatt, Kimberly T. Arnold, Elizabeth Dalianis) collected and analyzed the data. Maria Pajil-Battle and Nicole A. Vaughn conceived and designed the study. Jason Langheier and Caryn Roth contributed by providing their software tool, user-engagement metric and analysis of all text messages for all study participants; Nicole A. Vaughn, as well as each member of the research team (see above) including Paula J. Kalksma wrote and contributed substantially to the final product of this paper. Meg Grant contributed substantially to the implementation of the program and weekly lesson sessions at each church.

References

1. Ward, B.W.; Schiller, J.S.; Goodman, R.A. Multiple Chronic Conditions Among US Adults: A 2012 Update. *Prev. Chronic Dis.* **2014**, *11*, E62. [CrossRef] [PubMed]

2. Robert Wood Johnson Foundation Chronic Care: Making the Case for Ongoing Care. 2010. Available online: https://www.rwjf.org/en/library/research/2010/01/chroniccare.html (accessed on 23 June 2014).

3. Johns Hopkins Bloomberg, School of Public Health. Centers for Disease Control and Prevention C. NCHS Data on Obesity. 2013. Available online: http://www.cdc.gov/nchs/data/factsheets/factsheet_obesity.htm (accessed on 23 June 2014).

4. Go, A.S.; Mozaffarian, D.; Roger, V.L.; Benjamin, E.J.; Berry, J.D.; Blaha, M.J.; Dai, S.; Ford, E.S.; Fox, C.S.; Franco, S.; et al. American Heart Association Statistics Committee and Stroke Statistics Subcommittee. Heart disease and stroke statistics—2014 update: A report from the American Heart Association. *Circulation* **2014**, *129*, e28. [CrossRef] [PubMed]

5. Finkelstein, E.A.; Trogdon, J.G.; Cohen, J.W.; Dietz, W. Annual medical spending attributable to obesity: Payer-and service-specific estimates. *Health Aff.* **2009**, *28*, W822–W831. [CrossRef] [PubMed]

6. Center for Disease Control and Prevention National Diabetes Statistics Report. Available online: https://www.cdc.gov/diabetes/pdfs/data/statistics/national-diabetes-statistics-report.pdf (accessed on 1 November 2017).

7. Field, A.E.; Coakley, E.H.; Must, A.; Spadano, J.L.; Laird, N.; Dietz, W.H.; Rimm, E.; Colditz, G.A. Impact of overweight on the risk of developing common chronic diseases during a 10-year period. *Arch. Intern. Med.* **2001**, *161*, 1581–1586. [CrossRef] [PubMed]

8. Centers for Disease Control and Prevention. Chronic Disease Prevention and Health Promotion: Racial and Ethnic Approaches to Community Health (REACH). Available online: https://www.cdc.gov/chronicdisease/resources/publications/aag/reach.htm (accessed on 29 November 2016).

9. Centers for Disease Control and Prevention: Prevalence of Obesity Among Adults and Youth: United States, 2015–2016. Available online: https://www.cdc.gov/nchs/products/databriefs/db288.htm (accessed on 1 November 2017).

10. Centers for Disease Control and Prevention Vital Signs: African American Health. Available online: https://www.cdc.gov/vitalsigns/aahealth/index.html (accessed on 3 July 2017).

11. Philadelphia Department of Public Health. Community Health Assessment, Philadelphia, PA. In *Health*; Philadelphia Department of Public Health: Philadelphia, PA, USA, 2013. Available online: http://www.phila.gov/health/pdfs/chareport_52114_final.pdf (accessed on 15 May 2014).

12. The Daniel Fast. Available online: http://www.daniel-fast.com/ (accessed on 23 June 2014).

13. Bloomer, R.J.; Kabir, M.M.; Trepanowski, J.F.; Canale, R.E.; Farney, T.M. A 21 day Daniel Fast improves selected biomarkers of antioxidant status and oxidative stress in men and women. *Nutr. Metab.* **2011**, *8*, 17. [CrossRef] [PubMed]

14. Bloomer, R.; Kabir, M.M.; Canale, R.E.; Trepanowski, J.F.; Marshall, K.E.; Farney, T.M.; Hammond, K.G. Effect of a 21 day Daniel Fast on metabolic and cardiovascular disease risk factors in men and women. *Lipids Health Dis.* **2010**, *9*, 94. [CrossRef] [PubMed]

15. Alleman, R.J.; Harvey, I.C.; Farney, T.M.; Bloomer, R.J. Both a traditional and modified Daniel Fast improve the cardio-metabolic profile in men and women. *Lipids Health Dis.* **2013**, *12*, 114. [CrossRef] [PubMed]

16. Bloomer, R.J.; Gunnels, T.A.; Schriefer, J.M. Comparison of a Restricted and Unrestricted Vegan Diet Plan with a Restricted Omnivorous Diet Plan on Health-Specific Measures. *Healthcare* **2015**, *3*, 544–555. [CrossRef] [PubMed]

17. Trepanowski, J.F.; Bloomer, R.J. The impact of religious fasting on human health. *BMC Nutr.* **2010**, *9*. [CrossRef] [PubMed]

18. Gerber, B.S.; Stolley, M.R.; Thompson, A.L.; Sharp, L.K.; Fitzgibbon, M.L. Mobile phone text messaging to promote healthy behaviors and weight loss maintenance: A feasibility study. *Health Inform. J.* **2009**, *15*, 17–25. [CrossRef] [PubMed]

19. Steinberg, D.M.; Levine, E.L.; Askew, S.; Foley, P.; Bennett, G.G. Daily text messaging for weight control among racial and ethnic minority women: Randomized controlled pilot study. *J. Med. Internet Res.* **2013**, *15*. [CrossRef]

20. Patrick, K.; Raab, F.; Adams, M.A.; Dillon, L.; Zabinski, M.; Rock, C.; Griswold, W.; Norman, G. A text message–based intervention for weight loss: Randomized controlled trial. *J. Med. Internet Res.* **2009**, *11*. [CrossRef] [PubMed]

21. Sallis, J.F.; Grossman, R.M.; Pinski, R.B.; Patterson, T.L.; Nader, P.R. The development of scales to measure social support for diet and exercise behaviors. *Prev. Med.* **1987**, *16*, 825–836. [CrossRef]

22. Brownson, R.C.; Riley, P.; Bruce, T.A. Demonstration projects in community-based prevention. *JPHMP* **1998**, *4*, 66. [CrossRef] [PubMed]

23. Steptoe, A.; Pollard, T.M.; Wardle, J. Development of a measure of the motives underlying the selection of food: The food choice questionnaire. *Appetite* **1995**, *25*, 267–284. [CrossRef] [PubMed]

24. Blomain, E.S.; Dirhan, D.A.; Valentino, M.A.; Kim, G.W.; Waldman, S.A. Mechanisms of Weight Regain following Weight Loss. *ISRN Obes.* **2013**, *2013*. [CrossRef] [PubMed]

25. Burke, L.E.; Wang, J.; Sevick, M.A. Self-monitoring in weight loss: A systematic review of the literature. *J. Am. Diet. Assoc.* **2011**, *111*, 92–102. [CrossRef] [PubMed]

26. Wing, R.R.; Phelan, S. Long-term weight loss maintenance. *Am. J. Clin. Nutr.* **2005**, *82*, 222S–225S. [CrossRef] [PubMed]

## 12

Tackling the Consumption of High Sugar Products among Children and Adolescents in the Pacific Islands: Implications for Future Research

Katharine Aldwell [1,*], Corinne Caillaud [2], Olivier Galy [3] iD, Stéphane Frayon [3] iD and Margaret Allman-Farinelli [1] iD

[1] Charles Perkins Centre, University of Sydney, Sydney, NSW 2006, Australia;
    margaret.allman-farinelli@sydney.edu.au
[2] Faculty of Health Sciences and Charles Perkins Centre, University of Sydney, Sydney, NSW 2006, Australia;
    corinne.caillaud@sydney.edu.au
[3] Interdisciplinary Laboratory for Research in Education, EA 7483, School of Education,
    University of New Caledonia, Nouméa BP R4 98851, New Caledonia; olivier.galy@univ-nc.nc (O.G.);
    stephanefrayon@hotmail.com (S.F.)
*   Correspondence: katharine.aldwell@health.nsw.gov.au

Abstract: The Pacific Islands are experiencing an obesity epidemic with a rate of overweight and obesity as high as 80% among adults in some Pacific Island nations. Children and adolescents in the region are also affected by overweight and obesity, which is alarming due to the increased likelihood of remaining overweight as an adult. Research supports an association between poor diet and an increased risk of obesity and development of non-communicable diseases (NCDs). Excess consumption of free sugars is associated with poorer overall diet quality and increased risk of weight gain, chronic inflammation and dental caries. Traditional diets in the Pacific Islands are being supplemented with processed, high-sugar foods and beverages; thus, there is a clear need for effective interventions promoting positive dietary behaviors in the region. School and community based interventions offer an opportunity to promote positive behavior change among children and adolescents. This review aims to evaluate interventions targeting the consumption of high-sugar products in this population in the Pacific Islands.

Keywords: Pacific Islands; children; adolescents; sugar; intervention; Polynesian; Melanesian

1. Introduction

There are three broad geographical zones in the Pacific Islands: Micronesia, Melanesia and Polynesia [1]. The rate of overweight and obesity varies among Pacific Island countries and territories (PICTs) [2]. Tonga, Samoa and Kiribati report combined rates of adult overweight and obesity of as much as 80%, far exceeding the worldwide average [2]. Children and adolescents in the Pacific Islands are also impacted by overweight and obesity. The Global Burden of Disease study estimated a prevalence of overweight and obesity of up to 50% among boys and girls in Tonga, Samoa and Kiribati [3]. A study among nine thousand Fijian children aged 12–18 years found one quarter of participants were overweight or obese [4]. In 2011, Pacific leaders declared the obesity epidemic a health and economic crisis and threat to sustainable human development [5]. This region faces an increasing burden of non-communicable diseases (NCDs). Seven of the top ten countries/territories for prevalence of diabetes are Pacific Island nations [6]. Up to 80% of deaths in the region are related to NCDs [3,7].

Overweight and obesity and poor diet are primary risk factors for the development of NCDs [8]. Obesity during childhood and adolescence increases the likelihood of remaining above a healthy weight as an adult [8,9]. Childhood obesity is associated with several health conditions including increased risk of fracture, breathing difficulty, hypertension, early markers of cardiovascular disease (CVD), insulin resistance and depression [8]. The transition from childhood to adolescence involves increased independence, and formation of long-term dietary and lifestyle habits. Therefore, poor dietary behaviors developed during this period can significantly impact lifelong health [10,11]. Addressing poor dietary behaviors, before they become long-term habits, may prove effective in promoting sustainable behavior change and preventing weight gain [12].

Among various dietary factors related to weight gain, excess consumption of free sugars has been extensively researched. The term "free sugar" (sometimes referred to as added sugar) is the sugars added to foods and beverages during production and processing, in addition to the sugars naturally found in honey, syrups, fruit juices and fruit juice concentrates [13]. Current recommendations state that free sugars should comprise no more than 10% of total energy intake [14]. However, global dietary assessment studies suggest children and adolescents regularly exceed this recommendation [13,15–17]. Increased modernization, urbanization, economic development and market globalization in the Pacific Islands have driven a rapid nutrition transition towards consumption of processed and packaged foods [18–21]. Nations have become increasingly reliant upon imported produce, such as canned and preserved foodstuffs which has negatively impacted nutritional quality [20]. The rise of trans-national corporations and increased exposure to global food markets in the Pacific Islands has driven a nutrition transition towards consumption of more Westernized, processed foods and beverages [18,21,22]. The traditional Pacific diet is based on starchy root vegetables, such as taro or yams, and starchy fruits, such as breadfruit and banana. Other staples include seafood, non-starchy vegetables and other fruits [18]. This traditional dietary pattern contains little processed products and is low in free sugars. PICTs have become increasingly reliant on imported products high in free sugars. These products compete with domestic produce that have higher production costs and are less convenient [18,23]. Polished rice, processed breads and snack products are replacing traditional staples, meats are replacing seafood, and high sugar processed snacks are replacing fruit [24]. Studies among children and adolescents in PICTs have reflected this nutrition transition.

Excess consumption of free sugars has been linked with poor oral health, weight gain, chronic inflammation and the development of NCDs [25–29]. The significant increase in poor oral health among Pacific Islanders has been partially attributed to increased consumption of processed imported high sugar products [25]. Urban communities have shown higher prevalence of dental caries, which may be due to the ease of access to high-sugar products compared to those living in remote communities [25]. Sugar sweetened beverages (SSBs) have been a focus point for research with a large body of evidence supporting a relationship between excess consumption of free sugars and weight gain in both children and adults [14,27,28,30,31]. Decreased intake of dietary sugars is associated with significant weight loss and reduction in pro-inflammatory markers. Reducing consumption of SSBs and high-sugar products in early childhood and adolescence may have longer-term health benefits [29,31]. A small number of published dietary assessment studies in the Pacific Islands suggest consumption of SSBs and high-sugar snacks in this population is common, while fruit and vegetable intake is inadequate [17]. Interestingly, PICTs with higher rates of adolescent overweight and obesity have reported significantly higher rates of SSB consumption [19]. A study conducted in six Pacific Island nations involving more than ten thousand school-going adolescents found 40% of participants consumed one or more soft drinks per day. Only half of participants consumed the recommended serves of fruit and only one in three participants consumed more than three serves of vegetables per day [32]. Soft drink consumption was also associated with overweight and obesity [32]. Research in Tonga and Fiji has shown high-sugar foods and beverages are readily available and easy to access at school canteens [33]. Coupled with the intrinsic reward of sugary food and drinks (i.e., the taste of these products), the increased availability of high-sugar products can significantly enhance the acceptability and desirability of these products [34]. Clearly, effective strategies are needed to target consumption of products high in free sugars.

School and community based interventions may promote positive dietary behavior changes in children and adolescents. However, across the Pacific region, there is limited information on strategies that have been implemented in this population and whether they were successful in improving dietary behavior and reducing the risk of overweight and obesity. The aim of this review was to identify and evaluate the outcomes of school or community based programs that involved strategies targeting consumption of high-sugar products among children and adolescents in the Pacific Islands.

2. Methods

A literature search was conducted utilizing online research databases: Medline, Global Health, Science Direct and PubMed. A combination of search terms was used to identify relevant articles. Search terms are summarized in Table 1.

Table 1. Search terms used to generate relevant studies.

Topic	Term
Dietary exposure	Sugar OR added sugar OR sugar sweetened beverages, OR processed foods
Health	Overweight OR obesity
Setting	School OR community
Population	Children OR adolescent(s) OR Pacific Islands OR Polynesian OR, Melanesian OR Micronesian
Behavior	Behavior OR dietary behavior OR behavior change
Other	Intervention OR education OR nutrition education OR promotion

School or community based interventions that involved strategies to reduce consumption of high-sugar foods and beverages among children and adolescents were included. Studies were excluded if they were conducted outside of the Pacific Islands or targeted adults. Studies were also excluded if they didn't provide results of the intervention.

3. Results

Four published studies were identified that targeted consumption of high-sugar products among children and adolescents in the Pacific Islands. A summary of these studies is provided in Table 2. Overall, it was very difficult to identify studies that provided evaluations of outcome measures. Those that were identified included a small controlled trial in French Polynesia, an evaluation of Fiji's National School Canteen Guidelines and two larger studies from the Tongan and Fijian arms of the Pacific Obesity prevention in Communities (OPIC) program. Firstly, in 2005, the Fiji Ministries of Health and Education, and National Food and Nutrition Centre released the National Food and Nutrition Policy for Schools and School Canteen Guidelines. Schools were instructed to promote healthier school environments. For example, instructions were given on monitoring the quality of students' lunches to ensure they were 'healthy'. School canteens also provided healthy meals containing seasonal, fresh produce and remove unhealthy items (including SSBs and snacks high in free sugars and fats) from shelves [35,36]. Mandatory compliance to these guidelines began from early 2009. An evaluation of Fijian schools in 2010 found less than one fifth of assessed schools were compliant with guidelines [37]. Students who attended schools that were classed as 'adherent' were significantly less likely to be overweight or obese than students who attended 'non-adherent' schools [36,37].

Table 2. Summary of identified school and community based programs among children and adolescents in the Pacific Islands.

Authors	Name of Study	Participants	Intervention/Strategy	Results
Varman S. et al. (2013) [37]	-	230 Fijian primary schools	Healthy canteen guidelines regulating availability of energy-dense nutrient-poor foods and providing access to healthy products. The study sites were 230 primary schools in Fiji's Western Division.	33 (14%) schools had no canteen data. Of the 197 schools with canteen data, 31 (14%) schools were fully compliant
Gatti C. et al. (2015) [38]	Tubuai Island College Intervention	Intervention group: School students aged 10–18 years ($n = 240$). The group was divided based on attendance status: external collegians, half residents and full residents. Control group: School students aged 10–18 years ($n = 90$) from a neighboring island	5-month controlled trial set in the Tubuai Island college in French Polynesia. School nutrition program: aimed to offer healthier foods in the school canteen. Participants also received information on healthy lifestyles. Food sellers surrounding the college were encouraged to promote fruit, water and diet drink sales. Parents could also attend several sessions before, during and after the program to advice parents about benefits of healthy lifestyles. Physical activity program: 2–4 h of canoe training was implemented each week. Intervention groups were exposed to the intervention differently based on their attendance status. For example, external collegians did not eat in the school canteen whereas full residents at all meals at the school canteen. Control group received no intervention.	Weight increased significantly in all groups except for residents after 5 months of follow up. Intervention group had a significantly lower rate of weight gain than controls. Control group: adjusted weight gain was 4.2 kg (95% CI, 3.4–5.0) after 5 months. Intervention group adjusted difference in weight change was −3.4 kg (95% CI, −4.3 to −2.5). The proportion of adolescents who lost weight increased ($p < 0.001$) with exposure to healthy food and physical activity.
Fotu K.F. et al. (2011) [39]	Ma'alahi Youth Project	School students aged 11–19 years. (Intervention group at baseline $n = 1083$ and follow up $n = 815$. Comparison group at baseline $n = 1396$, follow up $n = 897$)	Tongan arm of the OPIC project. Intervention was conducted in three districts of the main island of Tongatapu (Houma, Nukunuku and Kolonga). School students attending all six secondary schools on the island of Vava'u were used as a comparison. Used social marketing approaches and community capacity building. Included school policies, community breakfasts, vegetable gardens, infrastructure provisions and activities, such as fun runs. Content varied by location. Baseline data collected between September 2005 and March 2006 with second baseline data collection in February and March 2007. Follow up data was collected between April and December 2008.	No significant difference in weight, BMI or prevalence of overweight/obesity between intervention and comparison groups. Adjusted weight (kg) difference was 0.05 ($p = 0.89$) and adjusted BMI difference was −0.02 ($p = 0.36$). Adjusted body fat percentage difference was −1.46 ($p < 0.001$). Intervention participants reported increased intake of SSBs (significantly greater than comparison groups).
Kremer P. et al. (2011) [40]	Healthy Youth Healthy Communities (HYHC)	Adolescents aged 13–18 years at baseline (Intervention group at baseline $n = 2670$ and follow up $n = 879$. Comparison group at baseline $n = 4567$ and follow up $n = 2069$)	Fijian arm of the OPIC project conducted over three school years (2006–2008) but with total of just over 2 years actual intervention exposure. Intervention conducted in Nasinu and three towns on the western side of Viti Levu were used as comparison regions. Multiple sites including faith-based organizations and schools. Intervention strategies included policy changes, education programs, and activities in schools and infrastructure changes. Content varied by location.	No significant difference in weight or BMI between intervention and comparison groups. The intervention group also reported poorer quality of life at follow up. Adjusted differences in weight (kg) and BMI were 0.05 ($p = 0.81$) and 0.10 ($p = 0.13$), respectively.

One of the key intervention features of the Tubuai Island College intervention was to improve the school canteen environment by offering healthy alternatives to high-sugar products [38]. Compared to control groups, those exposed to the intervention had a significantly reduced rate of weight gain [38]. The Ma'alahi Youth Project in Tonga and the Healthy Youth Healthy Communities project in Fiji were part of the OPIC program. These projects utilized multiple strategies including modifications to the school environment, education programs, activities in schools and policy changes. Results from both studies were not significant in reducing weight gain or promoting reduced consumption of high-sugar products [39–41].

4. Discussion

This review found a very small number of published school and community based programs that involved strategies targeting consumption of high-sugar products among children and adolescents in the Pacific Islands. Overall, the quality of the studies that were available was quite poor. Furthermore, while other interventions may have been implemented in this region, it is impossible to assess their impact due to the absence of quality, long-term publications of outcomes. Similar conclusions were drawn from a recent study evaluating school and community based NCD prevention programs worldwide [42].

The largest studies identified from the literature search originate from the Pacific OPIC program [39–41,43,44]. The OPIC program was originally conducted between 2004 and 2009. Its primary aims were to promote healthy eating (including reduced SSB and sugary snack consumption), physical activity and healthy weight in adolescents [43,44]. Four nations were involved in the project: Fiji, Tonga, New Zealand and Australia. A large component of the program involved using a community capacity building approach to promote healthy behaviors among communities in various settings including schools and churches. Community capacity building aims to enhance knowledge, skills, structures and systems in the environment to increase the ability of a community to deliver and sustain implementation of a program [40]. Unfortunately, available evaluations assessing the impact of the program suggest it was largely unsuccessful in reducing overweight and obesity and did not result in sustained healthy behavior changes among children and adolescents [39–41,43,44]. The OPIC program was limited by a lack of good quality, preliminary information to guide the development program components for each country [43,44]. One significant challenge identified by OPIC researchers was that the capacity of research staff was overstretched. This impacted the quality of data collected, and the records and results that were kept [44]. For example, the Healthy Youth Healthy Communities (HYHC) study in Fiji lost 59% of participants at follow-up, severely compromising data quality [40,41]. Furthermore, preliminary investigative studies looking at factors, such as socio-cultural influences on diet and lifestyle, were completed alongside the OPIC intervention components rather than prior to development of the study [43,44]. This reduced the capacity of researchers to consider the unique determinants of dietary behaviors in the study population. Exploring these determinants may have enabled researchers to target their strategies more effectively.

Various factors are known to determine dietary intake in children and adolescents. This includes individual characteristics, social and physical environmental influences and societal influences. Firstly, individual characteristics, such as attitudes, beliefs and knowledge, influence food choice [34,45]. There is limited data available on the perception of high-sugar foods and beverages in children and adolescents in the Pacific Islands. Studies in this population worldwide suggest the perceived 'healthiness' of a product may influence consumption [46]. This is important to note considering the way that many high-sugar products, such as sports drinks and energy drinks, are marketed. This age group often takes words and phrases commonly used in advertisements and on food packaging at face value (e.g., 'natural', 'refreshing' and 'hydrating') [47]. Addressing misconceptions about the healthiness of high-sugar foods and beverages may reduce desirability of these products. Self-perceived body weight and self-awareness of being overweight are also critical for weight loss and positive dietary changes [48]. A study among New Caledonian adolescents found half of overweight and obese adolescents underestimated their weight [48]. When coupled with factors, such as lack of access to healthy, traditional foods and beverages, this perception may result in increased intake of high-sugar products with poor nutritional quality [33].

Other individual characteristics, such as taste and preference, dominate food and beverage choices of children and adolescents [47]. The taste, texture and smell of high-sugar products are appealing and often increase their desirability [34]. However, this influence can be overridden by regulating access to these products [49]. Research in Tonga and Fiji has shown high-sugar foods and beverages are readily available and easy to access at school canteens [33]. While healthy canteen guidelines have been developed in some Pacific Island nations, such as Fiji, implementation and adherence to guidelines thus far has been limited [37]. It is up to governing bodies including ministries of health and national departments to ensure that school health policies are adhered to. Several other countries, such as the Cook Islands and Tonga, report having school food policies in place, but there are no published data on their impact, which makes it difficult to draw conclusions about the success or benefit of such programs [50]. A recent systematic review found that school nutrition policies targeting the reduction of SSBs significantly decreased consumption of SSBs among school students [51]. Interestingly, interventions that regulated access to SSBs in the school environment had the highest success rate in terms of reducing consumption of SSBs [51]. A review in the United States also found that students who attended schools with marketing bans on SSBs or limited availability in school canteens were less likely to drink these products [52]. However, another study from the United States found that SSB consumption was not significantly different. Interestingly, when availability was regulated at school, students compensated by drinking more SSBs outside of the school [53].

While regulating access to SSBs and high-sugar products in school may be an effective strategy, accessibility in other environments, such as the home, can also strongly influence intake. An Australian study in 2014 found that the strongest predictor of soft drink consumption among school aged children was availability in the home [54]. Including parents in future programs may facilitate positive changes in the home to reduce access to high-sugar products. This strategy has been successful in other countries, for example, the Health in Adolescents program in Norway. This program involved parents, providing strategies for improving accessibility and availability of healthy options at home. The program resulted in a significant reduction in SSB consumption and improvement of other dietary behaviors [55]. Providing access to healthy alternatives is vital to ensure positive dietary changes in this population. Research indicates that while many Pacific Island people prefer locally produced foods, they consume inferior imported products due to social and economic barriers to access [23]. The low cost and convenience of high-sugar products has promoted increased intake. The Tubuai Island College trial showed that providing access to healthier locally produced foods reduced the rate of weight gain in adolesecents [38]. Making healthy options, such as fresh fruits and vegetables available, must be incorporated into future programs.

Delivering interventions in school and community based settings, may be an effective means of promoting sustainability, facilitating intervention delivery and capacity for research outputs. For example, teachers or community members can be educated and engaged to facilitate components of an intervention. This can encourage maintenance of a program and balance the commitment of research members, teachers and the community. By utilizing local members of the community, researchers may also gain further insight into cultural or social trends that may influence the dietary habits of children and adolescents in the area. This method has been utilized with some success in other regions of the world, such as, the C3 program in the United States and the Dutch Obesity Intervention in Teenagers study. Both interventions utilized lessons targeting diet and lifestyle behaviors during class time with significant reductions in the consumption of SSBs for both studies [56,57]. Schools also offer the opportunity for social support. As a children transition into adolescents, peers may become more influential on dietary choices [58]. Interventions that involve collaboration with peers may be an effective strategy to promote behavior change. The fluids used effectively for living (FUEL) study in Canada used a peer educator approach to promote reduced consumption of SSBs among participants. Peer led groups significantly reduced their intake of SSBs compared to control groups at 3 months follow up [59]. Interventions that involve behavior change techniques and build self-management skills, such as self-monitoring, may also improve health behaviors including consumption of high-sugar products. One of the most frequently used behavior change techniques used in interventions is providing information about the health consequences of performing the behavior. Educational programs that explain to adolescents the consequences of excess consumption of free sugars via SSB and processed snack consumption may be beneficial. Educating children, while they are young about these consequences, may increase awareness and instill positive behaviors at earlier ages [51].

Consumption of SSBs and high-sugar products is not uniform across children and adolescents in the Pacific Islands. For example, a recent New Caledonian study found children and adolescents of Melanesian backgrounds and those living in a rural area were more likely to regularly consume SSBs [60]. Adolescents residing in rural locations were also more likely to be overweight or obese [60]. It is important that future programs target 'at risk' groups. Treatment programs for children and adolescents with obesity should also be considered along with obesity prevention programs. A large proportion of children and adolescents in the Pacific Islands are already above a healthy weight. Current evidence suggests that weight status can be improved through a variety of dietary regimes, including low carbohydrate, low fat or increased protein diets, intermittent fasting and even very low energy diet plans for adolescents with obesity [61]. While there is no 'one size fits all' dietary pattern for weight reduction, most of these diets ultimately result in reduced overall energy intake and reduction in consumption of free sugars [61].

Finally, while school and community based programs may promote healthy dietary habits, governments should also be responsible for implementing upstream strategies to improve the overall nutrition environment. Adopting taxes on the importation and sale of high-sugar products, such as SSBs, seems a beneficial strategy for decreasing the access to and availability of such products. Several nations have implemented taxes on SSBs and high-sugar foods (e.g., confectionary and processed snacks). Samoa has both import and domestic excise taxes on soft drinks applied since 1984. In Samoa, bottled water is now cheaper than soft drinks [20,50,62]. In 2002, French Polynesia introduced local and import taxes on all SSBs, confectionary and ice cream [50,62]. In 2006, Fiji placed an import tax and domestic excise tax on soft drinks. However, in 2007, domestic taxes were reduced, due to lobbying from the domestic soft drink industry [62]. In 2007, Nauru introduced a 30% import tax on sugar, confectionary, carbonated soft drinks, cordials, flavored milks and drink mixes [50,62]. Unfortunately, the impact of these taxes is largely unknown due to a lack of evaluation studies. A review of Samoan policies identified consumption of soft drinks in adults slightly decreased between 1991 and 2003 [62]. This suggests the taxes may have positively influenced dietary behavior; however, recent studies from the region are unavailable [62]. Conducting a large-scale evaluation of sugar taxes in the Pacific region would be valuable to determine whether these strategies are effective in producing positive behavior change in addition to producing revenue. Large-scale public health campaigns that involve digital communications and social media, such as the 'Change4Life' social marketing program in the United Kingdom, would also be beneficial. One key promotion in this campaign was 'smart swaps', which encouraged substitution of sugary drinks for non-sugar, diet drinks, milk or water. Purchase data from the promotional time period showed an 8.5% reduction in purchase of carbonated SSBs [13]. Implementing similar campaigns in the Pacific Islands may result in raised public awareness and reduced purchase of SSBs and high-sugar products.

The lack of quality published evaluations of school and community based programs implemented among children and adolescents in the Pacific Islands limits the ability to conclude which strategies may be useful to reduce the consumption of free sugars in this population. There is little good-quality longitudinal data from cohort studies among children and adolescents in the Pacific Islands, which makes it difficult to explore common dietary trends and compare to health outcomes in this population. While studies among children and adolescents worldwide offer insight into aspects that influence dietary behaviors, it would be useful to further evaluate differences between gender, age, ethnicity and geographic location in this population. Identifying whether there are any differences between these factors will allow for future programs to tailor strategies more effectively.

5. Conclusions

Children and adolescents in the Pacific Islands are at risk of developing a range of non-communicable diseases due to the rate of overweight and obesity in this region. Current research suggests this population frequently consumes free sugars via SSBs and high sugar snack foods. Research to date suggests there has been little success from school and community based interventions in reducing the consumption of high-sugar products in this population. The results of previous programs have highlighted the importance of conducting comprehensive preliminary assessments among target populations to inform the development process. To conclude, a combination of strategies ranging from school policies to nutrition education and behavior change interventions should be used to tackle the ongoing problem of excess consumption of free sugars among children and adolescents in the Pacific Islands. Governments have a responsibility to ensure health policies are adhered to and to implement other strategies, such as sugar taxes and public health initiatives, to achieve success in these programs.

Author Contributions: K.A. designed the review and drafted the article. All authors contributed to and approved the final manuscript.

Funding: This research received no external funding.

References

1. Hawley, N.L.; McGarvey, S.T. Obesity and diabetes in Pacific Islanders: The current burden and the need for urgent action. *Curr. Diabetes Rep.* **2015**, *29*, 1–10. [CrossRef] [PubMed]
2. Magnusson, R.S.; Patterson, D. How Can We Strengthen Governance of Non-communicable Diseases in Pacific Island Countries and Territories? *Asia Pac. Policy* **2015**, *2*, 293–309. [CrossRef]
3. Alwan, A. *Global Status Report on Noncommunicable Diseases*; World Health Organisation: Geneva, Switzerland, 2010.
4. Petersen, S.; Moodie, M.; Mavoa, H.; Waqa, G.; Goundar, R.; Swinburn, B. Relationship between overweight and health related quality of life in secondary school children in Fiji: Results from a cross-sectional population based study. *Int. J. Obes.* **2014**, *38*, 539–546. [CrossRef] [PubMed]
5. Pacific Community. Pacific NCD Crisis. 2011. Available online: http://www.spc.int/library/774-pacific-ncd-crisis.html (accessed on 10 November 2016).
6. Guariguata, L.; Whiting, D.; Hambleton, I.; Beagley, J.; Linnenkamp, U.; Shaw, J.E. Global estimates of diabetes prevalence for 2013 and projections for 2035. *Diabetes Res. Clin. Pract.* **2013**, *103*, 137–149. [CrossRef] [PubMed]
7. Parry, J. Pacific islanders pay heavy price for abandoning traditional diet. *Bull. World Health Organ.* **2010**, *88*, 484–485.
8. World Health Organisation. Obesity and Overweight. World Health Organisation, 2016. Available online: http://www.who.int/mediacentre/factsheets/fs311/en/ (accessed on 10 November 2016).
9. Verstraeten, R.; Roberfroid, D.; Lachat, C.; Leroy, J.L.; Holdsworth, M.; Maes, L.; Kolsteren, P.W. Effectiveness of preventive school-based obesity interventions in low- and middle-income countries: A systematic review. *Am. J. Clin. Nutr.* **2012**, *96*, 415–438. [CrossRef] [PubMed]
10. DiLorenzo, T.M.; Stucky-Ropp, R.; Van der Wal, J.S.; Gotham, H.J. Determinants of exercise among children II. A longitudinal analysis. *Prev. Med.* **1998**, *27*, 470–477. [CrossRef] [PubMed]
11. Hoelsher, D.M.; Evans, A.; Parcel, G.S.; Kelder, S.H. Designing effective nutrition interventions for adolescents. *J. Am. Diet. Assoc.* **2002**, *102* (Suppl. 3), S52–S63. [CrossRef]

12. Gill, T.; King, L.; Webb, K. *Best Options for Promoting Healthy Weight and Preventing Weight Gain in NSW*; State of Food and Nutrition NSW Series; NSW Centre for Public Health Nutrition: Sydney, Australia, 2005; pp. 1–116. Available online: http://sydney.edu.au/science/molecular_bioscience/cphn/pdfs/healthy_ weight_report.pdf (accessed on 15 October 2016).

13. Tedstone, A.; Anderson, S.; Allen, R. *Sugar Reduction. Responding to the Challenge*; Public Health England: London, UK, 2014; pp. 1–30. Available online: https://www.gov.uk/government/publications/sugar- reduction-responding-to-the-challenge (accessed on 10 November 2016).

14. World Health Organisation. *Sugars Intake for Adults and Children*; World Health Organisation: Geneva, Switzerland, 2015. Available online: http://apps.who.int/iris/bitstream/handle/10665/149782/9789241549028_eng.pdf? sequence=1 (accessed on 18 November 2016).

15. Australian Bureau of Statistics. *Australian Health Survey: Consumption of Added Sugars*; Australian Bureau of Statistics: Canberra, Australia, 2016; pp. 1–28. Available online: http://www.abs.gov.au/ausstats/abs@.nsf/ mf/4364.0.55.011 (accessed on 25 November 2016).

16. Lewesi, T. *Global School Based Student Health Survey*; Fiji Report; Fiji Ministry of Education, Ministry of Health & WHO: Suva, Fiji, 2013.

17. Wate, J.T.; Snowdon, W.; Millar, L.; Nichols, M.; Mavoa, H.; Goundar, R.; Kama, A.; Swinburn, B. Adolescent dietary patterns in Fiji and their relationships with standardised body mass index. *Int. J. Behav. Nutr. Phys. Act.* **2013**, *10*, 1–12. [CrossRef] [PubMed]

18. World Health Organisation. *Diet, Nutrition and the Prevention of Chronic Diseases*; World Health Organisation: Geneva, Switzerland, 2013. Available online: http://apps.who.int/iris/bitstream/handle/10665/42665/WHO_ TRS_916.pdf;jsessionid=1D022CA3365A0B974B27858F71D33849?sequence=1 (accessed on 10 November 2016).

19. Kessaram, T.; McKenzie, J.; Girin, N.; Merilles, O.E.A.; Pullar, J.; Roth, A.; White, P.; Hoy, D. Overweight, obesity, physical activity and sugar-sweetened beverage consumption in adolescents of Pacific Islands: Results from the global school-based student health survey and the youth risk behaviour surveillance system. *BMC Obes.* **2015**, *34*, 1–10. [CrossRef] [PubMed]

20. Snowdon, W.; Raj, A.; Reeve, E.; Guerrero, R.L.T.; Fesaitu, J.; Cateine, K.; Guignet, C. Processed foods available in the Pacific Islands. *Glob. Health* **2013**, *53*, 1–7. [CrossRef] [PubMed]

21. Thow, A.M.; Heywood, P.; Schultz, J.; Quested, C.; Jan, S.; Colagiuri, S. Trade and the Nutrition Transition: Strengthening Policy for Health in the Pacific. *Ecol. Food Nutr.* **2011**, *50*, 18–42. [CrossRef] [PubMed]

22. Moodie, R.; Stuckler, D.; Monteiro, C.; Sheron, N.; Neal, B.; Thamarangsi, T.; Lincoln, P.; Casswell, S. Profits and pandemics: Prevention of harmful effects of tobacco, alcohol and ultra-processed food and drink industries. *Lancet* **2013**, *381*, 670–679. [CrossRef]

23. Food Secure Pacific Working Group. Towards a Food Secure Pacific: Draft Framework for Action; Food Secure Pacific Working Group. 2010. Available online: lrd.spc.int/pubs/doc_download/1055-towards- a-food-secure-pacific-2011-2015- (accessed on 15 November 2016).

24. Hughes, R.G.; Lawrence, M. Globalisation, food and health in Pacific Island countries. *Asia Pac. J. Clin. Nutr.* **2005**, *14*, 298–306. [PubMed]

25. Cutress, T.W. Dental caries in South Pacific populations: A review. *Pac. Health Dialog* **2003**, *10*, 62–67. [PubMed]

26. Moynihan, P.; Petersen, P.E. Diet, nutriton and the prevention of dental diseases. *Public Health Nutr.* **2004**, *7*, 201–226. [CrossRef] [PubMed]

27. Malik, V.S.; Pan, A.; Willet, W.C.; Hu, F.B. Sugar-sweetened beverages and weight gain in children and adults: A systematic review and meta-analysis. *Am. J. Clin. Nutr.* **2013**, *98*, 1084–1102. [CrossRef] [PubMed]

28. Hu, F.B. Resolved: There is sufficient scientific evidence that decreasing sugar-sweetened beverage consumption will reduce the prevalence of obesity and obesity-related diseases. *Obes. Rev.* **2013**, *14*, 606–619. [CrossRef] [PubMed]

29. Sawani, A.; Farhangi, M.; Maul, T.M.; Parthasarathy, S.; Smallwood, J.; Wei, J.L. Limiting dietary sugar improves pediatric sinonasal symptoms and reduces inflammation. *J. Med. Food* **2018**, *21*, 527–534. [CrossRef] [PubMed]

30. Malik, V.S.; Schulze, M.B.; Hu, F.B. Intake of sugar-sweetened beverages and weight gain: A systematic review. *Am. J. Clin. Nutr.* **2006**, *86*, 274–288. [CrossRef]

31. Te Morenga, L.; Mallard, S.; Mann, J. Dietary sugars and body weight: Systematic review and meta-analyses of randomised controlled trials and cohort studies. *BMJ* **2013**, *346*, 1–25. [CrossRef] [PubMed]

32. Pengpid, S.; Peltzer, K. Overweight and obesity and associated factors among school-aged adolescents in six pacific island countries in Oceania. *Int. J. Environ. Res. Public Health* **2015**, *12*, 14505–14518. [CrossRef]

33. Mavoa, H.M.; McCabe, M. Sociocultural factors relating to Tongans' and Indigenous Fijians' patterns of eating, physical activity and body size. *Asia Pac. J. Clin. Nutr.* **2008**, *17*, 375–384. [PubMed]

34. Stevenson, C.; Dpherty, G.; Barnett, J.; Muldoon, O.T.; Trew, K. Adolescents' views of food and eating: Identifying barriers to healthy eating. *J. Adolesc.* **2007**, *30*, 417–434. [CrossRef] [PubMed]

35. Ministry of Education. *School Canteen Guidelines Summary*; Ministry of Education: Suva, Fiji, 2009. Available online: http://www.consumersfiji.org/upload/Campaigns/marketing%20of%20Junk%20Food/Summary%20Canteen%20Guidelines.pdf (accessed on 10 October 2017).

36. Ministry of Education, National Heritage, Culture & Arts. *National Food and Nutrition Policy for Schools*; N.H. Ministry of Education, Culture & Arts: Suva, Fiji, 2005; pp. 1–11.

37. Varman, S.; Bullen, C.; Taylor-Smith, K.; Van Den Bergh, R.; Kholagi, M. Primary school compliance with school canteen guidelines in Fiji and its association with student obesity. *Public Health Act.* **2013**, *3*, 81–84. [CrossRef] [PubMed]

38. Gatti, C.; Suhas, E.; Cote, S.; Laouan-Sidi, E.A.; Dewailly, E.; Lucas, M. Obesity and metabolic parameters in adolescents: A school-based intervention program in French Polynesia. *J. Adolesc. Health* **2015**, *56*, 174–180. [CrossRef] [PubMed]

39. Fotu, K.F.; Millar, L.; Mavoa, H.; Kremer, P.; Moodie, M.; Snowdon, W.; Utter, J.; Vivili, P.; Schultz, J.T.; Malakellis, M.; et al. Outcome results for the Ma'alahi Youth Project, a Tongan community-based obesity prevention programme for adolescents. *Obes. Rev.* **2011**, *12*, 41–50. [CrossRef] [PubMed]

40. Kremer, P.; Waqa, G.; Vanualailai, N.; Schultz, J.T.; Roberts, G.; Moodie, M.; Mavoa, H.; Malakellis, M.; McCabe, M.P.; Swinburn, B.A. Reducing unhealthy weight gain in Fijian adolescents: Results of the Healthy Youth Healthy Communities study. *Obes. Rev.* **2011**, *12* (Suppl. 2), 29–40. [CrossRef] [PubMed]

41. Waqa, G.; Moodie, M.; Schultz, J.; Swinburn, B. Process evaluation of a community-based intervention program: Healthy Youth Healthy Communities, an adolescent obesity prevention project in Fiji. *Glob. Health Promot.* **2014**, *20*, 23–34. [CrossRef] [PubMed]

42. Jourdan, D.; Christensen, J.; Darlington, E.; Bonde, A.H.; Bloch, P.; Jensen, B.B.; Bentsen, P. The involvement of young people in school- and community-based noncommunicable disease prevention interventions: A scoping review of designs and outcomes. *BMC Public Health* **2016**, *16*, 1–14. [CrossRef] [PubMed]

43. Swinburn, B.A.; Millar, L.; Utter, J.; Kremer, P.; Moodie, M.; Mavoa, H.; Snowdon, W.; McCabe, M.P.; Malakellis, M.; de Courten, M.; et al. The Pacific Obesity Prevention in Communities project: Project overview and methods. *Obes. Rev.* **2011**, *12*, 3–11. [CrossRef] [PubMed]

44. Schultz, J.; Utter, J.; Mathews, L.; Cama, T.; Mavoa, H.; Swinburn, B. The Pacific OPIC Project (Obesity Prevention in Communities): Action plans and interventions. *Pac. Health Dialog.* **2007**, *14*, 147–153. [PubMed]

45. Hattersley, L.; Irwin, M.; King, L.; Allman-Farinelli, M. Determinants and patterns of soft drink consumption in young adults: A qualitative analysis. *Public Health Nutr.* **2009**, *12*, 1816–1822. [CrossRef] [PubMed]

46. Bucher, T.; Collins, C.; Diem, S.; Siegrist, M. Adolescents' perception of the healthiness of snacks. *Food Qual. Preference* **2016**, *50*, 94–101. [CrossRef]

47. Battram, D.S.; Pattram, L.; Beynon, C.; Kurtz, J.; He, M. Sugar-sweetened beverages: Children's perceptions, factors of influence, and suggestions for reducing intake. *J. Nutr. Ed. Behav.* **2015**, *48*, 27–34. [CrossRef] [PubMed]

48. Frayon, S.; Cherrier, S.; Cavaloc, Y.; Wattelez, G.; Touitou, A.; Zongo, P.; Yacef, K.; Caillaud, C.; Lerrant, Y.; Galy, O. Misperception of weight status in the pacific: Preliminary findings in rural and urban 11 to 16 year olds of New Caledonia. *BMC Public Health* **2017**, *17*, 1–10. [CrossRef] [PubMed]

49. Hebden, L.; Hector, D.; Hardy, L.L.; King, L. A fizzy environment: Availability and consumption of sugar-sweetened beverages among school students. *Prev. Med.* **2013**, 416–418. [CrossRef] [PubMed]

50. Snowdon, W. Sugar sweetened beverages in Pacific Island countries and territories: Problems and solutions? *Pac. Health Dialog.* **2014**, *20*, 43–46. [PubMed]

51. Vezina-Im, L.A.; Beaulieu, D.; Belanger-Gravel, A.; Boucher, D.; Sirois, C.; Dugas, M.; Provencher, V. Efficacy of school-based interventions aimed at decreasing sugar-sweetened beverage consumption among adolescents: a systematic review. *Public Health Nutr.* **2017**, *20*, 2416–2431. [CrossRef] [PubMed]

52. Miller, G.F.; Sliwa, S.; Brener, N.D.; Park, S.; Merlo, C.L. School district policies and adolescents' soda consumption. *J. Adolesc. Health* **2016**, *59*, 17–23. [CrossRef] [PubMed]

53. Lichtman-Sadot, S. Does banning carbonated beverages in schools decrease student consumption? *J. Public Econ.* **2016**, *140*, 30–50. [CrossRef]

54. Australian National Preventive Health Agency. *Obesity: Sugar-Sweetened Beverages, Obesity and Health*; Commonwealth of Australia: Canberra, Australia, 2014.

55. Bjelland, M.; Hausken, S.E.S.; Bergh, I.H.; Grydeland, M.; Klepp, K.I.; Andersen, L.F.; Totland, T.H.; Lien, N. Changes in adolescents' and parents' intakes of sugar-sweetened beverages, fruit and vegetables after 20 months: Results from the HEIA study—A comprehensive, multi-component school-based randomized trial. *Food Nutr. Res.* **2015**, *59*, 1–9. [CrossRef] [PubMed]

56. Contento, I.R.; Koch, P.A.; Lee, H.; Sauberli, W.; Calabrese-Barton, A. Enhancing Personal Agency and Competence in Eating and Moving: Formative Evaluation of a Middle School Curriculum—Choice, Control and Change. *J. Nutr. Educ. Behav.* **2007**, *39* (Suppl. 5), 179–186. [CrossRef] [PubMed]

57. Van Nasau, F.; Singh, A.; Cerin, E.; Salmon, J.; van Mechelen, W.; Brug, J.; Chinapaw, M.J. The Dutch Obesity Intervention in Teenagers (DOiT) cluster controlled implementation trial: Intervention effects and mediators and moderators of adiposity and energy balance-related behaviours. *Int. J. Behav. Nutr. Phys.* **2014**, *11*, 1–11. [CrossRef] [PubMed]

58. Bruening, M.; MacLehose, R.; Eisenberg, M.E.; Nanney, M.S.; Story, M.; Neumark-Sztainer, D. Associations between sugar-sweetened beverage consumption and fast-food restaurant frequency among adolescents and their friends. *J. Nutr. Educ. Behav.* **2014**, *46*, 277–285. [CrossRef] [PubMed]

59. Lo, E.; Coles, R.; Humbert, M.L.; Polowski, J.; Henry, C.J.; Whiting, S.J. Beverage intake improvement by high school students in Saskatchewan, Canada. *Nutr. Res.* **2008**, *28*, 144–150. [CrossRef] [PubMed]

60. Frayon, S.; Cherrier, S.; Cavaloc, Y.; Touitou, A.; Zongo, P.; Wattelez, G.; Yacef, K.; Caillaud, C.; Lerrant, Y.; Galy, O. Nutrition behaviours and sociodemographic factors associated with overweight in the multi-ethnic adolescents of New Caledonia. *Ethn. Health* **2017**. [CrossRef] [PubMed]

61. Gow, M.L.; Ho, M.; Lister, N.L.; Garnett, S.G. Chapter 6. Dietary Interventions in the Treatment of Paediatric Obesity. In *Paediatric Obesity: Etiology, Pathogenesis and Treatment*; Humana Press: Totowa, NJ, USA, 2018.

62. Thow, A.M.; Quested, C.; Juventin, L.; Kun, R.; Khan, A.N.; Swinburn, B. Taxing soft drinks in the Pacific: Implementation lessons for improving health. *Health Promot. Int.* **2011**, *26*, 55–64. [CrossRef] [PubMed]

## 13

Oral Health Care in Hong Kong

Sherry Shiqian Gao * ⓘ, Kitty Jieyi Chen, Duangporn Duangthip, Edward Chin Man Lo and Chun Hung Chu ⓘ

Faculty of Dentistry, The University of Hong Kong, Hong Kong, China; kjychen@hku.hk (K.J.C.); u3001284@connect.hku.hk (D.D.); hrdplcm@hku.hk (E.C.M.L.); chchu@hku.hk (C.H.C.)
* Correspondence: gao1204@hku.hk

Abstract: Hong Kong, as a special administrative region of the People's Republic of China, is a metropolitan city in Asia with a population of approximately 7.4 million. This paper reflects the oral health care situation in Hong Kong. Water fluoridation was introduced in 1961 as the primary strategy for the prevention of dental caries. The fluoride level is currently 0.5 parts per million. Dental care is mainly provided by private dentists. The government's dentists primarily serve civil servants and their dependents, with limited emergency dental service for pain relief offered to the general public. Nevertheless, the government runs the school dental care service, which provides dental treatments to primary school children through dental therapists. They also set up an oral health education unit to promote oral health in the community. Hong Kong had 2280 registered dentists in 2017, and the dentist-to-population ratio was about 1:3200. The Faculty of Dentistry at the University of Hong Kong is the only institution to provide basic and advanced dentistry training programs in Hong Kong. Dental hygienists, dental surgery assistants, dental therapists, and dental technicians receive training as paradental staff through the university or the government.

Keywords: health care; oral health; dental caries; water fluoridation; dental education; Hong Kong

1. Introduction

Hong Kong is a metropolitan city located on the southeast coast of the People's Republic of China. It consists of 262 islands spanning a total area of 1054 square kilometers. As one of the special administrative regions of the People's Republic of China, Hong Kong enjoys a 'high degree of autonomy' under the 'one country, two systems' policy. It presents high international rankings in various aspects, such as the Human Development Index, quality of life, financial and economic competitiveness, economic freedom, and corruption perception. The Hong Kong dollar (HK$) has been pegged to the United States dollar (US$) since 1983, and the currency exchange rate is currently around US$ 1 = HK$ 7.8. In 2013, the per-capita gross domestic product (GDP) was about US$ 38,000 in Hong Kong, and the total expenditure on health was about 5.7% of GDP [1].

The population in Hong Kong steadily increased to around 7.4 million in 2017 [2]. The large majority of the population is Southern Chinese (91%), while Filipinos and Indonesians make up 5% of the population [3]. Similar to other countries, the aging of the population is an important demographic issue in Hong Kong. The proportion of elderly people aged 65 years or older was 17% in 2017, and is expected to rise to 27% in 2033. Around 11% of the population are below 15 years old, and 32% are 45 to 64 years old. The median age of the entire population was 42 in 2017 [4]. In addition, the mortality rate in 2016 was 6.4 per 1000 within the entire population, which is one of the lowest in the world. Similar to the situations in other developed countries, the infant mortality rate (1.5 per 1000 live births in 2015) and maternal mortality rate (1.6 per 100,000 live births in 2015) have decreased within the past few years [5]. Hong Kong also presents the highest life expectancy worldwide. The average life expectancy of males and females is 81.3 and 87.3 years, respectively [6]. Moreover, the number of medical doctors in Hong Kong is approximately 14,000, with the doctor-to-population ratio being around 1:520 [7].

2. Water Fluoridation

The domestic water supply can reach nearly the entire area of Hong Kong, including the rural parts and major remote islands. Water fluoridation was implemented in 1961 in Hong Kong and is considered the most significant strategy for the primary prevention of dental caries. The initial fluoride level was at 0.8 parts per million (ppm). In 1967, it was increased to 1.0 ppm. However, a survey found that a fluoride concentration of 1.0 ppm is excessive, and thus can lead to a high prevalence of dental fluorosis among 7- to 12-year-old children [8]. Dental fluorosis is an unaesthetic tooth defect caused by excessive intake of fluoride during enamel formation, which can result in the hypomineralization of tooth enamel. Therefore, in 1978, the fluoride concentration was reduced to 0.7 ppm, and in 1988, it was further adjusted to 0.5 ppm [8]. Dental fluorosis decreased accordingly because of the reduction of the fluoride level in water [9].

Since water fluoridation has been implemented, it has been beneficial to the local population's dental health [10]. In 1960, the caries experience in the mean decayed, missing (due to caries), and filled teeth for permanent teeth (DMFT) among 7- to 12-year-old Hong Kong children was 4.4 [8]. After water fluoridation was introduced, the mean DMFT was decreased to 1.5 in 1968. Further reductions were observed in 2001 (DMFT = 0.8) and 2011 (DMFT = 0.4) among 12-year-old children [11].

3. Oral Health Conditions

The prevalence of dental caries among 12-year-old children in Hong Kong was 23% in 2011. The caries experience in the mean DMFT was 0.4, which was the lowest worldwide [11]. Although the caries experience among 12-year-old children has decreased over the years, the dental caries status among preschoolers is unsatisfactory. A survey in 2017 reported that more than half of 5-year-old preschool children suffered from dental caries, and most of the caries were left untreated [12]. The caries experience in the mean decayed, missing (due to caries), and filled teeth for primary teeth was 2.7 [12]. The caries experience among the adult population was also considerable in Hong Kong. The mean DMFT of middle-aged people (35–44 years old) was 6.9, and 4% of them had root caries. Meanwhile, the elderly population (65–74 years old) presented a mean DMFT of 16.2, and 25% of them had root caries [11].

The periodontal condition deteriorated with age among Hong Kong people [11]. Most 12-year-old children (86%) had gingivitis. Calculus was prevalent (64%) among them [11]. Moving to the adults, only 1% of 35- to 44-year-old people had healthy gums. Eighty percent of them had bleeding gums surrounding at least half of their teeth, and 40% of them had deep pockets. In the elderly population (over 65 years old), it was found that almost all (97%) of them had bleeding gums, and more than half (60%) presented deep pockets [11]. Hence, the periodontal status indicates that people in Hong Kong need professional periodontal care, such as scaling and the polishing of teeth.

The incidence of oral cancer in Hong Kong was 5.5 per 100,000 among females and 12.2 per 100,000 among males in 2015. In addition, the mortality rate is 1.5 per 100,000 and 4.6 per 100,000 in females and males, respectively [13]. It is noteworthy that 18.6% of the males were daily cigarette smokers, whereas only 3.2% of the females were daily smokers [14]. In addition, the proportion of current drinkers in males was as twice as high as that in females [15]. The smoking and drinking situations may relate to the different incidences of oral cancer among males and females. Similar to the situations of other populations, squamous cell carcinoma is the most prevalent oral cancer in Hong Kong. The fundamental treatment of oral cancer is surgery followed by radiation therapy, which the government highly subsidizes. Oral complications, such as dry mouth and radiation caries, are common in patients undergoing long-term radiation therapy. Therefore, these patients need follow-up oral care to improve their quality of life.

4. Oral Health Practices

Daily oral health practices highly influence an individual's oral health condition. In Hong Kong, 95% of the population practice tooth brushing everyday [11]. Fluoridated toothpastes are common in the market. However, the majority of the population use toothpicks, rather than dental floss, for interdental cleaning. Although products for oral health care are widely available and accessible in Hong Kong, people's awareness and knowledge of oral health remains low. As a result, many people in Hong Kong consider dental diseases to be a low priority [10]. A survey conducted in Hong Kong reported that 73% of the respondents did not know about the signs and symptoms of dental erosion, and more than half of the participants (53%) could not distinguish dental erosion from dental caries [16].

5. Oral Health Care Systems

Dental service is mainly provided through the private sector in Hong Kong. Most of the dentists are working alone or under small groups of general practitioners. No regulation exists regarding the consultation and treatment fees that the government sets. Thus, huge variations in the services provided and fees charged may be observed within various clinics. Nevertheless, the Dental Council of Hong Kong has issued strict ethical guidelines for the advertisement of dental practices [17].

Apart from private practices, around 60 nongovernmental organizations (NGOs) in Hong Kong provide dental services. These NGOs are usually welfare organizations, religious groups, labor unions, or social service agencies. Basically, they do not receive subsidies from the government. Therefore, dental services are self-financed and/or covered with donations. Many NGO dental clinics provide similar dental services to those of private practices, but at a relatively lower price. The target population is usually people with low socioeconomic statuses or those from disadvantaged groups, such as the elderly and physically handicapped.

The government dental clinics that the department of health runs offer dental services mainly to civil servants, the dependents of civil servants, and civil servant pensioners. Limited emergency dental services for pain relief, such as tooth extractions, are provided to the public. The oral maxillofacial surgery and dental units under the department of health also provide emergency and specialist dental services, but only for referred patients or hospitalized patients with special oral health care needs.

Although the government provides limited dental care services, the department of health set up a dental health program for Hong Kong primary school children, named the School Dental Care Service (SDCS) [18]. This program was established in 1979 and is now running in nine SDCS clinics. It provides oral health education, dental examinations, preventive and basic restorative treatments for dental caries, and emergency dental services to children; however, orthodontic treatment and other advanced dental treatments are excluded. Professionally trained dental therapists provide these services under the supervision of government dentists. All primary school children (mostly aged 6–12 years) are eligible for SDCS, and the enrollment is voluntary through schools. A nominal enrollment fee of around US$ 2.50 (HK$ 20) per child is charged each year and covers all of the dental services that the child receives.

The department of health has also executed a health care voucher scheme for elderly individuals since 2008 [19]. This scheme is available for 65- to 69-year-old individuals who are eligible to apply for the Normal Old Age Allowance. Currently, this scheme provides 10 vouchers of around US$ 6 (HK$ 50) per entitled elderly individual annually. The vouchers can be used to cover dental costs in private clinics. Although the majority of elderly individuals appreciate this scheme, many of them still consider US$ 60 (HK$ 500) per year to be insufficient to subsidize their dental care expenses.

The department of health established an oral health education unit for oral health promotion to the general public [20]. The unit has been organizing various activities to promote oral health. Amongst them, the 'Love Teeth Campaign' is one of the most well-known oral health events in Hong Kong. This campaign was founded in 2011 [21]. Its aim is to raise awareness about oral health and to deliver information on preventing oral diseases. Related events are held every year, including lectures, consultation services, games, and oral health education for children. Apart from these events, oral-health-related messages are disseminated through local television, internet, radio, and newspaper advertisements, complemented by posters and banners displayed in public venues. The 'Love Teeth Campaign' is also conjoined with 'World Oral Health Day' to bring more international attention to the local event.

The oral health education unit has developed a dedicated website called 'Tooth Club' to disseminate information about oral health care through the internet to the general public [20]. The oral health education unit also distributes free materials for promoting oral health, such as pamphlets, brochures, posters, and video compact discs, to local schools and organizations from time to time. In addition, local schools and organizations can borrow various oral health education materials from the unit, such as games, models, and exhibits. The oral health education unit also provides a program called 'Brighter Smiles Playland', which is specially designed for 4-year-old children in local kindergartens and nursery schools. Through this program, children are expected to obtain and absorb oral health-related knowledge in an interactive way.

6. Dentist Profile

Dentists working in Hong Kong were all trained overseas before 1985. In 1980, under the requirements set by the General Dental Council of the United Kingdom, the Dental Studies at the University of Hong Kong (HKU, Hong Kong, China) admitted its first batch of dental students. After a five-year training course, 70 dental students graduated with Bachelor of Dental Surgery (BDS) degrees and began to practice in 1985. In 1982, the HKU Faculty of Dentistry was established and housed at the Prince Philip Dental Hospital (PPDH). So far, the HKU Faculty of Dentistry remains the only institution in Hong Kong that provides dental education. Since 2012, the training duration for BDS has been extended to six years. Completing a license examination prior to practicing is not required for those who graduated with BDS degrees from the HKU Faculty of Dentistry. Currently, around 70 BDS students are enrolled every year. More than 1600 dentists had trained under the HKU Faculty of Dentistry by April 2017. Dental graduates who have trained abroad can also practice dentistry in Hong Kong when they pass the license examination that the Dental Council of Hong Kong has established. Hong Kong had approximately 2280 registered dentists in 2017, and the dentist-to-population ratio was approximately 1:3200. In addition, approximately three-quarters of dentists practice in private dental clinics. Meanwhile, approximately one-fifth are enrolled in the government sectors. Dentists also work in NGOs or the HKU Faculty of Dentistry, or join the available postgraduate training program.

Apart from the undergraduate training, the HKU Faculty of Dentistry offers postgraduate clinical training in various dental specialties [22]. The College of Dental Surgeons of Hong Kong was established in 1993, which aimed to manage and promote postgraduate dental training and dental research. In Hong Kong, eight recognized specialties exist, including community dentistry, endodontics, family dentistry, oral and maxillofacial surgery, orthodontics, pediatric dentistry, periodontology, and prosthodontics [23]. Being a dental specialist requires at least six years of advanced training, which include a three-year master's degree (basic training) and three years of supervised specialty-related clinical practice (higher training). In 2017, the majority of dentists in Hong Kong were general practitioners, whereas around 12% of them were registered dental specialists.

7. Paradental Staff

Apart from dentists, paradental staff also work as an essential part of the dental team, which includes dental hygienists, dental surgery assistants, dental therapists, and dental technicians.

Dental hygienists are enrolled as professionals in Hong Kong. Their responsibilities include completing dental examinations; cleaning, scaling, and polishing of teeth; taking oral radiographs; applying topical fluorides and sealants; and providing oral health education. However, a dentist must have diagnosed the patient before a dental hygienist provides a service to him or her. In addition, a dentist must be available at all times on the premises when the dental hygienist is providing the prescribed dental procedures. A total of 424 dental hygienists were enrolled in 2016, and 210 of them were practicing [7]. A survey revealed that more than 90% of dental hygienists were working in the private sector in 2014 [24]. The PPDH began to offer a one-year training program for dental hygienists in the early 1980s. Since 2002, the program has been expanded to a two-year Higher Diploma in Dental Hygiene, which the Community College of HKU and the PPDH conjointly oversee.

Dental surgery assistants work closely with dentists in the clinic to provide dental services to patients. They are essential team members and are indispensable participants in four-handed operations in dental practices. The responsibilities of dental surgery assistants are not limited to chair side assisting; rather, they also complete appointment booking, receive patients, receive payments, maintain stock, provide oral health education, and sterilize instruments. Around 3800 dental surgery assistants were enumerated in 2014, and more than 85% of them worked in private dental clinics [24]. Dental surgery assistants in Hong Kong are not required to be enrolled. The Hong Kong Polytechnics provided a two-year full-time diploma program for dental surgery assistant training that started in 1980, but the program was discontinued in 1984. The department of health once trained dental surgery assistants through an in-service program, but it was also discontinued in the 1980s. So far, dental surgery assistant training programs are not standardized in Hong Kong. Various training courses are available in the market. The PPDH provides one-year full-time or two-year part-time certificate programs for dental surgery assistant training. Apart from these, commercial health institutions also offer training to dental surgery assistants. In addition, private dentists can hire lay persons for on-the-job training.

The department of health employs dental therapists, who also are not required to be enrolled. Most of them work in the SDCS. Their responsibilities include completing oral and radiographic examinations, providing preventive treatment (scaling, the application of topical fluoride and fissure sealants), providing basic dental treatment (fillings and extraction), and offering oral health education. All of the procedures that dental therapists perform should be completed under the supervision of a dentist. As of 2014, a total of 284 dental therapists were enumerated in Hong Kong [24]. Dental therapists were trained in a three-year in-service training program through the department of health starting in 1977. However, the training of dental therapists was later suspended because of the decrease in the birth rate from 2002 to 2015. However, in 2016, the training program was restarted and transformed into a one-year Advanced Diploma in Dental Therapy, held in the PPDH. Dental hygienists with diplomas are eligible to be enrolled in this program. Ten students are recruited every year.

Dental technicians (technologists) work mainly in dental manufactories or laboratories and are not required to be enrolled. As of 2014, more than 350 dental technicians were enumerated, and most of them (77%) worked in the private sector [24]. Dental technicians are responsible for manufacturing removable and fixed dental appliances, such as complete and partial dentures, inlays, crowns and bridges, orthodontic appliances, and oral and maxillofacial prostheses. The Hong Kong Polytechnics first provided a three-year, full-time diploma in dental technology in the late 1970s. Then, the training program was relocated to the PPDH in the 1980s. The PPDH now offers a two-year full-time Advanced Diploma in Dental Technology program for dental technicians. The technicians only work in the laboratory and provide no clinical care. This is different from other countries such as the United States and Canada (which have denturist), the United Kingdom (which has clinical dental technician), and Australia (which has dental prosthetist).

8. Discussion

The policy of the Hong Kong government on dental services is to raise public awareness of oral health and to encourage proper oral health habits through promotion and education. The government also set up SDCS in 1979 to provide basic and preventive dental care to primary school students. SDCS is a demonstration of a successful dental health program in Hong Kong. More than 95% of Hong Kong school children aged 6–12 years are joining SDCS. The caries experience of 12-year-old children gradually decreased after the introduction of the program [25]. In 2011, 12-year-old Hong Kong children enjoyed the lowest caries experience (DMFT = 0.4) worldwide, and most of the decayed teeth were restored (filled teeth, FT = 0.3) [11]. The dental care of SDCS is largely provided by dental therapists. Dental therapists, who used to be named dental nurses, were first proposed in New Zealand to address the high dental demands of children and the shortage of dentists [26]. The Hong Kong government had adopted this model from New Zealand by sending people there to receive training as dental therapist in the 1970s. Until recently, more than 53 countries have adopted the dental therapist model in their dental health care system to address dental needs. More than 14,000 dental therapists are presently working worldwide to provide dental care to the public [27]. There used to be a debate on whether the implementation of dental therapists improved the access to dental care or affected the quality of dental care. Nevertheless, reviews reported that the treatments provided by dental therapists were technically competent, safe, and effective, especially for children [28]. As for Hong Kong, the SDCS contributes to the low caries experience of the school children [11]. Thus, the adoption of dental therapists can be a promising strategy to lower the social burden of dental care and improve the oral health of the people under served.

Moreover, the government set up the oral health education unit to deliver oral health education to the public. The unit introduced the 'Brighter Smiles for the New Generation' program in 1993 to promote oral health for preschool children. This program also provides dental education to increase oral health care knowledge of kindergarten teachers and parents of the preschool children. Dental care service is mainly provided by private practitioners in Hong Kong. Because of the low dentist-to-population ratio and the limited available resources, more than half (51%) of Hong Kong preschoolers had early childhood caries experience. Furthermore, most of the affected children have never seen a dentist and the carious teeth were left untreated [12]. To address this severe problem, NGOs and the HKU Faculty of Dentistry have pioneered outreach dental care programs to manage dental caries using the atraumatic restorative technique and silver diamine fluoride therapy.

It is noteworthy that in the Hong Kong adult population, the number of decayed teeth presented as the smallest component in the DMFT score (0.7/6.9 or 10% in 35- to 44-year-olds and 1.3/16.2 or 8% in 65- to 74-year-olds), whereas the number of missing teeth due to caries presented as the highest component (3.4/6.9 or 49% in 35- to 44-year-olds and 12.7/16.2 or 78% in 65- to 74-year-olds) [11]. This might be a result of patients only seeking treatment when their affected teeth were in advanced disease stages, or because the patients' attitude to save and keep their teeth was poor.

9. Conclusions

Water fluoridation is the primary strategy for the prevention of dental caries in Hong Kong. The dentist-to-population ratio was around 1:3200 in 2017. Most dentists work as private practitioners. The department of health has established various programs and activities to promote oral health among different populations. Only one university in Hong Kong provides basic and advanced training programs in dentistry. Paradental staff members, such as dental hygienists, dental surgery assistants, dental therapists, and dental technicians, also receive training through the university or the government.

Author Contributions: S.S.G. prepared the manuscript; K.J.C., D.D., E.C.M.L., and C.H.C. critically reviewed the manuscript. All authors approved the final version of the manuscript to be submitted.

Acknowledgments: The authors would like to thank Kenneth Hui, Henry Luk, Richard Su, Rowena Chan, and Jenny Leung for providing information related to this article.

References

1. Statistics: Total Health Expenditure. Food and Health Bureau. Available online: http://www.fhb.gov.hk/statistics/en/dha/dha_summary_report.htm (accessed on 19 November 2017).
2. Hong Kong Statistics: Population. Census and Statistics Department. Available online: https://www.censtatd.gov.hk/hkstat/sub/so20.jsp (accessed on 19 November 2017).

3. Hong Kong—The Facts. Available online: https://www.gov.hk/en/about/abouthk/facts.htm (accessed on 19 November 2017).

4. Table 002: Population by Age Group and Sex. Census and Statistics Department. Available online: http://www.censtatd.gov.hk/hkstat/sub/sp150.jsp?tableID=002&ID=0&productType=8 (accessed on 19 November 2017).

5. Health Facts: Major Health Indicators. Department of Health. Available online: http://www.healthyhk.gov.hk/phisweb/en/healthy_facts/health_indicators/ (accessed on 19 November 2017).

6. Table 004: Vital Events. Census and Statistics Department. Available online: http://www.censtatd.gov.hk/hkstat/sub/sp150.jsp?tableID=004&ID=0&productType=8 (accessed on 19 November 2017).

7. Health Facts of Hong Kong, 2017 Edition. Available online: http://www.dh.gov.hk/english/statistics/statistics_hs/files/Health_Statistics_pamphlet_E.pdf (accessed on 19 November 2017).

8. Evans, R.W.; Stamm, J.W. Dental fluorosis following downward adjustment of fluoride in drinking water. *J. Public Health Dent.* **1991**, *51*, 91–98. [CrossRef] [PubMed]

9. Evans, R.W. Changes in dental fluorosis following an adjustment to the fluoride concentration of Hong Kong's water supplies. *Adv. Dent. Res.* **1989**, *3*, 154–160.

10. Chu, C.H.; Wong, S.S.; Suen, R.P.; Lo, E.C.M. Oral health and dental care in Hong Kong. *Surgeon* **2013**, *11*, 153–157. [CrossRef] [PubMed]

11. Oral Health Survey 2011. Department of Health. Available online: http://www.toothclub.gov.hk/en/en_pdf/Oral_Health_Survey_2011/Oral_Health_Survey_2011_WCAG_20141112_(EN_Full).pdf (accessed on 20 November 2017).

12. Chen, K.J.; Gao, S.S.; Duangthip, D.; Li, S.K.Y.; Lo, E.C.M.; Chu, C.H. Dental caries status and its associated factors among 5-year-old Hong Kong children: A cross-sectional study. *BMC Oral Health* **2017**, *17*, 121. [CrossRef] [PubMed]

13. Hong Kong Cancer Registry. Hospital Authority. Available online: http://www3.ha.org.hk/cancereg/tc/allages.asp (accessed on 20 November 2017).

14. Pattern of Smoking in Hong Kong. Tobacco Control Office, Department of Health. Available online: http://www.tco.gov.hk/english/infostation/infostation_sta_01.html (accessed on 7 March 2018).

15. Alcohol and Health: Hong Kong situation. Department of Health. Available online: http://www.dh.gov.hk/.english/pub_rec/pub_rec_ar/pdf/ncd_ap2/action_plan_2_alcohol%20and%20health%20HK%20situation_e.pdf (accessed on 7 March 2018).

16. Chu, C.H.; Pang, K.K.; Lo, E.C.M. Dietary behavior and knowledge of dental erosion among Chinese adults. *BMC Oral Health* **2010**, *10*, 13. [CrossRef] [PubMed]

17. Code of Professional Discipline for the Guidance of Dental Practitioners in Hong Kong. The Dental Council of Hong Kong. Available online: http://www.dchk.org.hk/docs/code.pdf (assessed on 20 November 2017).

18. School Dental Care Service. Department of Health. Available online: http://www.schooldental.gov.hk/wsmile/whatsnew_e.html (accessed on 20 November 2017).

19. Cheung, H.H.N.; Fong, S.T.S.; Lau, D.M.C.; Mak, R.L.Y.; Man, G.W.C.; So, K.M.K.; Tai, M.T.C.; Yee, S.Y.Y.; Yuen, C.H.C.; Wong, M.C.M. Health care voucher scheme and willingness to spend on dental care among Hong Kong elders. *Hong Kong Dent. J.* **2008**, *5*, 84–92.

20. Tooth club. Oral Health Education Unit. Available online: http://www.toothclub.gov.hk/en/en_index.html (assessed on 20 November 2017).

21. Love Teeth Campaign. Oral Health Education Unit. Available online: http://www.toothclub.gov.hk/en/teeth_2016.html (accessed on 20 November 2017).

22. Taught Postgraduate Programmemes, HKU Faculty of Dentistry. Available online: http://facdent.hku.hk/index.php/learning/tpg/ (accessed on 20 November 2017).

23. Ho, M.C.T.; Chung, A.Y.K.; Sit, E.K.F. An update on postgraduate dental education in Hong Kong and a comparison of three countries. *Hong Kong Dent. J.* **2008**, *5*, 60–66.

24. 2014 Health Manpower survey. Summary of the Characteristics of Healthcare Personnel Enumerated. Available online: http://www.dh.gov.hk/english/statistics/statistics_hms/sumohp14.html (assessed on 9 January 2018).

25. Lee, H.M.; Pang, H.H.; McGrath, C.P.; Yiu, C.K. Oral health of Hong Kong children: A historical and epidemiological perspective. *Hong Kong Med. J.* **2016**, *22*, 372–381. [CrossRef] [PubMed]

26. Friedman, J.W. The international dental therapist: History and current status. *J. Calif. Dent. Assoc.* **2011**, *39*, 23–29. [PubMed]

27. Nash, D.A.; Friedman, J.W.; Kardos, T.B.; Kardos, R.L.; Schwarz, E.; Satur, J.; Berg, D.G.; Nasruddin, J.; Mumghamba, E.G.; Davenport, E.S.; et al. Dental therapists: A global perspective. *Int. Dent. J.* **2008**, *58*, 61–70. [CrossRef] [PubMed]

28. Nash, D.A.; Friedman, J.W.; Mathu-Muju, K.R.; Robinson, P.G.; Satur, J.; Moffat, S.; Kardos, R.; Lo, E.; Wong, A.H.; Jaafar, N.; et al. A review of the global literature on dental therapists. *Community Dent. Oral Epidemiol.* **2014**, *42*, 1–10. [CrossRef] [PubMed]

## 14

Rescuing Suboptimal Patient-Reported Outcome Instrument Data in Clinical Trials: A New Strategy

Chengwu Yang [1],* (iD) and Kent E. Vrana [2]

[1]   Departments of Epidemiology and Health Promotion, College of Dentistry, New York University, New York, NY 10010, USA
[2]   Department of Pharmacology, College of Medicine, The Pennsylvania State University, Hershey, PA 17033, USA; kev10@psu.edu
*   Correspondence: chengwu.yang@nyu.edu

Abstract: *Background*: Psychometric instruments such as the Repeated Battery for the Assessment of Neuropsychological Status (RBANS) are commonly used under conditions for which they were not developed or validated. They may then generate troublesome data that could conceal potential findings. *Methods*: Based on a previously published refinement of the RBANS, we reanalyzed the data on 303 patients from two National Institutes of Health (NIH) trails in Parkinson's disease and contrasted the results using the original versus refined scores. *Results*: Findings from the original RBANS scores were inconsistent; however, use of the refined scores produced potential findings that were in agreement with independent reports. *Conclusion*: This study demonstrates that, for negative trials using instrument scores as primary outcomes, it is possible to rescue potential findings. The key to this new strategy is to validate and refine the instrument for the specific disease and conditions under study and then to reanalyze the data. This study offers a demonstration of this new strategy for general approaches.

Keywords: patient-reported outcome (PRO); clinical trials; instrument; measurement; scale; psychometrics; clinimetrics; Parkinson's disease; RBANS; factor analysis; placebo effect

---

1. Introduction

Since few health-related psychometric instruments have been "professionally developed" [1], it is common to see suboptimal instrument data in clinical trials. An example was the use of the Repeatable Battery for the Assessment of Neuropsychological Status (RBANS) [2] in two National Institutes of Health (NIH) Exploratory Trials in Parkinson's disease (NET-PD) [3,4]. The RBANS has been popular since its initial publication. According to Web of Science (Thomson Reuters; accessed 12 December 2017), the initial description of RBANS has been cited 472 times. Moreover, it has been translated and used in many other countries such as China [5], Japan [6], and Italy [7]. Its popularity may relate to its brevity. However, the original factor structure of RBANS was theory-driven [2], while multiple subsequent empirical studies have identified optimal factor structures that differ from the original (e.g., [8–14]). This has engendered significant concerns about the validity of the universal use of RBANS to assess cognitive function.

Two NET-PD trials tested four drugs for the treatment of movement impairment in PD: Creatine and Minocycline in FS1, and CoQ10 and GPI1485 in FS-TOO, indicating that Creatine and Minocycline might be promising [3,4]. The RBANS was used to assess cognition as a secondary outcome. Because we previously demonstrated that the original RBANS had not been validated for PD, it is not surprising that the RBANS assessments produced equivocal results [13]. Yet, we believe that better use of these problematic, but expensive, data is of critical and practical importance. We therefore set out to reanalyze the RBANS data from the two NET-PD trials based on the refined factor structure from our previous study [13], and then to contrast the results with those based on the original factor structure, in hope of rescuing potential findings.

2. Materials and Methods

2.1. Patients

The two NET-PD trials recruited 858 early untreated PD patients from 42 sites in North America, and randomized 413 participants into six arms. Details can be found in earlier publications [3,4]. In total, 339 finished the 12-month follow-up visit. RBANS data were collected at the baseline and 12-month follow-up visit. After the deletion of patients with missing values for the RBANS data and outliers as detected by the Malhanobis distance, 383 and 315 patients remained at baseline and follow-up. Since the change from baseline to follow-up in RBANS scores will be used as the primary outcome, only patients with complete RBANS data at both baseline and follow-up were included in the final analysis of this study. Therefore, 303 patients with complete RBANS data at both baseline and follow-up were analyzed.

2.2. The RBANS

The original RBANS has 12 items and offers scores on five cognitive domains [2]. Each of the first four domains is measured by two items, while the last domain is measured by four. In addition, the RBANS offers a total score based on the five domain scores (Figure 1A). However, these six original RBANS scores are neither valid nor reliable in the two NET-PD trials [13].

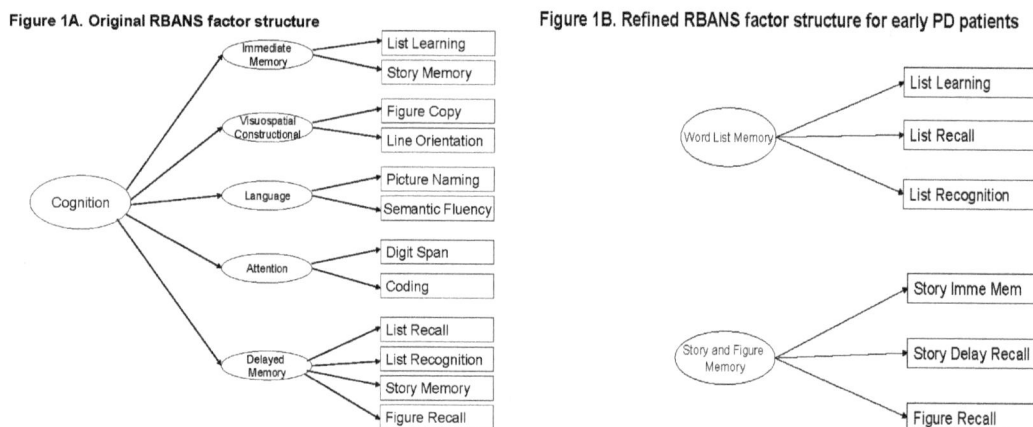

Figure 1. Factor structure of the RBANS: Original vs. refined for early PD patients.

Following psychometric analysis, we created a new instrument that retained half of the assessment items from the original RBANS and reorganized them into two domains [13]. The refined RBANS [13,15] for these trials has six items and offers scores on two new cognitive domains: word list memory (WLM) and story and figure memory (SFM), measured by three items each (Figure 1B). Specifically, six of the original RBANS items were excluded because they had low correlation with each other and the remaining six items [13]. The refined RBANS is valid and reliable for these specific patients, and makes clinical sense [13]. However, a unified total RBANS score based on these two domains was not supported by a two-level factor structure [13].

2.3. Statistical Analysis

Data from the two trials were analyzed separately and in parallel. The normality of each variable was checked in order to choose appropriate analysis approaches. Chi-square tests were applied to categorical data, and analysis of variance (ANOVA) or Kruskal-Wallis tests were applied to continuous data. Demographic and disease characteristics of the participants at baseline were summarized and compared across the three arms within each of the two trials. Preliminary comparisons of change from baseline on cognitive abilities as measured by the original and refined RBANS, within each of the two trials, were implemented. In comparing the original RBANS with the refined RBANS, we focused on providing consistent changes in cognitive scores. Comparing p-values would be flawed given the lack of power in these historical data (inadequate sample size) for assessing these secondary outcome measures [3,4]. Post hoc power analysis and sample size estimation were implemented to address the lack of power and small sample size issues. SPSS (Version 23, IBM Corp., Armonk, NY, USA) and SAS (Version 9.4, SAS Institute Inc., Cary, NC, USA) were used for data preparation and analysis. G*Power (Version 3.1.9.2, University of Düsseldorf, Düsseldorf, Germany) [16,17]) was used for post hoc power analysis and sample size estimation.

3. Results

Demographic and disease characteristics at baseline are summarized in Table 1.

Table 1. Demographic and disease characteristics of participants at baseline.

FS1 (n = 151)		1. Creatine (n = 46)	2. Minocycline (n = 52)	3. Placebo (n = 53)	p-Value
Age	Mean ± SD	61.0 ± 10.8	64.1 ± 10.5	60.7 ± 9.7	0.11
Education	Mean ± SD	15.4 ± 3.5	15.0 ± 2.9	15.2 ± 2.9	0.95
Gender	Male	32 (69.6%)	28 (53.9%)	34 (64.2%)	0.26
	Female	14 (30.4%)	24 (46.1%)	19 (35.8%)	
Race	White	43 (93.5%)	51 (98.1%)	49 (92.5%)	0.44
	Others *	3 (6.5%)	1 (1.9%)	4 (7.5%)	
Ethnicity	Not Hispanic or Latino	45 (97.8%)	51 (98.1%)	51 (96.2%)	0.99
	Others †	1 (2.2%)	1 (1.9%)	2 (3.8%)	
UPDRS Total Score (Parts I–III)	Mean ± SD	22.8 ± 8.9	23.7 ± 9.2	23.0 ± 10.3	0.78
Schwab and England Activities of Daily Living scale	Mean ± SD	92.9 ± 5.1	92.5 ± 6.4	94.5 ± 4.6	0.17
Tremor Dominant ‡	Yes	21 (45.7%)	25 (48.1%)	33 (62.3%)	0.19
	No	25 (54.3%)	27 (51.9%)	20 (37.7%)	
Hoehn and Yahr Staging	0	0	0	0	0.46
	1	27 (58.7%)	24 (46.1%)	27 (50.9%)	
	2	19 (41.3%)	28 (53.9%)	26 (49.1%)	
	3	0	0	0	
FS-TOO (n = 152)		1. CoQ10 (n = 50)	2. Minocycline (n = 50)	3. Placebo (n = 52)	p-Value
Age	Mean ± SD	61.1 ± 9.2	61.4 ± 10.9	61.4 ± 9.2	0.90
Education	Mean ± SD	15.6 ± 3.2	15.4 ± 3.0	15.4 ± 2.7	0.97
Gender	Male	31 (62.0%)	32 (64.0%)	38 (73.1%)	0.45
	Female	19 (38.0%)	18 (36.0%)	14 (26.9%)	
Race	White	47 (94.0%)	49 (98.0%)	47 (90.4%)	0.30
	Others *	3 (6.0%)	1 (2.0%)	5 (9.6%)	
Ethnicity	Not Hispanic or Latino	50 (100.0%)	48 (96.0%)	52 (100.0%)	0.21
	Others †	0	2 (4.0%)	0	
UPDRS Total Score (Parts I–III)	Mean ± SD	22.0 ± 9.6	20.8 ± 8.8	22.2 ± 9.1	0.67
Schwab and England Activities of Daily Living scale	Mean ± SD	92.9 ± 5.7	93.8 ± 4.4	93.1 ± 4.9	0.78
Tremor Dominant ‡	Yes	26 (52.0%)	31 (62.0%)	27 (51.9%)	0.50
	No	24 (48.0%)	19 (38.0%)	25 (48.1%)	
Hoehn and Yahr Staging	0	1 (2.0%)	0	0	0.96
	1	27 (54.0%)	28 (56.0%)	30 (57.7%)	
	2	21 (42.0%)	22 (44.0%)	22 (42.3%)	
	3	1 (2.0%)	0	0	

* Other races include Indian, Alaska Native, Asian, Black/African American, more than one race, and unknown or not reported. † Other ethnicities include Hispanic or Latino, and unknown or not reported. ‡ A PD patient was determined to be tremor dominant or not by using the method described by Jankovic et al. (1990) [18]. UPDRS: unified Parkinson's disease rating scale.

No statistically significant difference was detected at any of these characteristics among the two treatment groups and one placebo group within each of the trials, and characteristics are very similar within each of the two trials.

Preliminary comparisons of change from baseline on cognitive abilities are summarized in Table 2.

Table 2. Preliminary comparisons of change from baseline on cognitive abilities among treatment groups using the Repeated Battery for the Assessment of Neuropsychological Status (RBANS) scores: original vs. refined.

	RBANS Scores		Creatine (n = 46)		Minocycline (n = 52)		Placebo (n = 53)		p-Value
			Mean	SD	Mean	SD	Mean	SD	
	Original	IM	5.93	12.79	4.63	12.18	3.77	11.95	0.86
FS1		VC	−2.91	14.43	−7.29	18.37	−2.28	17.39	0.34
(n = 151)		La	−1.22	10.52	−2.94	9.33	0.53	9.34	0.09
		Att	0.63	13.17	−1.38	14.43	−0.94	12.48	0.87
		DM	2.09	13.49	−0.52	11.45	−2.28	14.28	0.26
		Total	1.39	9.77	−2.81	10.04	−0.94	9.81	0.14
	Refined	WLM	3.00	5.52	0.75	5.55	1.25	5.95	0.15
		SFM	1.11	7.91	0.87	7.36	0.11	6.25	0.95
	RBANS Score		CoQ10 (n = 50)		GPI1485 (n = 50)		Placebo (n = 52)		p-Value
			Mean	SD	Mean	SD	Mean	SD	
	Original	IM	0.60	10.24	0.18	10.41	0.19	14.98	0.82
FS-TOO		VC	−0.96	14.45	−5.72	16.90	−1.94	14.76	0.50
(n = 152)		La	1.44	9.55	−0.16	8.11	−1.60	8.38	0.13
		Att	−0.02	13.09	0.02	12.90	1.65	13.69	0.71
		DM	4.78	14.23	1.18	20.24	0.37	14.63	0.51
		Total	2.14	9.82	−1.16	10.43	−0.52	10.87	0.24
	Refined	WLM	0.10	4.71	0.60	4.92	0.52	6.12	0.80
		SFM	1.52	5.66	−0.12	6.86	−0.83	5.36	0.13

None of the pairwise comparisons of the refined RBANS scores was statistically significant (p-value not shown), mainly due to the small sample size; IM: Immediate Memory; VC: Visuospatial/Constructional; La: Language; Att: Attention; DM: Delayed Memory; WLM: Word List Memory; SFM: Story and Figure Memory [13].

When cognition is measured by the original six RBANS scores, there is no consistent trend over time. Out of the 36 changes, 17 (47.2%) are increased, 19 (52.8%) are decreased. Moreover, none of the six groups show consistency in the direction of change among the original six RBANS scores. For example, in the Creatine group, while four original RBANS scores show increases, the other two show decreases. In contrast, when cognition is measured by the two refined RBANS scores, the trend over time is much more consistent. Out of the 12 changes on refined RBANS scores, 10 (83.3%) show increases, and only two show a decrease, but both within one unit (−0.12, −0.83). None of the differences among groups, in change from baseline on either of the RBANS scores, is statistically significant ($p > 0.05$), because the study was underpowered. Clearly, however, the refined RBANS provides much more consistent data trends, and will therefore give greater insight into treatment outcomes.

Post hoc power analysis indicated that, in order to have 80% power to detect the difference shown on WLM between Creatine and Placebo (3.00 vs. 1.25, Cohen's d = 0.30 [19]), 178 patients per group would be needed. Given the current sample size of 50 per group, the statistical power to detect this difference was 31%. Since the effect size of Creatine on WLM was the largest, post hoc analysis on others would result in a larger required sample size or would show lower power at the current sample size.

4. Discussion

Given that suboptimal instrument data are commonly utilized in clinical trials, it is of great practical importance to better utilize these troublesome and expensive data in hope of rescuing important potential findings. This study offers a template for rescuing efforts through reanalyzing existing suboptimal instrument data. Findings from the two NET-PD trials that employed the unified Parkinson's disease rating scale (UPDRS) scores as the primary outcome indicated that two (Creatine, Minocycline) of the four tested drugs may be beneficial for PD patients [3], while the other two (CoQ10, GPI1485) may not [4]. Results from the present study indicate that, while using the original six RBANS scores showed no benefit of the treatments on cognitive ability as a secondary outcome, the use of the two refined RBANS scores may have produced a positive outcome had the sample sizes been larger (Table 2).

The inconsistencies in the trend among the original six RBANS scores are very troublesome. It is not easy to explain why a drug can help improve some cognitive abilities while impairing others (Table 2). This observation strengthens the conclusion that the RBANS was neither valid nor reliable in the two NET-PD trials studied here [13]. In contrast, the refined RBANS scores offer much more consistency in the trend, albeit in the absence of statistical significance. Most of the changes from baseline are increasing, indicating that the treatment is increasing each of the cognitive abilities. The increased outcomes in cognitive assessments offer more practical support for the validity and reliability of the refined RBANS in both trials [13].

Another advantage of the refined versus the original RBANS is indicated by the big differences in the standard deviations (SD) of the changes from baseline (Table 2). When using the original RBANS, the SDs are huge (e.g., for Creatine, Att has a mean of 0.65 and an SD of 13.17). However, after refinement, the SDs dropped substantially (e.g., for Creatine, WLM has a mean of 3.00 and an SD of 5.52.

Placebo effect [20] on the two refined RBANS scores is evidenced by the three increases in the two placebo groups. Participating in a clinical trial and receiving some kind of treatment may help patients feel better and can improve their cognition. However, these placebo effects are smaller than potential true treatment effects.

Lack of power due to the small sample size is the primary reason for potentially physiologically important, but statistically negative results. Had the sample size been large enough, these results should also be statistically significant. Future studies with appropriate sample size are therefore warranted.

Clearly, there are important limitations in this analysis related to statistical power. Take, for example, the observed differences on WLM between Creatine and Placebo in FS1 (details in Table 2). The observed difference was 3.00 for Creatine and 1.25 for Placebo, with Cohen's d as 0.30, which was between "small" and "medium" [19]. That is to say, the difference was clearly "clinically significant". However, due to the small sample size (46 in Creatine, 53 in Placebo, 99 total), the p-value was 0.15, and the difference was "statistically insignificant". This is a typical scenario when a study finding is "clinically significant", but "statistically insignificant", since the sample size is not big enough. However, clinical significance should be an important deciding factor for medical studies, not simply statistical significance, because "p-values do not measure evidence" [20] (p. 619). In addition, recent reports have re-emphasized the severe issue of p-driven research (e.g., [21]), including the American Statistical Association (ASA) statement on p-values [22]. What the present studies emphasize, however, is that a properly designed and validated instrument, combined with an appropriate sample size, can provide both clinical and statistical significance.

In clinical trials that use psychometric instruments, it is critical to validate or even refine the instruments for data collected before any formal statistical analysis. This is because most instruments are "not professionally developed" [1], and instrument validation is an "ongoing process" [23]. No instrument should be claimed to be "already validated"; rather, assessment instruments should be validated for the disease and population under study. Another good example appears a recent review on oral health-related quality of life (OHRQoL) instruments [24]. Other recent literature re-emphasizes the importance of sound psychometric properties of an instrument [25–27].

For negative trials that used instrument scores as primary outcomes, the present findings offer a path to rescuing potential findings: validating and refining the instruments and then reanalyzing the data based on the refined instrument scores. Our study offers a demonstration of the new strategy for this type of promising effort.

5. Conclusions

This study demonstrates that, for negative trials using instrument scores as primary outcomes, it is possible to rescue potential findings. The key to this new strategy is to validate and refine the instrument for the specific disease and conditions under study and then to reanalyze the data. This study offers a demonstration of this new strategy for general approaches.

Acknowledgments: This study was sponsored, in part, by the NIH (National Institute of Neurological Disorders and Stroke), U01NS043127, U01NS043128, and U10NS44415 through 44555, and by the National Institute on Aging (NIA) Resource Centers for Minority Aging Research (RCMAR) Grant 3P30 AG021677-02S1. We thank the NINDS NET-PD Investigators for the high-quality data collected in NET-PD FS1 and FS-TOO. The authors wish to acknowledge Barbara C. Tilley and Jay S. Schneider for their contributions to a poster presentation made at the 35th Annual Meeting of the Society for Clinical Trials (SCT), Philadelphia, Pennsylvania, 18–21 May 2014. Part of the materials in this study are contained within that poster.

Author Contributions: C.Y. conceived and designed the study, analyzed the data, and wrote the paper; K.E.V. contributed to conceiving the study and interpreting the results, and performed critical revision of the drafts.

References

1. Teresi, J.A.; Fleishman, J.A. Differential item functioning and health assessment. *Qual. Life Res.* **2007**, *16* (Suppl. 1), 33–42. [CrossRef] [PubMed]
2. Randolph, C.; Tierney, M.C.; Mohr, E.; Chase, T.N. The Repeatable Battery for the Assessment of Neuropsychological Status (RBANS): Preliminary Clinical Validity. *J. Clin. Exp. Neuropsychol.* **1998**, *20*, 310–319. [CrossRef] [PubMed]
3. NINDS NET-PD Investigators. A randomized, double-blind, futility clinical trial of creatine and minocycline in early Parkinson disease. *Neurology* **2006**, *66*, 664–671.
4. NINDS NET-PD Investigators. A randomized clinical trial of coenzyme Q10 and GPI-1485 in early Parkinson disease. *Neurology* **2007**, *68*, 20–28.
5. Xu, Y.; Lu, Z. Assessment and treatment of cognitive dysfunction in schizophrenia patient. *World Clin. Drugs* **2016**, *37*, 8–12.
6. Nakatsu, D.; Fukuhara, T.; Chaytor, N.S.; Phatak, V.S.; Avellino, A.M. Repeatable Battery for the Assessment of Neuropsychological Status (RBANS) as a Cognitive Evaluation Tool for Patients with Normal Pressure Hydrocephalus. *Neurol. Med. Chir.* **2016**, *56*, 51–61. [CrossRef] [PubMed]
7. Costaggiu, D.; Ortu, F.; Pinna, E.; Serchisu, L.; di Martino, M.L.; Manconi, P.E.; Mandas, A. RBANS: A valid tool for cognitive assessment of HIV-infected people on cART. *G. Gerontol.* **2015**, *63*, 268–273.
8. Carlozzi, N.E.; Horner, M.D.; Yang, C.; Tilley, B.C. Factor Analysis of the Repeatable Battery for the Assessment of Neuropsychological Status. *Appl. Neuropsychol.* **2008**, *15*, 274–279. [CrossRef] [PubMed]
9. Duff, K.; Langbehn, D.R.; Schoenberg, M.R.; Moser, D.J.; Baade, L.E.; Mold, J.; Scott, J.G.; Adams, R.L. Examining the Repeatable Battery for the Assessment of Neuropsychological Status: Factor Analytic Studies in an Elderly Sample. *Am. J. Geriatr. Psychiatry* **2006**, *14*, 976–979. [CrossRef] [PubMed]
10. Garcia, C.; Leahy, B.; Corradi, K.; Forchetti, C. Component Structure of the Repeatable Battery for the Assessment of Neuropsychological Status in Dementia. *Arch. Clin. Neuropsychol.* **2008**, *23*, 63–72. [CrossRef] [PubMed]
11. Torrence, N.D.; John, S.E.; Gavett, B.E.; O'Bryant, S.E. An Empirical Comparison of Competing Factor Structures for the Repeatable Battery for the Assessment of Neuropsychological Status: A Project Frontier Study. *Arch. Clin. Neuropsychol.* **2016**, *31*, 88–96. [CrossRef] [PubMed]
12. Vogt, E.M.; Prichett, G.D.; Hoelzle, J.B. Invariant Two-Component Structure of the Repeatable Battery for the Assessment of Neuropsychological Status (RBANS). *Appl. Neuropsychol. Adult* **2017**, *24*, 50–64. [CrossRef] [PubMed]

13. Yang, C.; Garrett-Mayer, E.; Schneider, J.S.; Gollomp, S.M.; Tilley, B.C. Repeatable battery for assessment of neuropsychological status in early Parkinson's disease. *Mov. Disord.* **2009**, *24*, 1453–1460. [CrossRef] [PubMed]

14. Wilde, M. The validity of the repeatable battery of neuropsychological status in acute stroke. *Clin. Neuropsychol.* **2006**, *20*, 702–715. [CrossRef] [PubMed]

15. Yang, C.; Schneider, J.; Tilley, B. Fix the left side of an equation: How to rescue positive findings from a clinical trial that used scales if they were wrong?—Illustration with an example. In Proceedings of the 35th Annual Meeting of the Society for Clinical Trials (SCT), Philadelphia, PA, USA, 18–21 May 2014.

16. Faul, F.; Erdfelder, E.; Lang, A.-G.; Buchner, A. G*Power 3: A flexible statistical power analysis program for the social, behavioral, and biomedical sciences. *Behav. Res. Methods* **2007**, *39*, 175–191. [CrossRef] [PubMed]

17. Faul, F.; Erdfelder, E.; Buchner, A.; Lang, A.G. Statistical power analyses using G*Power 3.1: Tests for correlation and regression analyses. *Behav. Res. Methods* **2009**, *41*, 1149–1160. [CrossRef] [PubMed]

18. Jankovic, J.; McDermott, M.; Carter, J.; Gauthier, S.; Goetz, C.; Golbe, L.; Huber, S.; Koller, W.; Olanow, C.; Shoulson, I.; Stern, M. Variable expression of Parkinson's disease: A base-line analysis of the DAT ATOP cohort. *Neurology* **1990**, *40*, 1529–1534. [CrossRef] [PubMed]

19. Cohen, J. Statistical power analysis. *Curr. Dir. Psychol. Sci.* **1992**, *1*, 98–101. [CrossRef]

20. Piantadosi, S. *Clinical Trials: A Methodologic Perspective*, 3th ed.; John Wiley & Sons: Hoboken, NJ, USA, 2017.

21. Nuzzo, R. Scientific method: Statistical errors. *Nature* **2014**, *506*, 150–152. [CrossRef] [PubMed]

22. Ronald, L.W.; Lazar, N.A. The ASA's Statement on *p*-Values: Context, Process, and Purpose. *Am. Stat.* **2016**, *70*, 129–133. [CrossRef]

23. Zumbo, B.D. Validity: Foundational Issues and Statistical Methodology. *Handb. Stat.* **2006**, *26*, 45–79.

24. Haag, D.G.; Peres, K.G.; Balasubramanian, M.; Brennan, D.S. Oral Conditions and Health-Related Quality of Life: A Systematic Review. *J. Dent. Res.* **2017**, *96*, 864–874. [CrossRef] [PubMed]

25. Zumbo, B.D.; Chan, E.K.H. (Eds.) *Validity and Validation in Social, Behavioral, and Health Sciences*; Social Indicators Research Series; Springer: New York, NY, USA, 2014.

26. American Academy of Clinical Neuropsychology (AACN). AACN practice guidelines for neuropsychological assessment and consultation. *Clin. Neuropsychol.* **2007**, *21*, 209–231.

27. American Educational Research Association (AERA); American Psychological Association (APA); National Council on Measurement in Education (NCME). *Standards for Educational and Psychological Testing*; AERA: Washington, DC, USA, 2014.

## 15

Strategies to Engage Adolescents in Digital Health Interventions for Obesity Prevention and Management

Stephanie R. Partridge [1,2,*] [iD] and Julie Redfern [1,3]

1 Faculty of Medicine and Health, Westmead Applied Research Centre, The University of Sydney, Westmead, NSW 2145, Australia; julie.redfern@sydney.edu.au
2 Faculty of Medicine and Health, Sydney School of Public Health, Prevention Research Collaboration, Charles Perkins Centre, The University of Sydney, Camperdown, NSW 2006, Australia
3 The George Institute for Global Health, The University of New South Wales, Camperdown, NSW 2006, Australia
* Correspondence: stephanie.partridge@sydney.edu.au

Abstract: Obesity is one of the greatest health challenges facing today's adolescents. Dietary interventions are the foundation of obesity prevention and management. As adolescents are digital frontrunners and early adopters of technology, digital health interventions appear the most practical modality for dietary behavior change interventions. Despite the rapid growth in digital health interventions, effective engagement with adolescents remains a pertinent issue. Key strategies for effective engagement include co-designing interventions with adolescents, personalization of interventions, and just-in-time adaptation using data from wearable devices. The aim of this paper is to appraise these strategies, which may be used to improve effective engagement and thereby improve the dietary behaviors of adolescents now and in the future.

Keywords: engagement; adolescents; obesity; diet; prevention; management

1. Introduction

The burden of obesity and its related comorbidities is one of the most significant health challenges facing today's youngest generation [1]. In 2016, 18% of the global population of children and adolescents had overweight or obesity and the prevalence of adolescent (10–19 years) overweight and obesity are increasing [2]. Weight gain during adolescence is associated with cardiovascular disease in later life [3,4]. Adolescents who gain weight and maintain a high body mass index (BMI) into adulthood, have higher odds of developing hypertension and systemic inflammation [3,5,6]. Management of obesity during adolescence is challenging as greater than 90% of adolescents with obesity will transition to adulthood remaining overweight or obese [7,8]. This is a significant concern as there are over 1.8 billion young people between the ages of 10 and 24 years, accounting for the largest generation in history [9]. Innovative, contemporary and engaging dietary interventions are needed to prevent and manage overweight and obesity, particularly in adolescents, whose specific needs are often unrecognized by healthcare providers.

Dietary interventions are the foundation of obesity prevention and management. Adolescents need engaging interventions, as they are not achieving dietary intake recommendations. This is concerning as poor nutritional behaviors are linked to one in five deaths, globally [10]. For example, in Australia in 2015, less than 1% of adolescents eat enough vegetables, less than 27% eat enough fruit, and less than 2% eat adequate amounts of high-calcium foods [11]. They were also the highest consumers of convenience foods, such as discretionary foods and sugar-sweetened beverages [12].

Adolescents face exposure to an overabundance of highly palatable convenience foods, which can result in excessive energy intake [13]. Such excess energy intake is often in combination with a decline in physical activity and an increase in sedentary behaviors during the transition from childhood to adolescence, thereby reducing their total energy expenditure [14]. The result is positive energy balance and subsequent weight gain. Weight gains of 1–5 kg per year, in addition to normal adolescent growth, can result from consuming as little as 84–418 kilojoules (kJ) (20–100 kilocalories (kcal)) per day more than expended [15,16]. Despite the debate about optimal macronutrient composition for weight management, national bodies have agreed achieving neutral or negative energy balance is the most critical factor affecting weight maintenance or loss, respectively [17,18]. It is therefore essential adolescents' dietary interventions for both obesity prevention and management are engaging and support sustainable long-term improvements in dietary behaviors.

There has been rapid growth in research using digital technologies for behavior change in the areas of physical activity, sedentary time and diet [19]. Digital behavior change interventions, defined as "a product or service that uses computer technology to promote behavior change" [20], use various technologies for delivery such as websites, social media, text messages, smartphones apps or wearable devices [20–22]. As adolescents are one of the highest users of technology [23], their online digital environment can be congested. It is, therefore, imperative researchers and clinicians are implementing strategies within the design and delivery of their digital health interventions to engage and capture the attention of adolescents effectively.

Given adolescents are technology frontrunners; digital health interventions appear to be a practical modality for dietary behavior change interventions for the prevention obesity [24–26]. We acknowledge digital interventions cannot replace the multifaceted treatment approached required for management of obesity in adolescents [27]. However, digital technologies show potential as an additional tool for weight-loss maintenance following obesity management [28–30]. In this paper we review the evidence supporting effective engagement in digital interventions as a critical factor in the adoption of healthy dietary behaviors in adolescents within the current "digital world" [31]. We then narratively review three key strategies that researchers and clinicians can use to promote engagement and thereby potentially increase the effectiveness of digital dietary interventions for the prevention of obesity and maintenance of weight-loss in adolescents. We selected three strategies, namely, co-design, personalization, and just-in-time adaptation, given the feasibility and practicality of these strategies for both researchers and clinicians working in obesity prevention and management.

2. Adolescents' and Their Digital World

Adolescence is the period of transition between childhood and adulthood, characterized by the complex interplay of biological growth, cognitive development and social role transitions [32,33]. Puberty is a key event in early adolescence resulting in rapid changes in body composition and subsequently dietary requirements [34]. The World Health Organisation (WHO) defines an adolescent as a person aged between 10–19 years [1]. Given the variability in onset and duration of puberty and the changing social environment, it has been suggested 10–24 years maybe more representative of the adolescent period [35]. Regardless, adolescence is a critical life stage to intervene for the establishment of healthy dietary behaviors and to ensure overall health and lower mortality risks in later life [7,8].

Inadequate nutrition, during adolescence, may compromise growth and development with long-term consequences, such as overweight and obesity. Adolescents have different nutritional needs according to their age, gender, stage of physical maturity and level of physical activity, however, requirements for all nutrients increases dramatically during puberty [36]. During adolescence, total energy (kilojoule, kJ), protein and some micronutrient requirements are lower than that of adults. However, per kilogram (kg) relative to their total body size, energy, macronutrients and micronutrients requirements are higher than that of adults [36]. Similarly, per kJ relative to their total energy requirements, macronutrients and micronutrients requirements are also higher than that of adults [36]. For example, boys aged 13 years usually require 29 milligrams (mg) of calcium per kg of body weight, compared to adult males, who need only 14 mg of calcium per kg of body weight [37]. It essential during this time of growth adolescents are consuming a nutrient dense diet and are forming healthy dietary behaviors and developing weight regulation strategies to carry forward into adulthood.

Engaging adolescents in obesity prevention or management programs to improve their dietary behaviors remains a crucial challenge. Adolescence is often a busy life stage. Along with school, adolescents' schedules can include additional activities such as study, extracurricular activities, part-time work and social events, all of which can complicate recruitment and engagement efforts. Current attrition rates for obesity management in children and adolescents are highly variable, suggesting between 27% and 73% of participants drop out of interventions [38]. There is emerging evidence suggesting researchers and clinicians need to initially engage adolescents by using positively framed messaging [39,40] with preferred weight terminology [41], as the stigma associated with being overweight or obese is a significant barrier for adolescents to seek out health services. Also, it is important to prioritize accessibility and enjoyment in the design phase of dietary interventions [39]. Digital technologies for obesity prevention and management can play a key role in addressing accessibly and enjoyment for adolescents, as well as to widely distribute positive messages to recruit adolescents.

The ubiquitous infiltration of technology in the lives of adolescents offers a potential opportunity for capitalizing on digital technology as a feasible and acceptable modality for dietary interventions to prevent and manage obesity. The current generation of adolescents ('Generation Z'), i.e., those born after 1995, are creating the most global youth culture in history and most have access to similar digital technologies. In Australia, over 90% of adolescents aged 14–17 years own a mobile phone, and 94% of those own a smartphone [42]. Adolescent smartphone ownership in Australia is higher than that of their counterparts in the United States (73%) and United Kingdom (69%) [42]. In developed countries, 83% of adolescents go online three or more times per day, text messaging is their primary form of mobile phone communication and they are one of the highest users of social media and smartphone applications ('apps') [23]. Digital health interventions for overweight and obesity in adolescents can result in improvements in BMI and lifestyle outcomes, including dietary behaviors, in the short-term (less than 6-months) [43–45]. Thus, adolescents are immersed in a 'digital world' and given the emerging short-term evidence this is likely to offer a further opportunity for incorporating dietary interventions into digital technologies.

3. Three Strategies for Effective Engagement with Digital Intervention

Effective engagement with digital health interventions is essential for effective behavior change. The complexity of engagement with digital interventions, which target various health-related behaviors has led to different conceptual models. A recent systematic review by Perski et al. [46], synthesized the literature on engagement and developed a conceptual framework of direct and indirect influences on engagement with digital health interventions. Moreover, in a recent publication by Yardley et al. [47], the authors presented a figure to conceptualize the closely linked and mediating relationship between engagement with digital technology and behavior change, at both micro and macro levels. In addition, Yardley and colleagues present a range of available methods to measure effective engagement [47]. Despite the current challenges about how to best define and measure engagement with digital health interventions [46,47], experts agree that effective intervention design requires a user-centered and iterative approach [47,48]. As well, researchers have identified behavior change techniques embedded within adolescent obesity prevention and management interventions which may contribute to effectiveness [40]. Considering this, we will now examine three strategies to increase effective engagement with digital health interventions to improve dietary behaviors. These interacting, user-centered strategies are co-design, personalization, and just-in-time adaptation. We present a conceptual illustration of these three strategies in Figure 1.

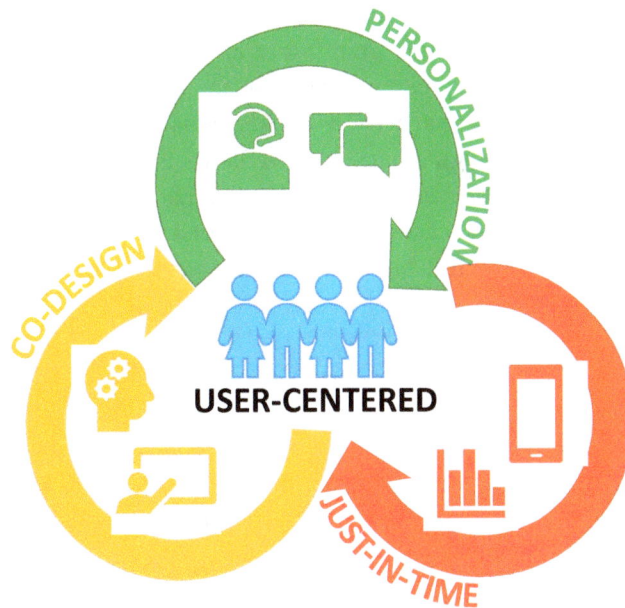

Figure 1. A conceptual illustration of the interaction between the three user-centered strategies, namely, co-design, personalization, and just-in-time adaptation.

3.1. Co-Design

Co-design or participatory design in public health is defined as the systematic co-creation, with those affected by the issues being studied, for the purpose of developing new strategies, programs, policies [49,50]. Co-design is an umbrella term used to describe the array of approaches that can be utilized to engage the end-users (i.e., those affected by the issue being studied) or other stakeholders in the research process [49]. Ideally co-design can be thought of as the 'golden thread' that runs through all stages of research, from design to implementation in real-world settings. It is the collective sum or a framework of these approaches which constitutes co-design, not the use of individual methods in isolation, such as focus groups or interviews [51]. However, given the rapid pace of digital technology development, and short research funding cycles, researchers and clinicians are using commercial apps for adolescent weight management that do not include evidence-based strategies and have not been co-designed with adolescents [52,53]. Considering adolescents are digital frontrunners, their lack of input into technologies to manage their own health and wellbeing is likely to result in ineffective levels of engagement.

Available frameworks [51] and findings from co-design research in adolescent mental health and primary care can guide the development of digital health interventions to address effective engagement with adolescent obesity prevention and management interventions. Two recent Australian research studies have described a co-design process to develop apps to improve young people's experience of seeing their general practitioner [54] and for self-monitoring and management mood symptoms in adolescents with depression [55]. A similarity of both studies throughout the co-design process was the identification of contrasting needs, motivations and intentions for the apps between researchers, clinicians, and adolescents [54,55]. However, the co-design method facilitated a process of mutual learning of each group's needs and expectations, with the emphasis on designing from the perspectives of the adolescent ('end user').

Two recent studies utilize co-design approaches for the development of digital technologies to address adolescent overweight and obesity [56,57]. Through a co-design process to develop a smartphone app to support weight and health management, Rivera et al. [56] were able to identify adolescents require personalized assistance with meal planning, including more convenient and efficient ways to plan meals and make healthier food choices throughout the day. This feature is not available in current commercial apps, which predominately focus on self-monitoring and caloric monitoring of food intake [58]. Moreover, Standoli et al. [57] found adolescents were interested in monitoring their daily activities by using wearable devices or clothing. However, the short lifespan of currently available commercial activity trackers was a significant barrier. The researchers and adolescents were able to co-design smart clothing items to monitor daily activities that were acceptable, personalized and met the needs of adolescents. Thus, these examples, albeit limited to smartphone apps, show co-design increases the likelihood of acceptable digital health technologies and subsequently may result in effective engagement in future interventions in both research and real-world settings.

3.2. Personalization

Personalization or tailoring is a common theme that emerges in the co-design process and also is a key component of effective dietary interventions [59,60]. Personalization in dietary interventions and healthcare in general, goes beyond recommending population-based guidelines to using such guidelines to develop individualized management plans [61]. As alluded to in our introduction, personalization is a key feature of the multifaceted face-to-face treatment approach required for management of obesity in adolescents [27,62]. At the present time, such personalization for obesity management is unlikely to be replicated fully in digital interventions. However, semi-personalization is presently achievable within digital interventions for obesity prevention and weight-loss maintenance following obesity management [63]. Digital interventions, such as text messaging programs, can provide semi-personalized messages to positively change individual lifestyle behaviors [64]. Large populations of people can also be targeted simultaneously, as text messages are a low-cost, convenient, and scalable method of health communication.

As text messaging remains a primary form of communication between adolescents, semi-personalized text messages, constructed carefully in collaboration with adolescents, have been shown to be a feasible and acceptable form of communication for obesity interventions [63,65,66]. High-quality evidence for the effect of text messages on BMI in both overweight and obesity adolescent populations is lacking [24,26]. The findings from two randomized controlled trials provide insights about the role of semi-personalized text messages in changing dietary behaviors and subsequently reducing in BMI. The multicomponent mobile health study in young adults by Allman-Farinelli et al. [67,68], used eight weekly motivational text messages based on the Transtheoretical Model of Behavior Change, whereby messages matched the stage-of-change for each lifestyle behavior at baseline. Text messages were delivered in conjunction with health coaching calls, a website and smartphone apps. Young adults in the intervention group weighed 3.7 kg (95% confidence interval (CI) -6.1, -1.3) less at 3-months, and 4.7 kg (95% CI -6.9, -1.8) less at 9 months [67] compared to their control counterparts. Further, intervention participants consumed more vegetables ($p = 0.009$), fewer sugary soft drinks ($p = 0.002$), and fewer energy-dense takeout meals ($p = 0.001$) compared to controls [68]. The process evaluation from the study found intervention participants valued the text messages and found the text messages increased their overall engagement with the program [69]. The study by Chow et al. used a multistep, iterative, mixed methods process with heart disease patients to develop text messages that provide semi-personalized information, motivation, and support to meet national guidelines for heart disease. Intervention participants significantly reduced their BMI at 6-months (-1.3 kg m^{-2} (95% CI -1.6, -0.9, $p < 0.001$) [22]. Moreover, a significantly higher proportion of intervention participants adhered to greater than four dietary guideline recommendations compared to the control group (93% vs. 75%, $p < 0.001$) [70]. Patients reported the semi-personalized text messages increased engagement and supported their behavior change [21]. Further research is required to see if the two semi-personalized text messages examples presented here can be applied to prevention of obesity or for weight-loss maintenance following obesity management in adolescent populations.

3.3. Just-in-Time-Adaptation

Just-in-time adaptive interventions are a form of personalized interventions that provide support relevant to an individual's changing behaviors and contexts over time [71]. The overall goal is to provide instantaneous contextual support for the targeted behaviors when the individual is most likely to be receptive. Just-in-time adaptive interventions use sensory data, e.g., a smartphone or smartwatch and momentary information directly from participants, e.g., ecological momentary assessments (EMAs), to send personalized feedback on targeted behaviors [72]. In these interventions, text messages commonly communicate the behavioral feedback. A recent systematic literature review of just-in-time-interventions found behavioral feedback that was always available, personalized, and practical resulted in significant positive behavioral changes [73].

Only a few studies have been conducted, which describing the potential role of interactive digital health interventions for adolescents [72,74]. One example is the KNOWME study, by Spruijt-Metz and colleagues, which demonstrated the feasibility and acceptability of a just-in-time adaptive intervention for overweight adolescents [72,75]. KNOWME study aimed to reduce sedentary behavior and promote physical activity. The pilot study showed adolescents decreased their sedentary time by 170.8 min per week compared to baseline ($p < 0.01$) and physical activity levels measured via accelerometers were found to be significantly higher after receiving text messages with feedback from the research team ($p < 0.01$) [72]. Pilot research by Garcia et al. [76] developed a feasible youth EMAs via a two-way text message system to collect information on daily activities, behaviors, and attitudes among adolescents. Adolescents live in an instantaneous and fast-paced digital environment. Therefore, such interventions show significant potential.

4. Conclusions

Engagement with digital health interventions is an important mediating factor to improve dietary behaviors and prevent and manage obesity in adolescents. The rapid development and diffusion of digital health interventions for adolescents has resulted in few interventions that are co-designed with end-users, personalized and provide real-time feedback. Incorporating such strategies may optimize the levels of engagement adolescents have with digital health interventions to improve their dietary behaviors. Strategies to increase engagement are not limited to those discussed in this narrative review. There are several other strategies that have the potential to increase engagement with digital interventions in other populations with different needs. Given the emerging body of evidence suggesting effective engagement with digital health interventions can mediate positive behavioral change, research efforts should be focused on incorporating engagement strategies throughout the research process and as well in real-world scaled up digital health interventions and programs.

Author Contributions: S.R.P. conceived the idea for the review and wrote the manuscript. J.R. provided supervision and mentoring in the form of discussions about the content and order of the review, as well as key ideas on areas of literature to include.

Funding: This research received no external funding.

Acknowledgments: J.R. is funded by a National Health and Medical Research Council Career Development Fellowship.

References

1. World Health Organization. Health for the World's Adolescents: A Second Chance in the Second Decade. Available online: http://apps.who.int/adolescent/second-decade/ (accessed on 12 December 2017).
2. Ng, M.; Fleming, T.; Robinson, M.; Thomson, B.; Graetz, N.; Margono, C.; Mullany, E.C.; Biryukov, S.; Abbafati, C.; Abera, S.F.; et al. Global, regional, and national prevalence of overweight and obesity in children and adults during 1980–2013: A systematic analysis for the global burden of disease study 2013. *Lancet* **2014**, *384*, 766–781. [CrossRef]

3.   Attard, S.M.; Herring, A.H.; Howard, A.G.; Gordon-Larsen, P. Longitudinal trajectories of BMI and cardiovascular disease risk: The national longitudinal study of adolescent health. *Obesity* **2013**, *21*, 2180–2188. [CrossRef] [PubMed]

4.   Doak, C.M.; Visscher, T.L.; Renders, C.M.; Seidell, J.C. The prevention of overweight and obesity in children and adolescents: A review of interventions and programmes. *Obes. Rev.* **2006**, *7*, 111–136. [CrossRef] [PubMed]

5.   Adams, K.F.; Leitzmann, M.F.; Ballard-Barbash, R.; Albanes, D.; Harris, T.B.; Hollenbeck, A.; Kipnis, V. Body mass and weight change in adults in relation to mortality risk. *Am. J. Epidemiol.* **2014**, *179*, 135–144. [CrossRef] [PubMed]

6.   Zheng, Y.; Manson, J.E.; Yuan, C.; Liang, M.H.; Grodstein, F.; Stampfer, M.J.; Willett, W.C.; Hu, F.B. Associations of weight gain from early to middle adulthood with major health outcomes later in life. *JAMA* **2017**, *318*, 255–269. [CrossRef] [PubMed]

7.   Gordon-Larsen, P.; Adair, L.S.; Nelson, M.C.; Popkin, B.M. Five-year obesity incidence in the transition period between adolescence and adulthood: The national longitudinal study of adolescent health. *Am. J. Clin. Nutr.* **2004**, *80*, 569–575. [PubMed]

8.   Patton, G.C.; Coffey, C.; Sawyer, S.M.; Viner, R.M.; Haller, D.M.; Bose, K.; Vos, T.; Ferguson, J.; Mathers, C.D. Global patterns of mortality in young people: A systematic analysis of population health data. *Lancet* **2009**, *374*, 881–892. [CrossRef]

9.   UNFPA. *The Power of 1.8 Billion—Adolescents, Youth, and the Transformation of the Future*; The United Nations Population Fund: New York, NY, USA, 2014.

10.   Forouzanfar, M.H.; Alexander, L.; Anderson, H.R.; Bachman, V.F.; Biryukov, S.; Brauer, M.; Burnett, R.; Casey, D.; Coates, M.M.; Cohen, A.; et al. Global, regional, and national comparative risk assessment of 79 behavioural, environmental and occupational, and metabolic risks or clusters of risks in 188 countries, 1990–2013: A systematic analysis for the global burden of disease study 2013. *Lancet* **2015**, *386*, 2287–2323. [CrossRef]

11.   Australian Bureau of Statistics. 4324.0.55.002—Microdata: Australian Health Survey: Nutrition and Physical Activity. Available online: http://bit.ly/2jkRRZO (accessed on 1 April 2017).

12.   Hardy, L.L.; Mihrshahi, S.; Drayton, B.A.; Bauman, A. *NSW Schools Physical Activity and Nutrition Survey (SPANS) 2015: Full Report*; NSW Department of Health: Sydney, Australia, 2016.

13.   Powell, L.M.; Szczypka, G.; Chaloupka, F.J. Trends in exposure to television food advertisements among children and adolescents in the united states. *Arch. Pediatr. Adolesc. Med.* **2010**, *164*, 794–802. [CrossRef] [PubMed]

14.   Pearson, N.; Braithwaite, R.E.; Biddle, S.J.H.; van Sluijs, E.M.F.; Atkin, A.J. Associations between sedentary behaviour and physical activity in children and adolescents: A meta-analysis. *Obes. Rev.* **2014**, *15*, 666–675. [CrossRef] [PubMed]

15.   Vandevijvere, S.; Chow, C.C.; Hall, K.D.; Umali, E.; Swinburn, B.A. Increased food energy supply as a major driver of the obesity epidemic: A global analysis. *Bull. World Health Organ.* **2015**, *93*, 446–456. [CrossRef] [PubMed]

16.   Hill, J.O. Can a small-changes approach help address the obesity epidemic? A report of the joint task force of the American society for nutrition, institute of food technologists, and international food information council. *Am. J. Clin. Nutr.* **2009**, *89*, 477–484. [CrossRef] [PubMed]

17.   Seagle, H.M.; Strain, G.W.; Makris, A.; Reeves, R.S. Position of the American Dietetic Association: Weight management. *J. Am. Diet. Assoc.* **2009**, *109*, 330–346. [PubMed]

18.   National Health and Medical Research Council. *Clinical Practice Guidelines for the Management of Overweight and Obesity in Adults, Adolescents and Children in Australia*; National Health and Medical Research Council: Melbourne, Australia, 2013.

19.   Müller, A.M.; Maher, C.A.; Vandelanotte, C.; Hingle, M.; Middelweerd, A.; Lopez, M.L.; DeSmet, A.; Short, C.E.; Nathan, N.; Hutchesson, M.J.; et al. Physical activity, sedentary behavior, and diet-related eHealth and mHealth Research: Bibliometric analysis. *J. Med. Int. Res.* **2018**, *20*. [CrossRef] [PubMed]

20.   Michie, S.; Yardley, L.; West, R.; Patrick, K.; Greaves, F. Developing and evaluating digital interventions to promote behavior change in health and health care: Recommendations resulting from an international workshop. *J. Med. Int. Res.* **2017**, *19*, e232. [CrossRef] [PubMed]

21. Redfern, J.; Santo, K.; Coorey, G.; Thakkar, J.; Hackett, M.; Thiagalingam, A.; Chow, C.K. Factors influencing engagement, perceived usefulness and behavioral mechanisms associated with a text message support program. *PLoS ONE* **2016**, *11*, e0163929. [CrossRef] [PubMed]

22. Chow, C.K.; Redfern, J.; Hillis, G.S.; Thakkar, J.; Santo, K.; Hackett, M.L.; Jan, S.; Graves, N.; de Keizer, L.; Barry, T.; et al. Effect of lifestyle-focused text messaging on risk factor modification in patients with coronary heart disease: A randomized clinical trial. *JAMA* **2015**, *314*, 1255–1263. [CrossRef] [PubMed]

23. Lenhart, A.; Duggan, M.; Perrin, A.; Stepler, R.; Rainie, H.; Parker, K. Teens, Social Media & Technology Overview. Available online: http://www.pewinternet.org/2015/04/09/teens-social-media-technology-2015/# (accessed on 6 December 2017).

24. Rose, T.; Barker, M.; Maria Jacob, C.; Morrison, L.; Lawrence, W.; Strommer, S.; Vogel, C.; Woods-Townsend, K.; Farrell, D.; Inskip, H.; et al. A systematic review of digital interventions for improving the diet and physical activity behaviors of adolescents. *J. Adolesc. Health* **2017**. [CrossRef] [PubMed]

25. Miller, M.; Damarell, R.; Bell, L.; Moores, C.; Miller, J. *Community-Based Approaches to Adolescent Obesity*; Sax Institute: Ultimo, Australia, 2017.

26. Keating, S.R.; McCurry, M.K. Systematic review of text messaging as an intervention for adolescent obesity. *J. Am. Assoc. Nurse Pract.* **2015**, *27*, 714–720. [CrossRef] [PubMed]

27. Steinbeck, K.S.; Lister, N.B.; Gow, M.L.; Baur, L.A. Treatment of adolescent obesity. *Nat. Rev. Endocrinol.* **2018**, *14*, 331–344. [CrossRef] [PubMed]

28. Lee, J.; Piao, M.; Byun, A.; Kim, J. A systematic review and meta-analysis of intervention for pediatric obesity using mobile technology. *Stud. Health Technol. Inf.* **2016**, *225*, 491–494.

29. Chaplais, E.; Naughton, G.; Thivel, D.; Courteix, D.; Greene, D. Smartphone interventions for weight treatment and behavioral change in pediatric obesity: A systematic review. *Telemed. J. E Health* **2015**, *21*, 822–830. [CrossRef] [PubMed]

30. Wickham, C.A.; Carbone, E.T. Who's calling for weight loss? A systematic review of mobile phone weight loss programs for adolescents. *Nutr. Rev.* **2015**, *73*, 386–398. [CrossRef] [PubMed]

31. Gibson, A.A.; Sainsbury, A. Strategies to improve adherence to dietary weight loss interventions in research and real-world settings. *Behav. Sci.* **2017**, *7*. [CrossRef]

32. Ahmed, S.P.; Bittencourt-Hewitt, A.; Sebastian, C.L. Neurocognitive bases of emotion regulation development in adolescence. *Dev. Cogn. Neurosci.* **2015**, *15*, 11–25. [CrossRef] [PubMed]

33. Peper, J.S.; Dahl, R.E. Surging hormones: Brain-Behavior interactions during puberty. *Curr. Dir. Psychol. Sci.* **2013**, *22*, 134–139. [CrossRef] [PubMed]

34. Patton, G.C.; Viner, R. Pubertal transitions in health. *Lancet* **2007**, *369*, 1130–1139. [CrossRef]

35. Sawyer, S.M.; Azzopardi, P.S.; Wickremarathne, D.; Patton, G.C. The age of adolescence. *Lancet Child Adolesc. Health* **2018**, *2*, 223–228. [CrossRef]

36. National Health Medical Research Council (NHMRC). *Australian Dietary Guidelines*; NHMRC: Canberra, Australia, 2013.

37. National Health and Medical Research Council. *Nutrient Reference Values for Australia and New Zealand Including Recommended Dietary Intakes*; Commonwealth of Australia: Canberra, Australia, 2006.

38. Skelton, J.A.; Beech, B.M. Attrition in paediatric weight management: A review of the literature and new directions. *Obes. Rev.* **2011**, *12*, e273–e281. [CrossRef] [PubMed]

39. Smith, K.L.; Straker, L.M.; McManus, A.; Fenner, A.A. Barriers and enablers for participation in healthy lifestyle programs by adolescents who are overweight: A qualitative study of the opinions of adolescents, their parents and community stakeholders. *BMC Pediatr.* **2014**, *14*. [CrossRef] [PubMed]

40. Martin, J.; Chater, A.; Lorencatto, F. Effective behaviour change techniques in the prevention and management of childhood obesity. *Int. J. Obes.* **2013**, *37*, 1287–1294. [CrossRef] [PubMed]

41. Puhl, R.M.; Himmelstein, M.S. Adolescent preferences for weight terminology used by health care providers. *Pediatr. Obes.* **2018**. [CrossRef] [PubMed]

42. Roy Morgan Research. Media Release: 9 in 10 Aussie Teens Now Have a Mobile. Available online: http://bit.ly/2bbuoAX (accessed on 20 September 2017).

43. Chen, J.L.; Wilkosz, M.E. Efficacy of technology-based interventions for obesity prevention in adolescents: A systematic review. *Adolesc. Health Med. Ther.* **2014**, *5*, 159–170. [CrossRef] [PubMed]

44. Turner-McGrievy, G.M.; Beets, M.W.; Moore, J.B.; Kaczynski, A.T.; Barr-Anderson, D.J.; Tate, D.F. Comparison of traditional versus mobile app self-monitoring of physical activity and dietary intake among overweight adults participating in an mHealth weight loss program. *J. Am. Med. Inf. Assoc.* **2013**, *20*, 513–518. [CrossRef] [PubMed]

45. Brannon, E.E.; Cushing, C.C. A systematic review: Is there an app for that? Translational science of pediatric behavior change for physical activity and dietary interventions. *J. Pediatr. Psychol.* **2015**, *40*, 373–384. [CrossRef] [PubMed]

46. Perski, O.; Blandford, A.; West, R.; Michie, S. Conceptualising engagement with digital behaviour change interventions: A systematic review using principles from critical interpretive synthesis. *Transl. Behav. Med.* **2017**, *7*, 254–267. [CrossRef] [PubMed]

47. Yardley, L.; Spring, B.J.; Riper, H.; Morrison, L.G.; Crane, D.H.; Curtis, K.; Merchant, G.C.; Naughton, F.; Blandford, A. Understanding and promoting effective engagement with digital behavior change interventions. *Am. J. Prev. Med.* **2016**, *51*, 833–842. [CrossRef] [PubMed]

48. Redfern, J.; Thiagalingam, A.; Jan, S.; Whittaker, R.; Hackett, M.L.; Mooney, J.; De Keizer, L.; Hillis, G.S.; Chow, C.K. Development of a set of mobile phone text messages designed for prevention of recurrent cardiovascular events. *Eur. J. Prev. Cardiol.* **2014**, *21*, 492–499. [CrossRef] [PubMed]

49. Cargo, M.; Mercer, S.L. The value and challenges of participatory research: Strengthening its practice. *Ann. Rev. Public Health* **2008**, *29*, 325–350. [CrossRef] [PubMed]

50. Andersson, N. Community-led trials: Intervention co-design in a cluster randomised controlled trial. *BMC Public Health* **2017**, *17*, 397. [CrossRef] [PubMed]

51. Hagen, P.; Collin, P.; Metcalf, A.; Nicholas, M.; Rahilly, K. *Participatory Design of Evidence-Based Online Youth Mental Health Promotion, Prevention, Early Intervention and Treatment*; Young and Well cooperative Research Centre: Melbourne, Australia, 2012.

52. Rivera, J.; McPherson, A.; Hamilton, J.; Birken, C.; Coons, M.; Iyer, S.; Agarwal, A.; Lalloo, C.; Stinson, J. Mobile apps for weight management: A scoping review. *JMIR mHealth uHealth* **2016**, *4*, e87. [CrossRef] [PubMed]

53. Schoffman, D.E.; Turner-McGrievy, G.; Jones, S.J.; Wilcox, S. Mobile apps for pediatric obesity prevention and treatment, healthy eating, and physical activity promotion: Just fun and games? *Transl. Behav. Med.* **2013**, *3*, 320–325. [CrossRef] [PubMed]

54. Webb, M.J.; Wadley, G.; Sanci, L.A. Improving patient-centered care for young people in general practice with a codesigned screening app: Mixed methods study. *JMIR mHealth uHealth* **2017**, *5*, e118. [CrossRef] [PubMed]

55. Hetrick, S.E.; Robinson, J.; Burge, E.; Blandon, R.; Mobilio, B.; Rice, S.M.; Simmons, M.B.; Alvarez-Jimenez, M.; Goodrich, S.; Davey, C.G. Youth codesign of a mobile phone APP to facilitate self-monitoring and management of mood symptoms in young people with major depression, suicidal ideation, and self-harm. *JMIR Ment. Health* **2018**, *5*, e9. [CrossRef] [PubMed]

56. Rivera, J.; McPherson, A.C.; Hamilton, J.; Birken, C.; Coons, M.; Peters, M.; Iyer, S.; George, T.; Nguyen, C.; Stinson, J. User-centered design of a mobile APP for weight and health management in adolescents with complex health needs: Qualitative study. *JMIR Form. Res.* **2018**, *2*, e7. [CrossRef]

57. Standoli, C.; Guarneri, M.; Perego, P.; Mazzola, M.; Mazzola, A.; Andreoni, G. A smart wearable sensor system for counter-fighting overweight in teenagers. *Sensors* **2016**, *16*, 1220. [CrossRef] [PubMed]

58. Chen, J.; Cade, J.E.; Allman-Farinelli, M. The most popular smartphone Apps for weight loss: A quality assessment. *JMIR mHealth uHealth* **2015**, *3*, e104. [CrossRef] [PubMed]

59. Adamson, A.J.; Mathers, J.C. Effecting dietary change. *Proc. Nutr. Soc.* **2004**, *63*, 537–547. [CrossRef] [PubMed]

60. Eyles, H.C.; Mhurchu, C.N. Does tailoring make a difference? A systematic review of the long-term effectiveness of tailored nutrition education for adults. *Nutr. Rev.* **2009**, *67*, 464–480. [CrossRef] [PubMed]

61. De Roos, B.; Brennan, L. Personalised interventions-a precision approach for the next generation of dietary intervention studies. *Nutrients* **2017**, *9*. [CrossRef] [PubMed]

62. Steinbeck, K.; Baur, L.; Cowell, C.; Pietrobelli, A. Clinical research in adolescents: Challenges and opportunities using obesity as a model. *Int. J. Obes.* **2008**, *33*, 2–7. [CrossRef] [PubMed]

63. Nguyen, B.; Shrewsbury, V.A.; O'Connor, J.; Steinbeck, K.S.; Hill, A.J.; Shah, S.; Kohn, M.R.; Torvaldsen, S.; Baur, L.A. Two-year outcomes of an adjunctive telephone coaching and electronic contact intervention for adolescent weight-loss maintenance: The Loozit randomized controlled trial. *Int. J. Obes.* **2013**, *37*, 468–472. [CrossRef] [PubMed]

64. Armanasco, A.A.; Miller, Y.D.; Fjeldsoe, B.S.; Marshall, A.L. Preventive health behavior change text message interventions: A meta-analysis. *Am. J. Prev. Med.* **2017**, *52*, 391–402. [CrossRef] [PubMed]

65. Woolford, S.J.; Barr, K.L.; Derry, H.A.; Jepson, C.M.; Clark, S.J.; Strecher, V.J.; Resnicow, K. OMG do not say LOL: Obese adolescents' perspectives on the content of text messages to enhance weight loss efforts. *Obesity* **2011**, *19*, 2382–2387. [CrossRef] [PubMed]

66. Woolford, S.J.; Clark, S.J.; Strecher, V.J.; Resnicow, K. Tailored mobile phone text messages as an adjunct to obesity treatment for adolescents. *J. Telemed. Telecare* **2010**, *16*, 458–461. [CrossRef] [PubMed]

67. Allman-Farinelli, M.; Partridge, S.R.; McGeechan, K.; Balestracci, K.; Hebden, L.; Wong, A.; Phongsavan, P.; Denney-Wilson, E.; Harris, M.F.; Bauman, A. A mobile health lifestyle program for prevention of weight gain in young adults (TXT2BFiT): Nine-Month outcomes of a randomized controlled trial. *JMIR mHealth uHealth* **2016**, *4*, e78. [CrossRef] [PubMed]

68. Partridge, S.R.; McGeechan, K.; Hebden, L.; Balestracci, K.; Wong, A.T.; Denney-Wilson, E.; Harris, M.F.; Phongsavan, P.; Bauman, A.; Allman-Farinelli, M. Effectiveness of a mHealth lifestyle program with telephone support (TXT2BFiT) to prevent unhealthy weight gain in young adults: Randomized controlled trial. *JMIR mHealth uHealth* **2015**, *3*, e66. [CrossRef] [PubMed]

69. Partridge, S.R.; Allman-Farinelli, M.; McGeechan, K.; Balestracci, K.; Wong, A.T.; Hebden, L.; Harris, M.F.; Bauman, A.; Phongsavan, P. Process evaluation of TXT2BFiT: A multi-component mHealth randomised controlled trial to prevent weight gain in young adults. *Int. J. Behav. Nutr. Phys. Act.* **2016**, *13*, 7. [CrossRef] [PubMed]

70. Santo, K.; Hyun, K.; de Keizer, L.; Thiagalingam, A.; Hillis, G.S.; Chalmers, J.; Redfern, J.; Chow, C.K. The effects of a lifestyle-focused text-messaging intervention on adherence to dietary guideline recommendations in patients with coronary heart disease: An analysis of the TEXT ME study. *Int. J. Behav. Nutr. Phys. Act.* **2018**, *15*, 45. [CrossRef] [PubMed]

71. Nahum-Shani, I.; Smith, S.N.; Spring, B.J.; Collins, L.M.; Witkiewitz, K.; Tewari, A.; Murphy, S.A. Just-in-time adaptive interventions (JITAIs) in mobile health: Key components and design principles for ongoing health behavior support. *Ann. Behav. Med.* **2018**, *52*, 446–462. [CrossRef] [PubMed]

72. Spruijt-Metz, D.; Wen, C.K.; O'Reilly, G.; Li, M.; Lee, S.; Emken, B.A.; Mitra, U.; Annavaram, M.; Ragusa, G.; Narayanan, S. Innovations in the use of interactive technology to support weight management. *Curr. Obes. Rep.* **2015**, *4*, 510–519. [CrossRef] [PubMed]

73. Schembre, S.M.; Liao, Y.; Robertson, M.C.; Dunton, G.F.; Kerr, J.; Haffey, M.E.; Burnett, T.; Basen-Engquist, K.; Hicklen, R.S. Just-in-Time feedback in diet and physical activity interventions: Systematic review and practical design framework. *J. Med. Int. Res.* **2018**, *20*, e106. [CrossRef] [PubMed]

74. Turner, T.; Spruijt-Metz, D.; Wen, C.K.; Hingle, M.D. Prevention and treatment of pediatric obesity using mobile and wireless technologies: A systematic review. *Pediatr. Obes.* **2015**, *10*, 403–409. [CrossRef] [PubMed]

75. Emken, B.A.; Li, M.; Thatte, G.; Lee, S.; Annavaram, M.; Mitra, U.; Narayanan, S.; Spruijt-Metz, D. Recognition of physical activities in overweight Hispanic youth using KNOWME Networks. *J. Phys. Act. Health* **2012**, *9*, 432–441. [CrossRef] [PubMed]

76. Garcia, C.; Hardeman, R.R.; Kwon, G.; Lando-King, E.; Zhang, L.; Genis, T.; Brady, S.S.; Kinder, E. Teenagers and texting: Use of a youth ecological momentary assessment system in trajectory health research with latina adolescents. *JMIR mHealth uHealth* **2014**, *2*, e3. [CrossRef] [PubMed]

## 16

The Healthfulness of Entrées and Students' Purchases in a University Campus Dining Environment

Krista Leischner [1], Lacey Arneson McCormack [1], Brian C. Britt [2], Greg Heiberger [3] and Kendra Kattelmann [1,*]

[1] Health & Nutritional Sciences Department, South Dakota State University, Brookings, SD 57007, USA; Krista.leischner@gmail.com (K.L.); Lacey.McCormack@sdstate.edu (L.A.M.)

[2] Journalism & Mass Communications Department, South Dakota State University, Brookings, SD 57007, USA; Brian.Britt@sdstate.edu

[3] Biology & Microbiology, South Dakota State University, Brookings, SD 57007, USA; Greg.Heiberger@sdstate.edu

* Correspondence: Kendra.Kattelmann@sdstate.edu

Abstract: The purpose of this study is to determine the availability of "more healthful" (MH) versus "less healthful" (LH) entrée items in the campus dining and if students' purchases are reflective of what is offered. This is an observational study in which purchases of the available entrée items in the campus dining at South Dakota State University in one academic year were collected and categorized as either MH or LH according to the American Heart Association guidelines. Chi-square tests were used to determine the differences between the proportion of purchased MH and LH versus those available. Odds ratio estimates with 95% confidence limits were used to determine the associations between the demographics and MH and LH purchases. Of the total entrée items available, 15.0% were MH and 85.0% were LH. In the fall, 8.0% of purchases were MH and 92.0% purchases were LH as compared to 8.9% MH and 91.1% LH in the spring. Whites were less likely than non-whites to purchase a MH entrée. Females were two times more likely to choose MH entrées than males. The campus dining offerings and students' purchases of entrees were primarily LH. Work with campus dining providers to create profitable, yet healthful, dining entrees is needed to improve the healthfulness of offerings.

Keywords: campus dining; food purchases; food environment; university dining environment; more healthful; less healthful

1. Introduction

Obesity has reached record levels and presents a major public health threat. Roughly one in three people nationally in the Unites States are currently obese, and the bodyweight of an average American adult is increasing at a rate of 0.9 kg (1.98 lbs.) per year [1,2]. An obese adult is defined as one with a body mass index (BMI) of greater than or equal to 30; BMI is measured by the ratio of mass in kilograms to height in meters squared [3]. Adult obesity is related to severe health consequences. This disease is detrimental to one's current health and also leads to complications in future well-being. Possible chronic health concerns resulting from obesity include stroke, sleep apnea, coronary heart disease, hypertension, type 2 diabetes, and dyslipidemia [3,4].

Unhealthy behaviors, such as decreased physical activity levels, increased sedentary time, and poor dietary intake develop during childhood and can continue through adolescence into adulthood [5]. A significant proportion of obese adults were previously obese as young adults (18–25 years) [5,6]. Moreover, young adults who attend college have been shown to gain between 1.8

and 4.1 kg (3.96–9.03 lbs.) annually [1]. Unhealthy weight gain can occur as a result of fluctuations in eating and exercise habits. The often stressful transition from home to college for many young adults can trigger alterations from a normally healthy lifestyle routine to one that promotes the onset of obesity [7]. Such lifestyle modifications, influenced by environmental, occupational, and behavioral changes typically include increased academic stress, increased alcohol intake, decreased physical activity, irregular sleep patterns, and poor dietary behaviors [7,8]. When combined with personal and environmental barriers, these lifestyle modifications can increase one's risk for the development of obesity. Personal barriers may include a student's lack of self-control when eating and a lack of motivation to increase healthful habits. An environmental barrier and the focus of this research, is the college dining environment and its relationship with unhealthful food purchases and dietary behaviors of students.

Elements common to the campus dining environment that may negatively affect dietary behaviors include a lack of availability to, and increased prices of, healthful food options and required campus meal plans [9,10]. On-campus dining facilities often offer meal options that cater toward students' busy school, social, work schedules, and food preferences; thus, many of these options include fast and convenient type foods. Although campus dining can be quick and easy, all too often, unhealthy fast food, oversized portions, and "all-you-can-eat" options are the norm [9,10]. Understandably, this environment can lead to excess energy consumption [10].

While previous studies have linked excess energy consumption to college student weight gain, little is known about the availability of less healthful foods and student purchases. Therefore, the purpose of this study is to determine the healthfulness of the entrée items and purchases of students in the campus dining environment. It is hypothesized that a higher availability of unhealthy foods will reflect a greater percentage of unhealthy foods purchased.

2. Materials and Methods

2.1. Study Design

This observational study was completed at South Dakota State University and used students' identification (ID) card data, which included demographic and food item purchasing information from the 2014–2015 school year. This study was conducted according to the guidelines laid down in the Declaration of Helsinki and all procedures involving human subjects were approved by Institutional Review Board, Human Subjects Committee at the university. The study was deemed exempt as the data was collected in a method that human subjects could not be identified, directly or through identifiers linked to the subjects.

First- and second-year college students were required to live in on-campus housing and purchase a campus dining meal plan. Students individually chose their meal plans at the beginning of the school year and used their student ID cards to make all on-campus food purchases during the fall 2014 and spring 2015 semesters; therefore, the data collected from the student ID cards were used to determine entrée purchases through the school year.

Permanent addresses of students were used to determine the degree of rurality of their home living environment. Students' zip codes were converted to counties using "Complete Zip Code Totals File" from the United States Census Bureau [11]. Each county was then assigned a Rural-Urban Continuum Code (RUCC) of one through nine, based on the population and proximity to a metro area. Counties assigned an RUCC of 8 or 9 were considered "completely rural or less than 2500 urban population and adjacent to a metro area" and "completely rural or less than 2500 urban population and not adjacent to a metro area", respectively. Due to the low degree of urbanization around the university where this data was collected, for the purposes of this study, RUCCs 8 and 9 were considered "completely rural" and RUCCs 1–7 were considered "not as rural". International students were excluded from the study, as their residences could not be assigned an RUCC.

The gender, race, and ethnicity data used in this study were obtained from the Integrated Postsecondary Education Data System (IPEDS) and included gender, Alaskan Native, American Indian, Asian, Black or African American, White, Hispanic or Latino, Multi-Racial, and Unknown. Due to the low frequency of American Indian, Asian, Black or African American, Hispanic or Latino, Multi-Racial, and Unknown, all were combined and categorized as non-white.

2.2. Food Items

A list of food items available for purchase was obtained from the campus dining provider and classified as entrées, snack foods and side dishes, drinks, or other. This study is limited to entrées that were purchased as individual items in the eating establishments on campus, which included the following categories of foods: Burger, Entrée Salad No Meat, Entrée Salad with Meat, Meat Entrée, Pizza/Calzone, Salad, Sandwiches/Pitas/Flatbreads/Wraps, Soup/Stew/Chili, Tacos/Nachos, and Vegetarian Entrée. A total of 662 food items were included in the final data set. At the time of the study, all but one eating establishment on campus priced entrees individually. The items from the all-you-can-eat cafeteria were not included in this analysis. At the time of the study, the all-you-can-eat-cafeteria, although open to all students, served primarily athletes.

To access nutrition information regarding the dining options on campus, dining services provider recommended the use of MyFitness Pal (MFP). As such, the online nutrient and calorie tracker was used to assign nutritional information to the majority of the food items. Researchers performed a preliminary search using the foodservice provider's name plus the specific food item. For those items that did not have the exact match in MFP, the closest best-fit option was chosen and that nutritional information was assigned to the item. If MFP did not have a close best-fit option available, the nutritional information was obtained from the branded vendor's website. Nutrition information selected for foods was reviewed and approved by a registered dietitian.

Food items were categorized by study personnel as either "more healthful" (MH) if the item met the American Heart Association (AHA) guidelines or "less healthful" (LH) if the item did not. The AHA's "Recommended Nutritional Standards for Procurement of Foods and Beverages Offered in the Workplace" required all entrées to meet the following limits: less than 500 kcal, less than 480 mg sodium, less than 10% saturated fat, and zero grams of trans fat per serving [12].

2.3. Analyses

The number of MH and LH entrées available and frequency purchased in the fall 2014 and spring 2015 semesters was determined. Chi-square tests were used to determine significant differences between the proportion of purchased MH and LH items versus those available during each semester and if the proportion of MH and LH purchases differed between semesters.

A logistic regression was used to determine the relationship between independent variables of demographics of students (completely rural versus not as rural, white versus non-white, and male versus female) and dependent variables of MH and LH purchases in the fall 2014 and spring 2015 semesters. Odds ratio estimates with 95% confidence limits were used to determine the differences between the various demographics and MH and LH purchases in fall versus spring semesters. All analyses were completed in SAS version 9.4 (2012). An alpha level of 0.05 was used for all statistical tests.

3. Results

3.1. Demographics

The individual entrée purchases of 5177 students were analyzed in the fall, while the entrée purchases of 4613 students were analyzed in the spring. Demographics of the students are shown in Table 1.

Table 1. Student demographics in the fall and spring semesters.

Demographic	Fall 2014 (*n* = 5177)	Spring 2015 (*n* = 4613)
	% (*n*)	% (*n*)
Degree of Rurality		
Completely Rural [1]	15.8% (818)	15.4% (712)
Not as Rural [2]	84.2% (4359)	84.6% (3901)
Race and Ethnicity [3]		
White	85.4% (4420)	84.2% (3883)
Non-White	14.6% (757)	15.8% (730)
Gender [3,4]		
Female	52.7% (2600)	52.1% (2249)
Male	47.3% (2334)	47.9% (2068)

[1] Includes students from counties assigned an RUCC of 8 or 9. RUCC 8 = "completely rural or less than 2500 urban population and adjacent to a metro area" and RUCC 9 = "completely rural or less than 2500 urban population and not adjacent to a metro area." [2] Includes students from counties assigned a RUCC of 1–7. RUCC 1–3 = metro counties and RUCCC 4–7 = more than 2500 urban population. [3] Race, ethnicity, and gender were from the Integrated Postsecondary Education Data System. [4] Frequencies differ due to missing data.

3.2. More Healthful versus Less Healthfull Purchases

The number of MH and LH entrée items available and purchased in the fall 2014 and spring 2015 semesters are shown in Table 2.

Table 2. More and less healthful entrée items available and purchased.

Entrée Item	Available [1] % (*n*)	Purchased	
		Fall % (*n*)	Spring % (*n*)
More Healthful [2]	15.0% (99)	8.0% (30,010) [4,5]	8.9% (21,934) [4,5]
Less Healthful [3]	85.0% (563)	92.0% (343,218) [5]	91.1% (225,293) [5]

[1] Availability of entrées was assumed to not differ between semesters. [2] Defined by the American Heart Association's Recommended Nutritional Standards for Procurement of Foods and Beverages Offered in the Workplace guidelines as entrée items with less than 500 kcal, less than 480 mg sodium, less than 10% saturated fat, and zero grams trans-fat. [3] Defined as foods that did not meet the American Heart Association's Recommended Nutritional Standards for Procurement of Foods and Beverages Offered in the Workplace guidelines. [4] Chi-square test for purchases are significantly different than expected, $p \leq 0.001$. Expected frequency is weighted based on the proportion of more versus less healthful products purchased. [5] Proportion of MH and LH entrée purchases between the fall and spring semesters differed significantly, $p < 0.0001$.

Of the total 662 entrée items available, 15.0% were MH and 85.0% were LH. In the fall, 8.0% of purchases were MH and 92.0% purchases were LH (χ^2 = 14,028.4, df = 1, $p < 0.0001$). In the spring, 8.9% of purchases were MH and 91.1% were LH (χ^2 = 7192.1, df = 1, $p < 0.0001$). There was a statistically significant difference in proportion of MH and LH entrée purchases between the fall and spring semesters (χ^2 = 134.0, df = 1, $p < 0.0001$), with the proportion of MH purchases increasing from 8.0% in the fall to 8.9% in the spring.

3.3. Relationships between Student Demographics and Purchases

The relationship between students' demographics and their MH versus LH food purchases are shown in Table 3. Higher odds ratios indicate that when individuals within the specified groups purchased an entrée, it was more likely to be MH. There was no statistical difference between completely rural and not as rural student purchases in the fall; however, in the spring, for each purchase made by someone from a completely rural population, it was slightly more likely to be a MH entrée (OR = 1.06, 95% CI [1.02, 1.10]). Whites were less likely than non-whites to purchase a MH entrée in both fall and spring semesters (OR = 0.84, 95% CI [0.81, 0.88] in the fall and OR = 0.79, 95% CI

[0.75, 0.84] in the spring). Females were two times more likely to choose MH options than males in both the fall (OR = 1.97, 95% CI [1.92, 2.02]) and spring (OR = 2.26, 95% CI [2.20, 2.33]) semesters.

Table 3. Relationship between demographics of students and more versus less healthful entrée purchases in the fall and spring semesters.

Demographic	Fall 2014	Spring 2015
	OR (95% CI) [4]	OR (95% CI)
Degree of Rurality		
Completely Rural [1] Versus Not as Rural [2]	0.99 (0.96–1.03)	1.06 (1.02–1.10)
Race and Ethnicity [3]		
White Versus Non-White	0.84 (0.81–0.88)	0.79 (0.75–0.84)
Gender		
Female Versus Male	1.97 (1.92–2.02)	2.26 (2.20–2.33)

[1] Includes students from counties assigned a Rural-Urban Continuum Code (RUCC) of 8 and/or 9. RUCC 8 = "completely rural or less than 2500 urban population and adjacent to a metro area." RUCC 9 = "completely rural or less than 2500 urban population and not adjacent to a metro area." [2] Includes students from counties assigned a RUC code of 1–7. RUCC 1–3 = metro counties and RUCC 4–7 = more than 2500 urban population. [3] Compared to Whites; no purchases were reported for Alaskan Natives due to missing data; no comparisons were completed with Pacific Islanders due to the low frequency. [4] OR = Odds Ratio and CI = Confidence Interval.

4. Discussion

This study examined the availability of LH foods in the campus dining environment and potential relation to purchases of these foods by students. The lack of MH entrée items (15.0%) and overabundance of LH available entrée items (85.0%) suggests the campus dining environment lacks encouragement of healthy dietary behaviors among college students at this university. These results suggest that the environment may influence students' purchases and that offering a low percentage of MH entrées may result in even fewer MH purchases. These findings are consistent with those reported by Tseng and colleagues in a similar campus study [13]. Tseng reported that of the 314 available entrée items, 88.0% were considered "unhealthful" and the remaining 12.0% were considered "healthful" options as categorized by the Nutrition Environment Measures Survey for campus dining [13].

Campus dining facilities need to run their operations profitably. If healthy food does not sell, foodservice operations have little incentive to offer different options. The findings in this study lay the groundwork for future research to determine why young adults, who are at an increased risk for weight gain, are surrounded by unhealthy foods and how their purchases of these foods may impact their weight over time. It was shown that a large percentage of the foods in the campus dining environment evaluated were considered LH, and the majority of students' purchases were considered LH. Purchases reflected what was offered, suggesting that, in order to make an impact on college students' dietary behaviors, the campus dining environment may be important. This impact of the environment on dietary behaviors is supported by the Social Ecological Model (SEM), a program-planning framework suggesting there are different levels of influence (individual, interpersonal, organizational, community, and public policy) on one's dietary behaviors [14]. Each influence is related to the next, with the broadest influences at the public policy level. Applying the SEM framework to a college students' food purchases, the campus dining environment falls under the third level (organizational), suggesting the environment strongly impacts a student's purchases [15]. Findings by Greaney and colleagues address the levels of the SEM influencing college students' dietary behaviors and stated students identified lack of healthy foods served at dining facilities, easy access to unhealthy foods and fast-food restaurants, and expensive healthful options as barriers to eating healthy in the campus dining environment [16].

In summary, as stated by Horacek, the college dining environment, does not simply feed college students, but has the potential to be highly impactful in the dietary behaviors of college students [17].

Hanks and colleagues at Cornell University have extensively studied adolescents' healthful food purchases at the high school level and have determined a lunch room that makes healthier options convenient increases purchases of those healthier options [18]. Although a younger age group, these findings may also be applied to the campus dining environment as college students have reported 'a lack of time' as a barrier to healthful food choices [19]. Interventions that provide food cost incentives for healthier foods [20] and/or free fruits and vegetables college cafeterias [21] reported modest increase in selection of healthier foods. Nutrition labeling [22,23], nutrition messaging [24], and nutrition information at point of purchase [25,26] have been reported to enhance healthier choices in college dining environments. The type of eating establishment may influence the healthfulness of choices by college campus students. Horacek et al. [27] evaluated the healthfulness of campus eating establishments and reported that among fast food, sit down, cafeteria and take-out establishments that cafeterias were offered healthier options and environment than the other establishments. The entrées evaluated and reported in this paper were offered in franchised kiosk-type eating (fast food), sit down, and take out.

Other notable findings were that non-whites versus whites and females versus males made more MH purchases in both semesters. Females were two times more likely to choose MH options than males. This study was not designed to determine the cause of these differences. However, these differences do support the potential importance of inclusion of culturally appropriate and gender specific programing in interventions developed to improve the dietary choices of college students.

A strength of this study is the analysis of the healthfulness of entrée purchases (373,228 in the fall semester and 247,227 purchases in the spring semester) from a large population of college students. Additionally, because actual food purchases of students were analyzed using sales records, limitations common to self-reported food data were avoided. Assuming the purchased foods were eaten, this form of data collection provides an objective representation of typical eating patterns, with greater accuracy than that of self-reported data for this age group [28]. Lastly, the food purchasing data was collected over a significant period of time (academic school year) versus a shorter period of time, thereby providing a stable representation of purchasing activity rather than one prone to short-term behavioral fluctuations.

Although this study is a strong contributor to the literature addressing the healthfulness of students' purchases, the results need to interpreted in the context of the limitations. First, this was an observational study collecting the card purchases of students through the academic year and, in order to correlate food purchases with dietary behaviors, it was assumed that the purchased foods were consumed. Likewise, this study did not track students' off-campus purchases or those at the all-you-care-to-eat dining hall; therefore, only the entrée purchases from on-campus à la carte dining facilities were acknowledged. In addition, the reported nutritional information classifying items as MH and LH was highly dependent on (1) the foodservice provider's product name, (2) available items in MFP, and (3) the accuracy of the nutritional information in MFP. It was also assumed that the available items did not change between semesters, as foods were offered on fixed or cycle menus. This study occurred in a comprehensive public university that offers bachelors and graduate degrees in a Midwestern state, and 85.4% of the students were white, which may limit the generalizability to other education settings and populations.

5. Conclusions

This study addresses the healthfulness of the campus dining options offered in relation to the healthfulness of students' purchases. Purchases of the students were reflective of what was offered which consisted of primarily less healthful entrée items. Implications for research and practice include the further study of the environment, inclusion of the campus dining providers in the research assessment and intervention and efforts to tailor to the specific audience. Since females tended to have healthier purchases, obesity prevention efforts at the college level should include tailoring towards males. Interventions aiming to improve the dietary behaviors of college students should consider targeting the campus dining environment and public policies (versus only the individual). Future research for obesity prevention interventions should include collaborations with campus dining providers in programming to create profitable, yet healthful, campus dining environments. The relationship between a primarily healthful environment and students' purchases ought to then be measured to determine if an environment consisting of mainly MH foods correlates with an increase in students' purchases of MH items.

Acknowledgments: This Project was partially supported by the Agriculture and Food Research Initiative Grant No. 2014-67001-21851 from USDA National Institute for Food and Agriculture, "Get Fruved:" A peer-led, train-the-trainer social marketing interventions to increase fruit and vegetable intake and prevent childhood obesity. No funds were received to cover the costs of publishing in open access.

Author Contributions: Greg Heiberger and Lacey McCormack collected data, Krista Leischner and Brian Britt analyzed data, Kendra Kattelmann and Krista Leischner wrote the manuscript. All authors reviewed and provided significant input to writing the manuscript to interpretation of results, discussion and conclusion of the manuscript.

References

1. Dennis, E.A.; Potter, K.L.; Estabrooks, P.A.; Davy, B.M. Weight gain prevention for college freshmen: Comparing two social cognitive theory-based interventions with and without explicit self-regulation training. *J. Obes.* **2012**, *2012*, 803769. [CrossRef] [PubMed]

2. Ogden, C.L.; Carroll, M.D.; Kit, B.K.; Flegal, K.M. Prevalence of childhood and adult obesity in the United States, 2011–2012. *JAMA* **2014**, *311*, 806–814. [CrossRef] [PubMed]

3. Lorenzini, A. How much should we weigh for a long and healthy life span? The need to reconcile caloric restriction versus longevity with body mass index versus mortality data. *Front. Endocrinol.* **2014**, *5*, 121. [CrossRef] [PubMed]

4. What Are the Health Risks of Overweight and Obesity? National Heart, Lung, and Blood Institute Web Site. Updated 13 July 2012. Available online: https://www.nhlbi.nih.gov/health/health-topics/topics/obe/risks (accessed on 20 July 2016).

5. Desai, M.N.; Miller, W.C.; Staples, B.; Bravender, T. Risk factors associated with overweight and obesity in college students. *J. Am. Coll. Health* **2008**, *57*, 109–114. [CrossRef] [PubMed]

6. Guo, S.; Huang, C.; Maynard, L.M.; Demerath, E.; Towne, B.; Chumlea, W.C.; Siervogel, R.M. Body mass index during childhood, adolescence and young adulthood in relation to adult overweight and adiposity: The Fels Longitudinal Study. *Int. J. Obes.* **2000**, *24*, 1628–1635. [CrossRef]

7. Crombie, A.P.; Ilich, J.Z.; Dutton, G.R.; Panton, L.B.; Abood, D.A. The freshman weight gain phenomenon revisited. *Nutr. Rev.* **2009**, *67*, 83–94. [CrossRef] [PubMed]

8. Wengreen, H.J.; Moncur, C. Change in diet, physical activity, and body weight among young-adults during the transition from high school to college. *Nutr. J.* **2009**, *8*, 32. [CrossRef] [PubMed]

9. Freedman, M.R.; Rubinstein, R.J. Obesity and food choices among faculty and staff at a large urban university. *J. Am. Coll. Health* **2010**, *59*, 205–210. [CrossRef] [PubMed]

10. Levitsky, D.A.; Halbmaier, C.A.; Mrdjenovic, G. The freshman weight gain: A model for the study of the epidemic of obesity. *Int. J. Obes.* **2004**, *28*, 1435–1442. [CrossRef] [PubMed]

11. Bureau USC. County Business Patterns: 2014. United States Census Bureau Web Site. Updated June 2016. Available online: http://www.census.gov/data/datasets/2014/econ/cbp/2014-cbp.html (accessed on 20 July 2016).

12. Recommended Nutrition Standards for Procurement of Foods and Beverages Offered in the Workplace. American Heart Associate Web Site. 2016. Available online: https://www.heart.org/idc/groups/heart-public/@wcm/@adv/documents/downloadable/ucm_320781.pdf (accessed on 5 November 2015).

13. Tseng, M.; DeGreef, K.; Fishler, M.; Gipson, R.; Koyano, K.; Neill, D.B. Assessment of a university campus food environment, California, 2015. *Prev. Chronic Dis.* **2016**, *13*, 150455. [CrossRef] [PubMed]

14. Lytle, L. Examining the etiology of childhood obesity: The IDEA study. *Am. J. Community Psychol.* **2009**, *44*, 338–349. [CrossRef] [PubMed]

15. Story, M.; Kaphingst, K.M.; Robinson-O'Brien, R.; Glanz, K. Creating healthy food and eating environments: Policy and environmental approaches. *Annu. Rev. Public Health* **2008**, *29*, 253–272. [CrossRef] [PubMed]

16. Greaney, M.L.; Less, F.D.; White, A.A.; Dayton, S.F.; Riebe, D.; Blissmer, B.; Shoff, S.; Walsh, J.R.; Greene, G.W. College students' barriers and enablers for healthful weight management: A qualitative study. *J. Nutr. Educ. Behav.* **2009**, *41*, 281–286. [CrossRef] [PubMed]

17. Horacek, T.M.; Erdman, M.B.; Byrd-Bredbenner, C.; Carey, G.; Colby, S.M.; Greene, G.W.; Guo, W.; Kattelmann, K.K.; Olfert, M.; Walsh, J.; et al. Assessment of the dining environment on and near the campuses of fifteen post-secondary institutions. *Public Health Nutr.* **2013**, *16*, 1186–1196. [CrossRef] [PubMed]

18. Hanks, A.S.; Just, D.R.; Smith, L.E.; Wansink, B. Healthy convenience: Nudging students toward healthier choices in the lunchroom. *J. Public Health* **2012**, *34*, 370–376. [CrossRef] [PubMed]

19. Nelson, M.C.; Kocos, R.; Lytle, L.A. Understanding the perceived determinants of weight-related behaviors in late adolescence: A qualitative analysis among college youth. *J. Nutr. Educ. Behav.* **2009**, *41*, 287–292. [CrossRef] [PubMed]

20. Michels, K.B.; Bloom, B.R.; Riccardi, P.; Rosner, B.A.; Willett, W.C. A study of the importance of education and cost incentives on individual food choices at the Harvard School of Public Health cafeteria. *J. Am. Coll. Nutr.* **2008**, *27*, 6–11. [CrossRef] [PubMed]

21. Lachat, C.K.; Verstraeten, R.; De Meulenaer, B.; Menten, J. Availability of free fruits and vegetables at canteen lunch improves lunch and daily nutritional profiles: A randomised controlled trial. *Br. J. Nutr.* **2009**, *102*, 1030–1037. [CrossRef] [PubMed]

22. Nikolaou, C.K.; Hankey, C.R.; Lean, M.E.J. Preventing weight gain with calorie-labeling. *Obesity* **2014**, *22*, 2277–2283. [CrossRef] [PubMed]

23. Bergen, D.; Yeh, M.C. Effects of energy-content labels and motivational posters on sales of sugar sweetened beverages: Stimulating sales of diet drinks among adult study. *J. Am. Diet. Assoc.* **2006**, *106*, 1866–1869. [CrossRef] [PubMed]

24. Peterson, S.; Duncan, D.P.; Null, D.B.; Roth, S.L.; Gill, L. Positive changes in perceptions and selections of healthful foods by college students after a short-term point-of-selection intervention at a dining hall. *J. Am. Coll. Health* **2010**, *58*, 425–431. [CrossRef] [PubMed]

25. Turconi, G.; Bazzano, R.; Roggi, C.; Cena, H. Helping consumers make a more conscious nutritional choice: Acceptability of nutrition information at a cafeteria. *J. Am. Coll. Health* **2012**, *60*, 324–330. [CrossRef] [PubMed]

26. Buscher, L.A.; Martin, K.A.; Crocker, S. Point-of-purchase messages framed in terms of cost, convenience, taste, and energy improve healthful snack selection in a college foodservice setting. *J. Am. Diet. Assoc.* **2001**, *101*, 909–913. [CrossRef]

27. Horacek, J.M.; Yildrim, E.D.; Simon, M.; Byrd-Bredbenner, C.; White, A.A.; Shelnutt, K.P.; Olfert, M.D.; Morrell, J.; Mathews, A.; Kidd, T.; et al. Development and validation of the Full Restaurant Evaluation Supporting a Healthy (FRESH) Dining Environment Audit. *J. Hunger Environ. Nutr.* **2018**. [CrossRef]

28. Driskell, J.A.; Schake, M.C.; Detter, H.A. Using nutrition labeling as a potential tool for changing eating habits of university dining hall patrons. *J. Am. Diet. Assoc.* **2008**, *108*, 2071–2076. [CrossRef] [PubMed]

## 17

Academic Palliative Care Research in Portugal: Are We on the Right Track?

Alexandra Pereira [1,2,*] (iD), Amélia Ferreira [1,2] and José Martins [3]

[1] Community Care Unit of Lousada, Rua de Santo Tirso 70, Meinedo, Lousada, 4620-848 Porto, Portugal; amelia.leite.ferreira@gmail.com

[2] Abel Salazar Biomedical Institute, R. Jorge de Viterbo Ferreira 228, 4050-313 Porto, Portugal

[3] Nursing School of Coimbra, 3046-841 Coimbra, Portugal; jmartins@esenfc.pt

* Correspondence: alemnap@gmail.com

Abstract: Background: The narrow link between practice, education, and research is essential to palliative care development. In Portugal, academic postgraduate publications are the main booster for palliative care research. Methods: This is a bibliometric study that aims to identify Portuguese palliative care postgraduate academic work published in electronic academic repositories between 2000 and 2015. Results: 488 publications were identified. The number of publications has increased, especially in the last five years. The most frequently used method was quantitative, healthcare professionals were the most studied participants, and psychological and psychiatric aspects of care comprised the most current theme. Practice-based priorities are financial costs and benefits of palliative care, awareness and understanding of palliative care, underserved populations, best practices, communication, and palliative care in nonhospital settings. Conclusion: The number of palliative care postgraduate academic publications has increased in Portugal in the past few years. There is academic production in the eight domains of quality palliative care and on the three levels of recommendation for practice-based research priorities. The major research gaps in Portugal are at the system and societal context levels.

Keywords: palliative care; end-of-life care; research

1. Introduction

Changing demographic trends, such as an ageing population and increased life expectancy, in addition to medical and scientific advances accentuate the need to develop, evaluate, and research palliative care [1,2].

Palliative care is an approach for addressing the needs of individuals with life-threatening illnesses from a holistic, interdisciplinary perspective [3]. Estimates show that 19 million people need palliative care worldwide each year, 69% of which are older adults. Although the majority (78%) of adults in need of palliative care belong to low- and middle-income countries, the highest rates of those in need of palliative care per 100,000 adults are found in higher-income countries [4].

In recent years, palliative care research has evolved from care targeting patients with cancer to a care approach relevant for patients with diverse life-limiting conditions [5], therefore the scope of palliative care research is now wider. In spite of that, research in this field is still challenging, due to the sensitive nature of the topic and patients with complex and unstable symptoms [6]. Palliative care research has a fundamental role in informing evidence-based clinical practice, service development, education, and policy, and it is needed to improve service delivery and optimise patients' quality of life [7,8].

With a population of 10 million, Portugal is the 7th most ageing country in the world [9] and is one of the countries with the highest rates of adults in need of palliative care [4]. Estimates show that Portugal needs 133 palliative care home teams, 102 hospital support teams, 28 palliative care units, and 46 hospices [10]. To date, according to the Portuguese palliative care directory, there are 20 palliative care home teams, 34 support teams, and 33 palliative care units. Comprising 18 districts and 2 autonomous regions, Portugal has an unequal distribution of palliative care teams: 10 districts don't have home care teams and 3 districts don't have a hospital support team or a palliative care unit [11]. Therefore, although Portugal is considered to have a generalized provision of palliative care [12], there still are inequities in the distribution of and access to palliative care [13].

Recently, the Portuguese palliative care strategic plan recognized education and research as two important vectors for palliative care development [14]. In 2003, the Council of Europe recommended that postgraduate training and education should be established in every country to ensure that every health professional is able to deliver palliative care in an insightful and culturally sensitive manner [15]. In Portugal, the first master's course in palliative care emerged in 2002 at the University of Lisbon [16]. The offer of postgraduate education and training in this area has increased: five other master's courses are now available [17]. The first doctoral program in palliative care was created in 2016 at the University of Porto.

The narrow link between practice education and research can enable the development of palliative care knowledge, identify research priorities, and contribute to evidence-based practice [18]. Education and practice are often identified as barriers to the development of palliative care [19–21], but, in fact, the gap between education research and practice might also be considered a problem that should be addressed as a complex and differentiated phenomenon [22], as significant knowledge gaps impede palliative care effectiveness. Educational research is essential to provide evidence for practice and practitioners can enrich research by posing adequate research questions. Thus, integrating the needs of palliative care practitioners with scientific expertise is likely to generate proposals for innovative studies that will ultimately improve practice [23]. In 2015, 10 recommendations for palliative care research to address knowledge gaps were published. These practice-based research priorities were clustered into three categories: (1) research to improve individual-level palliative care practice, (2) research to improve system-level palliative care practice and capacity, and (3) research on societal context for palliative care. These categories are mapped onto three domains that palliative care aims to affect: (1) the care that practitioners provide to patients and families, (2) palliative care organization and delivery, and (3) the popular, political, and social understanding and reception of palliative care [23].

Country reviews and bibliometric studies of palliative care research are motivated by a recognition of the importance of evidence in supporting decision-makers to meet the challenges that palliative care faces [24]. This is a current practice in research in different countries [24–26]. In Portugal, academic postgraduate publications are still the main booster for palliative care research, and thus, this bibliometric study aims to identify all Portuguese palliative care postgraduate academic works published in electronic academic repositories between 2000 and 2015 and to analyse their alignment with the internationally identified research priorities in palliative care. The research questions are:

(1) How many postgraduate academic works related to palliative care were published between 2000 and 2015 in Portugal? By which health professions?

(2) How many studies were undertaken?

(3) What designs were used and what populations were studied?

(4) What areas/themes were studied? Are they aligned with the identified research priorities in palliative care?

2. Materials and Methods

2.1. Design

This is a bibliometric study. Bibliometric methods are established as scientific specialties and are an integral part of research evaluation methodology, especially within the scientific and applied fields [27]. Bibliometrics is the application of quantitative analysis and statistics to publications [28], in this case, postgraduate academic research. We have chosen this method because we intend to obtain an overview of Portuguese postgraduate academic research related to palliative care. This way we can highlight a lack of evidence in certain areas that might help researchers to develop subsequent studies. Therefore, we haven't made a critical appraisal of the articles or a synthesis of findings as conventionally required. The ethical procedures were guaranteed through rigorous methodology compliance and respect for the ethical principles that guide health research.

2.2. Search Strategies

This bibliometric study was undertaken to identify palliative care postgraduate academic research produced in Portugal. The following academic repositories were researched: Catholic University of Portugal, Coimbra Nursing School, Fernando Pessoa University, ISCTE-IUL, ISPA, Lusíada University, Lusófona University, Open University, Polytechnic Institute of Bragança, Polytechnic Institute of Castelo Branco, Polytechnic Institute of Oporto, Polytechnic Institute of Santarém, Polytechnic Institute of Viana do Castelo, Polytechnic Institute of Viseu, RCAAP, Technical University of Lisbon, New University of Lisbon, University of Algarve, University of Aveiro, University of Azores, University of Beira Interior, University of Coimbra, University of Évora, University of Lisbon, University of Oporto, and UTAD. The search terms used were "palliative care" or "end-of-life care" or "terminal care" in the following repository fields: subject or description or keyword.

2.3. Inclusion and Exclusion Criteria

Publications were selected based on the following inclusion criteria: (1) academic publications related to a master or a PhD, (2) academic publications relevant within the palliative care field, and (3) published between 2000 and 2015. Publications that were based on opinion or commentary or that were editorials, conference abstracts, or research papers were excluded.

2.4. Data Extraction

All postgraduate academic publications were exported to an Excel database and duplicates were removed. A data extraction protocol was developed. Results were analysed by two independent researchers to confirm the inclusion criteria. After the initial extraction by one of the researchers, the data extracted were cross-checked by the other researcher; consequently, all data were double-checked. When there was disagreement between the two researchers, a third researcher was invited to contribute an opinion to reach a consensus.

The data extracted from each included publication were as follows: author, author's profession, author's gender, year of publication, repository of publication, type of academic publication, research method, study participants, setting of care, and themes. Themes were decided a priori and were categorized after reading the abstracts according to the eight domains of quality palliative care: structure and processes of care; physical aspects of care; psychological and psychiatric aspects of care; social aspects of care; spiritual, religious, and existential aspects of care; cultural aspects of care; care of the imminently dying patient; ethical and legal aspects of care [29]. During the data extraction process, we added four other categories: lived experience of patients, lived experience of caregivers, lived experience of health professionals, and study of specific groups (for instance: diabetic patients, dementia patients, children). Recommendations for practice-based research priorities for palliative care were used to classify all studies [23]. After all the data were extracted, all postgraduate academic publications were categorized by the region corresponding to the repository. The author's profession was confirmed by research on the electronic registration of Portuguese professional orders.

3. Results

A flow diagram with the selection of cases is detailed in Figure 1. Overall, 28 repositories and 1980 studies were identified, after removing six studies that were duplicates. Also, 173 studies were excluded as they did not correspond to postgraduate academic publications. The titles and abstracts of the remaining 1807 studies were reviewed. This resulted in 1319 studies being excluded as they did not meet the inclusion criteria. The final review included 488 studies that were published in the electronic academic repositories during the period under examination.

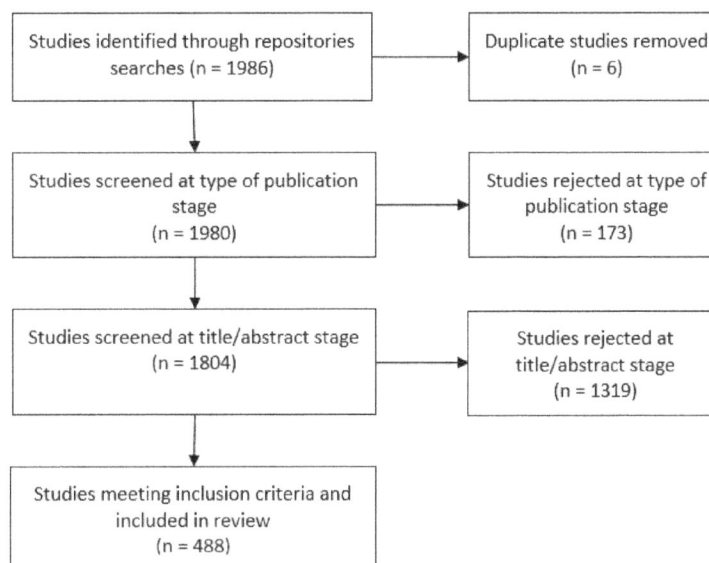

Figure 1. Selection and review process.

From the 488 studies identified, 19.9% were published on the University of Oporto's repository, followed by the Catholic University's repository (17.8%), and the University of Lisbon's repository (15.8%) (Table 1).

Table 1. Distribution of scientific production by repository (*n* and %).

Repository	*n*	%
Catholic University	87	17.8
Coimbra Nursing School	3	0.6
Fernando Pessoa University	4	0.8
ISCTE-IUL	6	1.2
ISPA	10	2.0
Lusíada University	1	0.2
University Lusófona	1	0.2
Open University	7	1.4
Polytechnic Institute of Bragança	16	3,3
Polytechnic Institute of Castelo Branco	49	10.0
Polytechnic Institute of Oporto	5	1.0
Polytechnic Institute of Santarem	8	1.6
Polytechnic Institute of Viana do Castelo	29	5.9
Polytechnic Institute of Viseu	12	2.5
RCAAP	10	2.0
Technic University of Lisbon	1	0.2
University Nova	7	1.4
University of Algarve	9	1.8
University of Aveiro	21	4.3
University of Azores	3	0.6
University of Beira Interior	7	1.4
University of Coimbra	18	3.7
University of Évora	1	0.2
University of Lisbon	1	0.2
University of Madeira	1	0.2
University of Oporto	97	19.9
UTAD	1	0.2
Total	488	100

Regarding the region of the country where the university was located, there was a predominance of the northern (38.9%) and southern regions (37.7%) (Table 2).

Table 2. Distribution of scientific production by region (*n* and %).

Country Region	*n*	%
Azores	3	0.6
Centre	110	22.5
Madeira	1	0.2
North	190	38.9
South	184	37.7
Total	488	100

The majority of authors were female (86.5%). Regarding the profession of the author, the majority were nurses (63.3%), followed by physicians (9.2%). It was not possible to identify the profession of the author in 8.6% of the studies (Table 3).

Table 3. Characteristics of authors.

Category	*n*	%
Gender		
Female	422	86.5
Male	66	13.5
Total	488	100
Profession		
Dentist	4	0.8
Gerontologist	6	1.2
Physician	45	9.2
Nurse	309	63.3
Occupational Therapist	5	1.0
Other	4	0.8
Pharmacist	3	0.6
Physiotherapist	12	2.5
Psychologist	35	7.2
Social worker	16	3.3
Sociologist	3	0.6
Speech Therapist	4	0.8
Unknown	42	8.6
Total	488	100

There was an upward trend in the number of postgraduate academic studies published from 2009 to 2015 (94.1%). The oldest study was published in 2000. There was an absence of publications in 2001 and 2002 (Figure 2).

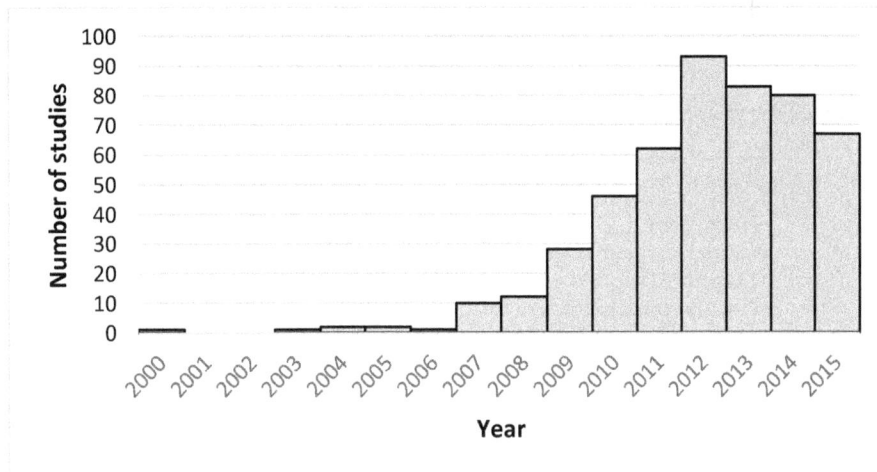

Figure 2. Number of studies per year (*n*).

In terms of academic degree, 95.3% of the studies were published at the master's degree level and 4.7% were published at the PhD degree level. In Portugal, a master's degree can be obtained by a scientific dissertation, project work, or internship report [30]. In terms of type of academic publication, 68.9% were master's dissertations, 18.6% were internship reports, 7.4% were research projects, and 5.1% were PhD theses (Table 4). Also, 51.0% of the postgraduate academic publications studies were not from a specific palliative care master's or PhD degree, which shows that palliative care is a transversal theme of study in many healthcare-related courses.

Table 4. Distribution of scientific production by type of academic publication (*n* and %).

Type of Academic Publication	*n*	%
Internship reports	91	18.6
Master's dissertation	336	68.9
PhD theses	25	5.1
Research projects	36	7.4
Total	488	100

Master's dissertations and PhD theses were classified according to the research method described in the abstracts as shown in Table 5. Quantitative methods were used in 48.2% of the studies, followed by qualitative methods (31.0%).

Table 5. Distribution of scientific production by type of research methods (*n* and %).

Type of Research Method	*n*	%
Measurement/methodology	13	3.6
Mixed methods	19	5.3
Other methods	10	2.8
Qualitative	112	31.0
Quantitative	174	48.2
Reviews	28	7.7
Unclassifiable	5	1.4
Total	361	100

In terms of study participants, the majority of publications involved healthcare professionals and/or healthcare students (32.1%), followed by patients (25.8%) and caregivers (17.7%). Also, a mixed population was studied in 7.5% of publications (Table 6). Only 3.3% of publications were related to paediatric palliative care.

Table 6. Distribution of scientific production by type of study participants (*n* and %).

Type of Study Participants	n	%
Caregivers	64	17.7
Caregivers and health professionals	6	1.7
Documentation	40	11.1
General population	1	0.3
Health professionals and/or students	116	32.1
Other	3	0.8
Patients	93	25.8
Patients and caregivers	6	1.7
Patients and health professionals	6	1.7
Patients, caregivers and health professionals	9	2.5
Unclassified	17	4.6
Total	361	100

Regarding the setting of research, we were able to classify 72.0% of publications. The investigation took place in a hospital setting in 47.9% of publications, followed by the community setting (11.1%), long term care setting (9.4%), hospital and community setting (2.2%), and resident home setting (1.4%).

The themes most frequently described in the 361 postgraduate academic publications were psychological and psychiatric aspects of care (19.4%), followed by structure and processes of care (19.1%) and physical aspects of care (15.5%). An additional nine themes were identified and we were unable to classify six publications (Table 7).

Table 7. Distribution of scientific production by areas of focus (*n* and %).

Areas of Focus	n	%
Care of the imminently dying patient	9	2.5
Cultural aspects of care	2	0.6
Ethical and legal aspects of care	26	7.2
Lived experience of caregiver	26	7.2
Lived experience of health professional	39	10.8
Lived experience of patient	10	2.8
Physical aspects of care	56	15.5
Psychological and psychiatric aspects of care	70	19.4
Social aspects of care	13	3.6
Specific groups	20	5.5
Spiritual, religious, and existential aspects of care	15	4.2
Structure and processes of care	69	19.1
Unclassified	6	1.6
Total	361	100

According to the level of practice-based research priority, most postgraduate academic publications were at the individual level (61.5%), meaning that the aim was to study the care that individual practitioners provide patients and families. The least represented level was the societal context for palliative care (5.0%). We were unable to classify 1.7% of the publications (Table 8).

Table 8. Distribution of scientific production by level of research priority recommendation (*n* and %).

Level of Research Priority Recommendation	*n*	%
Individual-level palliative care practice	222	61.5
System-level palliative care practice and capacity	115	31.9
Societal context for palliative care	18	5.0
Unclassified	6	1.7
Total	361	100

The two most represented research priority recommendations were at the individual level of palliative care practice: symptom management (29.1%) and decision-making (23.3%). The third most represented was education and training for palliative care providers (13.0%) at system-level palliative care practice (Table 9).

Table 9. Distribution of scientific production by research priority recommendation (*n* and %).

Research Priority Recommendation	*n*	%
Individual-level palliative care practice		
Communication	21	5.8
Decision-making	84	23.3
Symptom management	105	29.1
Best practices	12	3.3
System-level palliative care practice and capacity		
Nonhospital settings	28	7.8
Education and training for palliative care providers	47	13.0
Palliative care across the span of serious illness and the end of life	40	11.1
Societal context for palliative care		
Awareness and understanding of palliative care	11	3.0
Financial costs and benefits of palliative care	3	0.8
Underserved and vulnerable populations	4	1.1
Unclassified	6	1.7
Total	361	100

4. Discussion

Country bibliometric studies of palliative care research are becoming a current practice in different countries as they support decision-making and can help researchers to identify potential lack of evidence in certain areas. We found three recent European studies, developed in Scotland [24], Ireland [25], and Sweden [26], that used a methodology similar to that in our study. Although it might seem odd to compare scientific publication production between countries, we have decided to do so in order to compare the Portuguese reality to countries that follow the same European guidelines yet have greater tradition and development in the palliative care field. There are also two Portuguese studies with which we will compare our results: one is from 2011 [31] and the other one, which is only nursing related, is from 2016 [32].

The findings from this bibliometric study show a considerable increase in palliative care postgraduate academic publications, particularly in the last five years. Today, there are almost nine times more postgraduate publications than the number reported until 2010 [31] and almost double the number of postgraduate publications reported in a bibliometric study until 2014, although this last one was only nursing related [32].

These results might be linked to several factors that have supported the development of palliative care in Portugal. Firstly, there has been an increase in the availability of postgraduate education related to palliative care and the possibility to join various scholarship programs. Secondly, there has been profuse public discussion surrounding palliative care in Portugal: TV debate programs have been made and research results have been diffused through various media channels. Thirdly, several government initiatives and laws have been implemented, including a recent publication of the Portuguese palliative care strategic plan that aims to foster awareness of the importance of palliative care and the creation of palliative care teams [14]. Lastly, there have been private funding initiatives to open palliative care home teams. These two last factors are also related to job market opportunities and might have had a direct influence on the increase in the number of people seeking specific palliative care education.

The fact that the majority of publications are from the north and south universities' repositories is not surprising, as the two largest Portuguese cities are located in those regions and the majority of specific palliative care postgraduate courses are also offered there. Furthermore, there is evidence that postgraduate academic research is originating from different types of health courses, and, in similar vein, palliative care research papers are being published in a range of journals [33]. These results show that palliative care is an area of interest for a large portion of healthcare professionals from different backgrounds, even if the master's or PhD course they are attending is not directly linked to the palliative care field.

The authors were predominantly nurses, followed by physicians. This is consistent with other Portuguese results [32]. The Swedish review showed the same tendency [26]. Although the composition of palliative care teams varies depending on needs and resources, the presence of physicians and nurses is constant and essential. The relation between nursing and palliative care is not new. In fact, Virginia Henderson said that palliative care "was the essence of nursing" [34]. Perhaps the fact that palliative care and nursing both maintain a commitment to the care of the whole person [35] may attract nurses to pursue the study of palliative care. Also, in Portugal, the recent government initiatives and the public discussion regarding palliative care has brought renewed attention to this area, which might be considered as a job opportunity. On the other hand, nursing postgraduate education has some tradition in Portugal: the master's degree has existed since 1991 and the PhD degree since 2000. Even so, several other professions were found that reflect the multidisciplinary nature of palliative care. This multidisciplinary approach is fundamental to developing a consensus on the clinical definitions and guidelines for complex conditions and to provide comprehensive care [36]. This approach obliges their members to develop and share knowledge and skills that contribute to the overall functioning of the team [37].

In terms of design methods, the majority of the studies were descriptive and used a quantitative approach. Most quantitative studies were cross-sectional, using a small sample size. Also, few multicentre studies were found. This is consistent with other Portuguese results [31,32]. Similar results were obtained in Scotland and Ireland [24,25]. In Sweden, the qualitative approach was more commonly used [26]. Although the qualitative approach might be considered more holistic and humanized, in consideration of the nature of the studied themes it is understandable that the quantitative approach is more prevalent as palliative care research in Portugal is still a relatively new field. There is a lack of intervention studies in Portugal due to the fact that palliative care research can involve sensitive topics as well as ethical issues related to patients and families in vulnerable conditions [6]. In fact, these factors, in addition to the difficulty of achieving adequate sample sizes in a heterogeneous group of patients with chronic and incurable diseases, reduce the power of the studies and their follow-up periods, and so the "gold standard" of randomized trials is not necessarily applicable [8]. For these reasons, researchers usually employ alternative research methodologies, including observational studies with a large sample size and a valid methodology, in an attempt to improve palliative care research [38]. Commonly, postgraduate academic research is time constrained and usually limited in duration from a few months to one year in a master's degree and up to three or four years in a PhD degree. Therefore, the utilization of a more accessible population can be a reason for why most publications have health professionals and students as study participants. Curiously, the Scottish review showed a preference for patient-related research [24]. There have also been few methodological studies (3.6%) conducted in Portugal. This type of study would be important for the development of adequate measurement instruments to improve the possibility to assess quality palliative-care-related indicators [39]. The lack of reliable instruments is one of the factors that hinder the assessment of quality indicators in palliative care [40].

Themes were categorized through abstract reading, and so the quality of abstracts may have influenced the categorization. It is important to reflect upon abstract quality in postgraduate academic research as it is an essential tool for the reader as it is for the author. The formatting and content of abstracts in academic research might be one barrier preventing a wider dissemination and use of research [41]. The three most prevalent themes that were found in our study were psychological and psychiatric aspects of care, structure of care, and physical aspects of care. From our point of view, and regarding the domains of quality palliative care [29], these themes are related to two dimensions: patient and family, and healthcare professionals. The first one is related to the following subthemes: patient and family needs assessment, symptom management, and grief/bereavement counselling. The second dimension is related to the following subthemes: education and training, and the emotional impact of work. Although similar country bibliometric studies use different classifications to categorize themes, it is possible to conclude that the results are similar. Symptom management was the most researched theme in Sweden [26], the second most researched in Ireland [25], and the third most researched in Scotland [24]. In the 2011 Portuguese study, medical care was the most researched theme [31]. We also discovered that only 5.5% of the publications were related to specific groups. In the Irish review this was the most researched theme [25]. In our study, 3.3% of the publications were related to children. In the Scottish review this was the 13th most researched theme [24]. Even so, we consider that these results are consistent with Portuguese practice, as paediatric palliative care is still an underdeveloped area in Portugal [42], and only in the past two years has attention been brought to this subject with the creation of a national group and the opening of the first paediatric palliative care unit in the north of Portugal.

The majority of publications were related to the hospital setting. Scotland has similar results, although the Portuguese results are more than double (47.9% versus 23.0%). In Sweden, the most common setting was home care. This might indicate that in Portugal, the healthcare system is hospital-centred. Recent studies show that, in spite of the fact that the majority of Portuguese people would prefer to die at home [43], most deaths occur in a hospital setting [44]. This subject has been discussed extensively in Portugal and the palliative care strategic plan highlights the importance of palliative care home teams, as a recent Cochrane review shows that home palliative care increases the chance of dying at home and reduces the symptom burden, without impacting on caregiver grief [45].

One of the aims of this study was to compare the results with the recommendations for practice-based research priorities for palliative care [23]. Although these recommendations were made in the United States, they have been adopted in the Portuguese palliative care strategic plan [14]. We found that there is postgraduate academic research production at the three levels of recommendations, but the majority is done at the individual level. This level includes the study of patients and families and the way that direct bedside practice is provided. In Portugal, palliative care emerged in the 1990s through pioneer initiatives and only a decade later did the first government initiative appear, so it was expected that most postgraduate academic research would be done at this level. Even so, a considerable number of studies were conducted at the system level of care practice and capacity, partly due to the research on education and training of palliative care providers. As we observed earlier, due to time constraints, many postgraduate academic research is done using health professionals and students as participants. Production at the societal context level is still low, whereby only 18 such studies were produced. Development of studies at this level of research is needed to improve the awareness and understanding of palliative care, to understand its financial cost and benefits, and to better understand underserved vulnerable populations. This is essential to improve the access to and distribution of palliative care in Portugal. Apart from the recommendations at the societal context level, major gaps in the postgraduate academic research in palliative care in Portugal are: best practices, communication, and palliative care in nonhospital settings.

5. Conclusions

This study provided baseline evidence of postgraduate academic research in Portugal over the last 15 years. The amount of postgraduate academic research has been increasing, especially in the last five years. The majority of postgraduate academic research was developed by nurses. A mix of research methods was identified, with a predominance of quantitative studies. Most postgraduate academic research is hospital-centred and the most studied population comprises healthcare professionals. In spite of that, several studies targeted patients. Most studied themes were the psychological and psychiatric aspects of care, structure and processes of care, and physical aspects of care. The current bibliometric study identified several palliative care research gaps, especially at the system and societal context levels. Practice-based priorities research in Portugal are: financial cost and benefits of palliative care, awareness and understanding of palliative care, underserved and vulnerable populations, best practices, communication, and palliative care in nonhospital settings.

The research undertaken was clearly limited by the fact that only electronic academic repositories were included. Although there might be a few publications in nonelectronic repositories, we believe that their inclusion would not be significantly relevant to the present study results. The keywords choice used on research might also be considered a limitation. Also, the poor quality of some abstracts might be considered a limitation during the data extraction.

We suggest that authors should improve the formatting and content of abstracts, as a poor-quality abstract can prevent a wider dissemination and use of research. We also suggest that domains of quality palliative care are used to classify themes/areas of focus in similar studies so that it is possible to obtain more comparable results in future research. A follow-up bibliometric study is recommended in a few years' time.

Author Contributions: A.P. and A.F. conceived and designed this bibliometric study. A.P. and A.F. performed the full-text reviews. Findings of the reviews were discussed among all authors. A.P. and A.F. wrote the paper supervised by J.M.

Funding: No funding has been received to facilitate the completion of this work.

Acknowledgments: To Jessica Oliveira and Laura Davies for the careful revision of this paper.

References

1. Williams, A.M.; Crooks, V.A.; Whitfield, K.; Kelley, M.; Richards, J.; DeMiglio, L.; Dykeman, S. Tracking the evolution of hospice palliative care in Canada: A comparative case study analysis of seven provinces. *BMC Heal. Serv. Res.* **2010**, *10*, 147–162. [CrossRef] [PubMed]

2. Davies, E.; Higginson, I.J. *Palliative Care: The Solid Facts*; World Health Organization: Copenhagen, Denmark, 2004.

3. World Health Organization. Definition of Palliative Care. Available online: http://www.who.int/cancer/palliative/definition/eu/ (accessed on 10 June 2018).

4. Worldwide Palliative Care Alliance; World Health Organization. *Global Atlas of Palliative Care at the End of Life*; Worldwide Palliative Care Alliance: London, UK, 2014.

5. World Health Organization. National Cancer Control Programs Programmes, Policies and Behavioral Guidelines. Available online: http://www.who.int/cancer/media/en/408.pdf (accessed on 10 June 2018).

6. Higginson, I.J. Research challenges in palliative and end of life care. *BMJ Support. Palliat. Care* **2016**, *6*, 2–4. [CrossRef] [PubMed]

7. LeBlanc, T.W.; Kutner, J.S.; Ko, D.; Wheeler, J.L.; Bull, J.; Abernethy, A.P. Developing the evidence base for palliative care: Formation of the palliative care research cooperative and its first trial. *Hosp. Pract.* **2010**, *38*, 137–143. [CrossRef] [PubMed]

8. Visser, C.; Hadley, G.; Wee, B. Reality of evidence-based practice in palliative care. *Cancer Biol. Med.* **2015**, *12*, 193–200. [CrossRef] [PubMed]

9. Department of Economic and Social Affairs of United Nations—Population Division. World Population Ageing 2017. Available online: http://www.un.org/en/development/desa/population/theme/ageing/WPA2017.shtml (accessed on 31 July 2018).
10. Capelas, M.L.V. Cuidados paliativos: Uma proposta para Portugal. *Cad. Saúde* **2009**, *2*, 51–57.
11. Associação Portuguesa de Cuidados Paliativos. Diretório Nacional de Cuidados Paliativos. Available online: http://www.apcp.com.pt/ (accessed on 31 July 2018).
12. Lynch, T.; Connor, D.; Clark, D. Mapping levels of palliative care development: A global update. *J. Pain Symptom Manag.* **2013**, *45*, 1094–1106. [CrossRef] [PubMed]
13. Observatório Português do Sistema de Saúde. Relatório Primavera 2017. Available online: http://opss.pt/wp-content/uploads/2018/06/Relatorio_Primavera_2017.pdf (accessed on 30 June 2018).
14. Comissão Nacional de Cuidados Paliativos. Plano Estratégico para o Desenvolvimento dos Cuidados Paliativos Biénio 2017–2018. Available online: https://www.sns.gov.pt/wp-content/uploads/2016/09/Plano-Estrat%C3%A9gico-CP_2017-2018-1-1.pdf (accessed on 30 June 2018).
15. Council of Europe. Recommendation Rec (2003) 24 of the Committee of Ministers to Member States on the Organisation of Palliative Care. Available online: https://www.coe.int/t/dg3/health/Source/Rec(2003)24_en.pdf (accessed on 25 June 2018).
16. Neto, I.G. Palliative care development is well under way in Portugal. *Eur. J. Palliat. Care* **2010**, *17*, 278–281.
17. A3ES. Acreditação de Ciclos de Estudo. Available online: http://www.a3es.pt/pt/acreditacao-e-auditoria/resultados-dos-processos-de-acreditacao/acreditacao-de-ciclos-de-estudos (accessed on 25 June 2018).
18. Hanks, G.; Kaasa, S.; Forbes, K. Research in palliative medicine. In *Oxford Textbook of Palliative Medicine*, 4th ed.; Hanks, G., Cherny, N., Christakis, N., Eds.; Oxford University Press: Oxford, UK, 2011.
19. Sigurdardottir, K.R.; Haugen, D.F.; Van der Rijt, C.C.; Sjøgren, P.; Harding, R.; Higginson, I.J.; Kaasa, S.; PRISMA. Clinical priorities, barriers and solution in end-of-life cancer care research across Europe. Report from a workshop. *Eur. J. Cancer* **2010**, *46*, 1815–1822. [CrossRef] [PubMed]
20. Mousing, C.A.; Timm, H.; Lomborg, K.; Kirkeyold, M. Barriers to palliative care in people with chronic obstructive pulmonary disease in home care: A qualitative study of the perspective of professional caregivers. *J. Clin. Nurs.* **2018**, *27*, 650–660. [CrossRef] [PubMed]
21. Lynch, T.; Clark, D.; Centeno, C.; Rocafort, J.; Flores, L.A.; Greenwood, A.; Praill, D.; Brasch, S.; Giordano, A.; De Lima, L.; et al. Barriers to the development of palliative care in the countries of Central and Eastern Europe and the Commonwealth of Independent States. *J. Pain Symptom Manag.* **2009**, *37*, 305–315. [CrossRef] [PubMed]
22. Vanderlinde, R.; Braak, J. The gap between educational research and practice: Views of teachers, school leaders, intermediaries and researchers. *Br. Educ. Res. J.* **2013**, *36*, 299–316. [CrossRef]
23. Pillemer, K.; Chen, E.K.; Riffin, C.; Prigerson, H.; Schultz, L.; Reid, M.C. Practice-based research priorities for palliative care: Results from a research-to-practice consensus workshop. *Am. J. Public Health* **2015**, *105*, 2237–2244. [CrossRef] [PubMed]
24. Finucane, A.M.; Carduff, E.; Lugton, J.; Fenning, S.; Johnston, B.; Fallon, M.; Clark, D.; Spiller, J.A.; Murray, S.A. Palliative and end-of-life care research in Scotland 2006–2015: A systematic scoping review. *BMC Palliat. Care* **2018**, *17*, 19. [CrossRef] [PubMed]
25. McIlfatrick, S.J.; Murphy, T. Palliative care research on the island of Ireland over the last decade: A systematic review and thematic analysis of peer reviewed publications. *BMC Palliat. Care* **2013**, *12*, 33. [CrossRef] [PubMed]
26. Henoch, I.; Carlander, I.; Holm, M.; James, I.; Sarenmalm, E.K.; Hagelin, C.L.; Lind, S.; Sandgren, A.; Öhlén, J. Palliative care research—A systematic review of foci, designs and methods of research conducted in Sweden between 2007 and 2012. *Scand. J. Caring Sci.* **2016**, *30*, 5–25. [CrossRef] [PubMed]
27. Ellegaard, O.; Wallin, J. The bibliometric analysis of scholarly production: How great is the impact? *Scientometrics* **2015**, *105*, 1809–1831. [CrossRef] [PubMed]
28. Thomson Reuters. White Paper Using Bibliometrics: A Guide to Evaluating Research Performance with Citation Data. Available online: http://ips.clarivate.com/m/pdfs/325133_thomson.pdf (accessed on 10 August 2018).
29. Ferrell, B.; Connor, S.R.; Cordes, A.; Dahlin, C.M.; Fine, P.G.; Hutton, N.; Leenay, M.; Lentz, J.; Person, J.L.; Meier, D.E.; et al. The national agenda for quality palliative care: The National Consensus Project and the National Quality Forum. *J. Pain Symptom Manag.* **2007**, *33*, 737–744. [CrossRef] [PubMed]

30. Diário da República. Decreto-lei 115/2013. Available online: https://dre.pt/web/guest/pesquisa/-/search/ 498487/details/maximized (accessed on 25 June 2018).

31. Santos, M.; Capelas, M. Palliative care research in Portugal. *Cad. Saúde* **2011**, *4*, 63–69.

32. Ferreira, M.A.; Pereira, A.M.; Martins, J.C.; Barbieri-Figueiredo, M.C. Palliative care and nursing in dissertations and theses in Portugal: A bibliometric study. *Rev. Esc. Enferm. USP* **2016**, *50*, 313–319. [CrossRef] [PubMed]

33. Payne, S.A.; Turner, J.M. Research methodologies in palliative care: A bibliometric analysis. *Palliat. Med.* **2008**, *22*, 336–342. [CrossRef] [PubMed]

34. Coyle, N. Introduction to palliative nursing care. In *Oxford Textbook of Palliative Nursing*; Ferrell, B., Coyle, N., Eds.; Oxford University Press: Oxford, UK, 2010; pp. 3–12.

35. Rosa, W.E.; Hope, S.; Matzo, M. Palliative nursing and sacred medicine: A holistic stance on entheogens, healing and spiritual care. *J. Holist. Nurs.* **2018**. [CrossRef] [PubMed]

36. Choi, B.C.; Pak, A.W. Multidisciplinarity, interdisciplinarity and transdisciplinarity in health research, services, education and policy: 1. Definitions, objectives, and evidence of effectiveness. *Clin. Investig. Med.* **2006**, *29*, 351–364.

37. McCloskey, J.C. The discipline hearts of a multidisciplinary team. *J. Prof. Nurs.* **1995**, *11*, 202. [CrossRef]

38. Benson, K.; Hartz, A.J. A comparison of observational studies and randomized, controlled trials. *N. Engl. J. Med.* **2000**, *342*, 1878–1886. [CrossRef] [PubMed]

39. Capelas, M.; Vicuna, M.; Rosa, F. Quality assessment in palliative care—An overview. *Eur. J. Palliat. Care* **2013**, *20*, 196–198.

40. Benítez, M. Outcome evaluation in palliative care. *Med. Clin.* **2004**, *123*, 419–420. [CrossRef]

41. Hahs-Vaughn, D.L.; Onwuegbuzie, A.J. Quality of abstracts in articles submitted to a scholarly journal: A mixed methods case study of the journal research in the schools. *Libr. Inf. Sci. Res.* **2010**, *32*, 53–61. [CrossRef]

42. Lacerda, A.; Gomes, B. Trends in cause and place of death for children in Portugal (a European country with no pediatric palliative care) during 1987–2011: A population based study. *BMC Pediatr.* **2017**, *17*, 215.

43. Gomes, B.; Higginson, I.J.; Calanzani, N.; Cohen, J.; Deliens, L.; Daveson, B.A.; Bechinger-English, D.; Bausewein, C.; Ferreira, P.L.; Toscani, F.; et al. Preferences for place of death if faced with advanced cancer: A population survey in England, Flanders, Germany, Italy, the Netherlands, Portugal and Spain. *Ann. Oncol.* **2012**, *23*, 2006–2015. [CrossRef] [PubMed]

44. Gomes, B.; Sarmento, V.; Ferreira, P.L.; Higginson, I.J. Epidemiological study of place of death in Portugal in 2010 and comparison with the preferences of the Portuguese population. *Acta. Med. Port.* **2013**, *26*, 327–334. [PubMed]

45. Gomes, B.; Calanzani, N.; Curiale, V.; McCrone, P.; Higginson, I.J. Effectiveness and cost—Effectiveness of home palliative care services for adults with advanced illness and their caregivers. *Cochrane Database Syst. Rev.* **2013**, *6*. [CrossRef] [PubMed]

## 18

Taking Another Look: Thoughts on Behavioral Symptoms in Dementia and Their Measurement

Diana Lynn Woods [1,*] **and Kathleen Buckwalter** [2]

[1] School of Nursing, Azusa Pacific University, Azusa, CA 91702, USA
[2] College of Nursing, University of Iowa, Iowa City, IA 52242, USA; kathleen-buckwalter@uiowa.edu
* Correspondence: dwoods@apu.edu

Abstract: This article proposes taking another look at behavioral symptoms of dementia (BSDs) both from a theoretical perspective that informs research and practice and from a measurement perspective. We discuss why this rethinking of behaviors impacts current models of care and our ability to better detect outcomes from interventions. We propose that BSDs be viewed from a pattern perspective and provide some suggestions for how to identify and measure these patterns that can influence the timing and type of intervention. Evidence suggests that BSDs are complex, sequential, patterned clusters of behavior recurring repeatedly in the same individual and escalate significantly without timely intervention. However, BSDs are frequently viewed as separate behaviors rather than patterns or clusters of behaviors, a view that affects current research questions as well as the choice, timing, and outcomes of interventions. These symptoms cause immense distress to persons with the disease and their caregivers, trigger hospitalizations and nursing home placement, and are associated with increased care costs. Despite their universality and that symptoms manifest across disease etiologies and stages, behaviors tend to be underrecognized, undertreated, and overmanaged by pharmacological treatments that may pose more harm than benefit.

Keywords: reconceptualization; behavioral symptoms; measurement; clustering

1. Introduction

Evidence suggests that behavioral symptoms of dementia (BSDs) are complex, sequential, patterned clusters of behavior recurring repeatedly in the same individual and escalate significantly without timely intervention [1]. However, BSDs are frequently viewed as separate behaviors rather than patterns or clusters of behaviors, a view that affects current research questions as well as the choice, timing, and outcomes of interventions. Behavioral symptoms are a hallmark of dementia, representing a heterogeneous group of non-cognitive manifestations [2], commonly occurring in most persons with dementia and across disease stages and etiologies. These symptoms are often more devastating than the cognitive deficits and are frequently associated with poorer quality of life, caregiver distress, more time in caregiving, and increased hospitalizations and nursing home placements.

Despite their prevalence and negative consequences for individuals, families, and care systems (IFCS), behavioral symptoms remain under-detected, undertreated, and overmanaged by pharmacological treatments that may cause more harm than benefit and do not address symptoms most problematic to IFCS. Although nonpharmacologic treatments are promising, they continue to be underutilized.

This paper argues for rethinking how we conceptualize, define, and measure behavioral symptoms of dementia in terms of clusters and patterns, as opposed to single behaviors. This reconceptualization may significantly impact current models of care as well as the ability to evaluate treatment outcomes.

2. Current Thinking about Behavioral Symptoms

Six main foci are used to briefly discuss earlier and current conceptualizations of behavioral symptoms: early definitions and views of origin, disciplinary traditions, biomedical views, behavior as a form of communication, the Dementia Initiative perspective, and Kitwood's person-centered, personhood-oriented view [3].

The authors acknowledge that there are a variety of other conceptualizations, such as the Kales, Gitlin, and Lykestos framework used in a recent scoping review of the evidence base for determinants of selected individual BSDs including agitation, apathy, psychosis, depression, and aggression [4].

The intent of this section, however, is only to highlight selected prominent approaches to BSDs that provide background information we regard as foundational to rethinking behaviors as patterns or clusters, rather than to present an exhaustive or systematic review that evaluates the merits of each approach or favors one conceptualization over another. The way one conceptualizes BSDs influences the way in which behaviors are examined and measured, as well as the type of interventions developed and the manner in which care is provided.

How behavioral symptoms are conceptualized and defined has changed over time, and still varies today. An early definition of the term "behavioral disturbance" referred to "a behavioral or psychological syndrome or a pattern associated with subjective distress, functional disability or impaired interactions with others in the environment" [5], which evolved to behavioral and psychological symptoms of dementia (BPSDs) [6]. BSDs affect almost all persons with dementia (PWDs) at some point over the course of their illness [7], tend to fluctuate, and seldom occur in isolation [8]. Most perspectives, as reflected in the early definition above, are deficit-oriented, viewing BSDs in a negative light, as something to be "fixed" or eliminated. More recently, investigators have argued for understanding the meaning of actions and behaviors rather than pathologizing them [9].

Definitions also vary according to disciplinary traditions. Recognizing that dementia is not a disease of cognition alone, Donnelly [10] referred to BSDs as "non-cognitive neuropsychiatric symptoms" (NPSs). Included in this conceptualization are behaviors such as aggression, agitation, depression, anxiety, delusions, hallucinations, apathy and disinhibition, sleep disturbances, and executive dysfunction [2,11].

Biomedical models emphasize that BSDs arise from measurable anatomical and biochemical changes such as the association of agitation with bilateral orbitofrontal and left anterior cingulated tangles [12]. Moreover, from this perspective, neurochemical changes, alterations in neural structure and genetics, are emphasized. For example, using neuroimaging, Poulin and colleagues [13] found that aggressive behavior was associated with amygdala atrophy, while Berlow and colleagues [14] found that anxiety, sleep disorders, and aberrant motor behavior was associated with increased white matter hyperintensities. Furthermore, Boronni and colleagues [15] found sleep disturbances and delusions associated with catechol-O-methyl transferase (COMT) in the Dopamine pathway. Suffice it to say that, while imaging has helped to potentially locate neuroanatomical areas associated with behavioral symptoms, they do not fully explain the origin or clusters of behaviors.

In contrast to the biomedical conceptualization of BSDs that emphasizes the role of neurochemical, neuropathological, and genetic factors [7], multidisciplinary participants in the Dementia Initiative [16] preferred the term "behavioral expressions," which has fewer paternalistic connotations, a less negative orientation, and favors a person-centered approach to dementia care. This term also reflects an understanding that behaviors may be expressions of unmet needs that a person with dementia is unable to communicate [17,18]. An earlier but related conceptualization [3] sought to keep the PWD at the forefront of care, fostering their wellbeing rather than considering BSDs as a negative consequence of dementia. From this perspective, caregivers strive to respectfully provide meaningful activities focusing on retained strengths and interests rather than losses.

In their recent scoping review, Kolanowski and colleagues noted, "Nursing has a rich history of conceptualizing BPSD as expressions of unmet needs within frameworks, where a number of pathophysiologic, psychological, and environmental determinants are hypothesized to underlie BPSD" that have guided research [4]. They caution, however, that intervention studies based on these frameworks have seldom found large effect sizes. One early conceptual model of care for persons with dementia, the Progressively Lowered Stress Threshold Model, developed by a nurse clinician and scientist, noted that all behavior has meaning [18] and that behavior is a form of communication. Further, behaviors may arise when levels of stimuli, both external such as large groups and loud noises, and internal, such as pain or hunger, exceed the person with dementia's ability to tolerate stress. Care management strategies are therefore aimed at knowing what environments, factors or people escalate individual stress and keeping those factors in balance, and intervening before they may be disturbing to the person with dementia. Experts have long agreed that the inability of PWDs to express what they want to say or to verbally communicate concepts such as pain, loneliness, and boredom can lead to frustration, feeling upset, and agitation that is often communicated by body language, gestures, actions, and behaviors [19].

The Need-Driven Dementia-Compromised Behavioral Model (NDB), also developed from a nursing perspective and set forth by Algase and colleagues [17], posits the need to change our view of behaviors as "problematic" or "disturbing" to one of understandable expression of unmet needs, reflecting the interaction of stable background factors and environmental triggers. The NDB Model was extended by Kovach, Noonan, Schlidt, and Wells [20] to include consequences of need-driven behaviors in PWDs, or expressing needs behaviorally rather than verbally. Inherent in these nursing approaches to care of PWDs is also the need to support and educate caregivers, both formal and informal, and to treat them and the person with dementia as respected adults.

3. Etiology of Behaviors

Conceptualization of BSDs depends on the perspective of the origin of these behaviors. Many agree that cognitive impairment alone does not explain the etiology of behaviors. A variety of factors are believed to contribute to BSDs [4], including changes in the brain (biological factors), psychosocial factors such as high levels of premorbid anxiety or depression, and situational stressors such as pain, fatigue, and confusing stimuli [7,21]. As patients with dementia experience heightened vulnerability to their environment, behavioral symptoms may result from the confluence of multiple, some potentially modifiable, interacting factors including internal (e.g., pain, fear), [22] or external (e.g., over-stimulating environment, complex caregiver communications) features [23].

Single BSDs such as wandering [24,25], aggressive behavior [26,27], and disruptive vocalization [28,29] have been extensively studied. Early work by Hall and Buckwalter [18], based on clinical observations, suggested that BSDs were related to a progressively lowered stress threshold (PLST). Other explanations for BSDs have included the idea that behaviors may be driven by an individual's inability to express a need (or Need Driven Behavior, NDB) [17], resulting in behaviors such as restlessness, problematic vocalization, and wandering. More recent work by Whall et al. [26] and Algase et al. [25] examined factors underlying aggressive behavior (AB) and wandering [30,31]. Whall et al. found that AB was related to three factors: gender, stage of dementia as measured by the Mini Mental State Exam (MMSE) [32], and the degree of pre-morbid personality agreeableness. Algase et al. found that wandering differs from restlessness and is potentially related to a disordered frontal lobe. Environmental stressors may act as triggers in vulnerable individuals. All of these models have implicit/explicit characterizations of BSDs that subsequently influence research and practice.

4. Conceptualizing and Characterizing Patterns in BSDs/Behaviors Occurring in Clusters

Although numerous investigators have studied BSDs and have viewed them from a variety of perspectives as noted earlier [24–26,29,33–37], there remains little understanding of its complex organization. Research suggests that more than a third (38%) of PWDs have purposeless activity such as restlessness that is repetitive in nature, and 29–45% [29,38] exhibit problematic vocalization [39]. Although only a third (32%) of behaviors of behaviors occur alone, more than double that amount, or 66.4%, co-occur [15], and 18% co-occur within the same hour [39]. These behaviors can have significant consequences; for example, restlessness is strongly associated with reduced caregiver quality of life and premature nursing home (NH) placement [40].

Non-pharmacological interventions are currently recommended for BSDs [41] based in part on the premise that these behaviors arise as a consequence of the PWD's response to stress [18]. Two main approaches to reducing stress through nonpharmacological means are offered. The first assumes that stress can be relieved by relaxation and engendering a relaxation response; the second focuses on triggers. Both of these approaches address internal (pain, fear, sleep) and external factors (the environment and complex caregiver communication). First, researchers have studied the effects of treatments believed to produce relaxation, such as individualized music [42] calming touch [43], and aromatherapy [44,45]. Overall these interventions have demonstrated small to moderate effects with a short or unknown duration of action [46,47]. In addition, there is great within-group variation in response to treatment, a finding that has remained unexplained.

The second approach has focused on identifying BSD triggers, so that the intervention can address them. This research was guided by the assumption that given their decreased cognitive abilities, PWDs have difficulty processing environmental stimuli, including those arising from social interactions, and that if triggers can be identified and blocked, BSDs will be reduced [18,48,49]. For example, Radgneskog et al. [50] found that an increased number of BSDs was related to loss of control over a situation and loss of independence in addition to environmental noise and invasion of personal space.

The quality of interactions with people has also been studied as a trigger for BSDs, with equivocal results. For example, studies have shown that the likelihood of BSD onset during periods of verbal interaction with staff is reduced for some residents but increased for others and that the frequency and quality of social interactions with other residents, family, and visitors is negatively correlated with problematic vocalizations [51,52]. Kolanowski and Litaker [53] found a positive relationship between the number of social interactions and the number of BSDs, suggesting that an inappropriate amount of interaction might elicit BSDs, because too little or too much interaction may frustrate PWDs, thereby leading to further BSDs [51].

Herman and Williams [54] and Williams and Herman [23] examined the effect of elderspeak, an intergenerational communication style between staff and residents frequently associated with demeaning language. They found a significant co-occurrence between the use of elderspeak and resistiveness to care. While somewhat promising, these and similar studies have been limited by small samples, small effect sizes, and large intergroup variability. Hence, while the association between triggers and BSDs has been examined over the past 40 years, understanding the contribution of various triggers to BSDs remains elusive.

Recurrences of BSDs vary considerably within and between individuals. This variability is a major methodological block to the establishment of an analytic technique to reliably assess the severity, change, and temporality of BSDs [55,56]. Without the ability to meaningfully characterize BSDs, the relationship between these complex behavioral patterns and other factors, such as the environment or personality traits, remain difficult to detect reliably. Further, a recent systematic review of the literature looked at the incidence and persistence of 11 different BSDs (called BPSD in the published article), and found differences in the longitudinal courses of different behaviors and symptoms [57].

Despite numerous studies of interventions to treat BSDs, no approaches have emerged as robust treatments. Treatment effects are small, and individual response patterns vary [58]. Some speculate [59] that the development of effective interventions is compromised by measurement problems [29]. This problem is related to how we have conceptualized BSDs, contributing to our inability to quantify BSDs in ways that allow for detection of subtle behavior changes that might signify intervention responses.

The way we conceptualize behavioral symptoms is important as this continues to influence models of care, research methodologies and to guide clinical practice. This understanding has led to a focus on the quantification of frequency and severity of symptoms, devaluing the context in which a behavior occurs, particularly as we now appreciate the important role environmental factors can play in contributing to and reducing or resolving BSDs. Similarly, enduring habits, personality traits, life experiences, co-morbid conditions, and their treatment can influence what types of behaviors occur [60].

5. Measurement Issues/Problems

Accurate measurement of behaviors is essential for clinicians and researchers alike for a number of reasons. They must be able to track dementia progression, monitor the effectiveness of pharmacologic and nonpharmacologic interventions, and examine correlates of caregiver outcomes such as burden and coping. The importance of reliably capturing behaviors is evident, and yet there is no "gold standard" measure or methodology for operationalizing behaviors, despite the fact that for more than two decades clinicians and researchers have argued for a "brief, conceptually and psychometrically sound method for assessing behavioral problems in patients with dementia" [61] (p. 622). Years ago, Davis and colleagues [62] noted that variations in definition and measurement across studies have hampered efforts to draw meaningful conclusions about behaviors in dementia. Comments that remain true today. As van Derlinde and colleagues note [63] (p. 95), "Better measurements of these symptoms are needed to improve knowledge of their prevalence, associations and management." This need is echoed by Kolanowski et al. [4] (p. 516) who argue that the wide variety of symptoms associated with BSDs "are often measured inconsistently and imprecisely as one construct."

The ABC model of behavior (antecedent–behavior–consequence) [48,49,64] describes BSDs as single troublesome, or unsafe behaviors ("target behaviors") that usually emerge following a stressful event or stimuli. This perspective has heavily influenced BSD research. Under this single behavior approach, some researchers [34,65] have conceptualized BSDs as comprised of clusters or subtypes of disturbing or potentially dangerous behaviors. The single-behavior approach to studying BSDs has been used extensively including research on wandering [24,25,33], aggressive behavior [27], and problematic vocalizations (yelling) [28,29,66,67].

Most measures of BSDs, using the single behavior approach, rely on frequency (presence or absence) of the target behavior. The Cohen Mansfield Agitation Inventory (CMAI) [35] is the most widely used instrument for measuring BSDs. Moreover, this approach is not sensitive to the subtlety and discrete data that is needed to potentially characterize behaviors. Rarely considered in this type of measurement is that the absence of a behavior can also mean (as frequently happens with use of psychotropic drugs), that the target behavior is absent, but so are functional behaviors, (i.e., the PWD is somnambulant). Another factor complicating measurement using the single behavior approach is that data are often elicited using proxy reporting (family caregivers and/or nursing personnel), using scales such as the BEHAVE-AD [68]. While there is efficiency in this approach in terms of time, it is fraught with problems since caregivers' recall of BSDs is strongly influenced by their psychological state and needs [69].

Using a Functional Analysis Checklist (FAC), a checklist that uses the ABC model of behavior, James and colleagues [70] assessed the ability of 76 staff members to indicate situations and settings that triggered challenging behaviors. Each pair of staff rated antecedents. Results indicated that staff agreement was poor related to what may be triggering these challenging behaviors. James and colleagues concluded that training about systematic observation and reporting on the nature of behaviors may result in higher agreement scores. Another issue may be the reliance on a priori assumptions, such as are evident in the ABC model, rather than using observed quantitative data and an algorithmic approach to assessing the clustering of behaviors.

Two major sources of error are possible: caregiver exaggeration, where the caregiver reports an increased number of events, and caregiver denial, where the few or benign behavior problems are not reported [71,72]. In addition, caregivers' reports can be unstable from hour to hour and day to day, changing as their own needs change. Another problem is that scales such as the BEHAVE-AD take a global approach to measurement. Because they rely on recall, behaviors are "lumped" together over a specified time period (e.g., yesterday, or in the last week), even though studies show that BSDs have temporal patterns [73–75], meaning that they vary in more or less predictable ways throughout the day. Lumping leads to a lack of specificity with the loss of temporal variation. In addition, the recall of one behavior at one time may be considered sufficient for a global categorization of "displaying BSDs", but not for determining the temporal or individual variation.

Researchers have long recognized these limitations. For example, Cohen-Mansfield further refined the CMAI by developing the Agitated Behavior Mapping Instrument (ABMI) for use with direct observation [35]. While an improvement over informant reporting, this scale measures only the frequency of a behavior and not the intensity, remaining focused on single target behaviors [69]. That BSDs are characterized by intensity as well as frequency is rarely considered. Intensity is defined as the troublesomeness of the behavior. Yelling, for example, is more troublesome than mumbling or picking at the bedclothes. The only scales to date that rate both the frequency and the intensity of BSDs using direct observation are the Agitated Behavior Rating Scale (ABRS) [76] and the refined version of the Modified Agitated Behavior Rating Scale (mABRS) [77]. For example, with vocalization, mumbling is scored at an intensity of 1, while yelling is scored at an intensity of 3. Direct observation allows for specificity about the type, intensity, and frequency of behavior and permits exploration of temporal variation.

While current conceptualizations of BSDs include the concept of behavioral patterns, measuring these patterns remains challenging [78]. Two types of patterns have been considered: temporal patterns and patterns of escalation. Both patterns have been acknowledged and examined for the past several years using a variety of methods in an attempt to determine the time of peak behavior, albeit using aggregated data, and instruments designed to be used in cross-sectional studies [69]. Previous examination has been limited by the statistical methods and computer technology available as well as the breadth of accessible data.

Patterns of escalation describe an increase in (usually frequency and less commonly intensity) a specific behavior. For example, vocalization may progress from repeating a word to screaming. Several researchers have described a sequence of behavioral escalation that has clear starting and ending points, calm behavior progressing to violence. Behavior that follows an "ideal" sequence from verbal agitation escalating to verbally aggressive behavior suggests a linear pattern. The reverse, de-escalation, is assumed but rarely described. Less severe/intense behaviors are placed lower on the continuum, while more severe/intense behaviors are higher [1]. Escalation can also proceed from one behavioral category to another, suggesting that these patterns are more complex, increasing in variability while co-occurring [78,79].

Temporality, the period of time within which a behavior changes, can be demonstrated in the case of vocalization. This behavior may begin as repetitive mumbling and escalate to louder calling, then yelling within a period of 20–40 min [1]. Viewed from this perspective, a model of escalation predicts that PWDs initially demonstrate low-intensity BSDs, which, when they continue over time, may escalate to a more severe behavior. However, in contrast to the "ideal" escalation/de-escalation pattern, Woods et al. [1] examined patterns of escalation of BSDs using videotaped data, finding that the "ideal" pattern was rarely observed. Rather, patterns moved back and forth between behavioral categories rather than escalating within categories in a linear fashion. This suggests that patterns escalate in frequency and intensity as well as complexity (i.e., an increase in variability among co-occurring behaviors).

To further confound measurement issues there is a great deal of intra- and interindividual variability in the expression and frequency of behaviors among persons with dementia. Certainly behaviors are not consistently expressed by all PWDs and commonly fluctuate over the course of the illness as well as during the day (diurnal variation). Thus, while a particular instrument may capture behaviors in the early disease stages, it may not be valid later on in the disease or be sufficiently sensitive to clinical change. For example, in the early stages, personality changes, apathy, decreased capability to manage instrumental activities of daily living and irritability are common. As the dementia progresses, behaviors often become more disruptive and psychiatric symptoms may emerge, including aggression, wandering, paranoia, hallucinations, and delusions. By the late or final stages of the illness, PWDs are frequently bedbound and too debilitated to express many of the aforementioned behaviors. Bharucha and colleagues [80] suggest that it is particularly difficult to capture low-frequency high-impact behaviors over time. Other factors that can complicate the measurement of behaviors include bias in raters and scoring, a lack of bench-marking studies, construct slippage, and shifting domains [62].

Other measurement issues include attempts to integrate multiple, distinct constructs into one measure. For example, early conceptually challenged scales measured not only behaviors but also activities of daily living and cognition [80]. Further, many symptoms may overlap in conditions such as depression and apathy, agitation, and aggression.

The validity of instruments that rely on responses from the person with dementia may be compromised by their sensory loss (visual/hearing) or perceptual and cognitive deficits [80]. Other tools for which data is provided by proxy informants (e.g., clinical staff and family caregivers) can be affected by factors such as inadequate training in assessment or devaluing of the importance of careful documentation of behaviors [80]. Their own stress levels and emotional health, as well as their relationship to the person with dementia, may also affect the soundness of caregiver evaluations.

6. Analysis Issues/Problems

Studying patterns of BSDs is hampered by measurement as well as the analysis strategies used. In the study of temporal patterns, for example, to establish peak times of BSDs, single behaviors or several behaviors tend to be summed, aggregated, and analyzed using ANOVA for repeated measures, thus limiting the ability to detect clustered behavior patterns across time. However, data show [24,25, 29,33,75,79] that recurrences of BSDs vary considerably within and between individuals. While data aggregation may demonstrate differences in response between groups, individual variation within subjects across time is lost.

Measuring individual variability may be key to the timing of interventions [55,56] and to answering the question: will this intervention work for this person? [81]. Another method used extensively to determine behavioral complexity and temporal patterns using direct observational data is lag sequential analysis (LSA) [82].

This analytic method examines the probability that a behavior will be followed by another behavior of interest and has been used to detect behavioral recurrence and temporal patterns such as those seen in persons with self-injurious behavior (SIB) [83] in persons with disabilities [36] and to a limited extent in persons with dementia exhibiting BSDs [1]. While this type of analysis allows examination of both the persistence of a behavior (behavior remaining the same within a period of time) and transition, or a change from one state (intensity) to another, a major limitation is the assumption that a temporal window can be specified, for example that the behavior occurs every 20 min. Any behavior that does not fall into this temporal window will be missed.

7. Rethinking BSDs

Given the acknowledged problems with measurement, the authors propose that BSDs, rather than always being single events, are complex, non-sequential, non-random, patterned clusters of behavior that recur repeatedly in the same person [1,59,78]. These behavior patterns vary by the number of clusters in a specific time period, the level of intensity of behaviors contained in the clusters, and the number of different clusters displayed in a specific time period. We conceptualize escalation as behaviors becoming more frequent, but also becoming more complex (increased in variability among co-occurring behaviors) and more intense (more troublesome) over time [1]. These patterned clusters of behavior may be linked together in predictable ways. As recently noted by Kovach in an editorial commenting on gerontological nursing research trends and needs [84] (p. 228), "When symptoms co-occur or occur in clusters, there may be important interactions and influences on health and the treatment needed."

Therefore, escalation involves behavioral chains that begin with benign behaviors and culminate in the target behavior that can be very disruptive to family and staff caregivers. For example, particularly troublesome behaviors like yelling may be accompanied by benign behaviors (e.g., fidgeting and tapping) that may actually be part of a pattern of escalation. One reason for the failure of studies of BSD triggers to have definitive results may be that measurement begins at the point when the target behavior (e.g., yelling) occurs, although a trigger may have precipitated a behavioral chain that begins with the appearance of more benign behaviors and escalates to the target behavior. Other distinguished nurse scientists have come to this conclusion in other clinical populations. For example, Woods and colleagues [85] utilized more innovative analytic techniques, such as Group Based Trajectory Modelling and Latent Class Analysis, to elucidate how menopausal symptoms cluster and are associated with specific single nucleotide polymorphisms (SNPs) [86].

Current conceptualizations of BSDs, bound by disciplinary perspectives, have been somewhat limiting to date. As emphasized earlier, the way we conceptualize behavioral symptoms is important as this continues to influence models of care and research methodologies and to guide clinical practice. They have also led to measures that focus on the quantification of frequency and severity, devaluing the context in which a behavior occurs. The latter is particularly unfortunate as both research findings and theoretical developments have noted the powerful role environmental factors can play in contributing to BSDs. When such measures are used in a supportive manner, and consider the context, they may reduce and resolve behaviors. Similarly, long-standing habits, personality traits, life experiences, co-morbid conditions, and their treatment can also influence what types of behaviors occur [60]. For these reasons, we need to reconceptualize behavioral symptoms. This reconceptualization is germane to models of care because the models that we use, whether implicit or explicit, profoundly affect our practice.

Research outcomes that are more sensitive and that enable us to target us to target interventions more precisely are needed. The more precise we are in describing the phenomenon, the more precise and timely the intervention, thus leading to improved clinical outcomes. This need has also been recognized by Kolanowski et al. [4], who support more funding for the development of measures that will have more precision to capture the characteristics of BSDs, attending to the context in which those behaviors occur.

8. Alternative Measurement Strategy: Principles of Measurement

Consistent with our conceptualization of BSDs, we suggest using a pattern recognition software strategy such as THEME™ software [87] to detect complex, non-random behavior patterns that do not necessarily occur in a proscribed sequence within a person. THEME™ makes no a priori assumptions about the characteristics of the behavior patterns. Rather, it allows the data to inform the patterns, providing a more accurate characterization of temporal behavior patterns, behavior complexity and escalation. THEME™ detects the complexity, frequency, and interrelationships of behavior patterns, and then quantifies these factors within person, providing a method of detecting within individual sequential and non-sequential temporal patterns (T-patterns) of related behavior clusters (chains) that are not obvious to the trained observer or identifiable by traditional sequential methods [87,88].

Initially, this pattern recognition software identifies significant (non-random) recurrences of any two behaviors, such as low intensity restlessness or vocalization. These patterns are incorporated into more complex patterns. For example, behaviors such as vocalization and restlessness at a high intensity, combined with other behaviors such as tapping and banging, interacting with a staff member, and then being left alone, can constitute a complex behavior pattern. Escalation measured in this way shows behavior clusters that include behaviors of low intensity becoming more complex and different behaviors of higher intensity. A further description of this methodology can be found in Woods et al. [78].

Utilizing this method has several advantages. It (a) is not constrained by implicit assumptions about the behaviors of interest, (b) allows the data to inform the resultant patterns, a process that is more inductive than deductive; (c) results in a more accurate characterization of behavior patterns, and (d) captures nuances in pattern escalation that cannot be detected by a trained observer or identifiable using traditional sequential methods. Once the behavior clusters have been identified and quantified, these data can be transferred into a statistical software package such as SPSS for further analysis, such as the calculation of within individual percent of patterns containing high-intensity behavior. Individual characteristics can then be compared and behavior change over time and individual patterns of response can be identified.

Limitations to the use of this software include the use of humans to collect the data using prior definitions of behaviors, issues similar to those noted previously in the paper. Questions include what the definitions of behaviors are, whether they are being observed, and what data is input and by whom? This is true if human beings are completing all of the observations but does not necessarily apply if the data are gathered by motion sensors and other types of technology such as Kinect by Microsoft, which does not require collection by human beings. Algorithms are currently being devised and tested, similar to those within THEME, to "read" the data and flag potential issues. These areas are in development and show promise for the future.

Pattern recognition software can contribute significantly to the detection and characterization of BSDs. The following are examples of what might be an expected result from different interventions.

8.1. Example of Pharmacological Intervention

THEME™ can detect behavioral subtlety in temporal patterns of behavioral clusters. Once these clusters are detected and quantified, pharmacological interventions can be specifically targeted and timed to alter these detected behavioral clusters of high-intensity behavior. The intervention can then be tested such that an expected outcome would be a decrease in the percentage of complex behaviors containing high-intensity behavior, which would create a more sensitive measure for determining the dosage and timing of pharmacological treatments.

8.2. Example of Nonpharmacological Intervention

Nursing home settings are complex environments [89], and the level of noise and crowding may increase environmental press leading to BSDs [90]. Using THEME™, the pattern of temporal behavioral clusters can be quantified and related to environmental complexity at baseline. If an intervention is applied to decrease environmental complexity, the effect could be reflected in a decrease in complex patterns of behavioral clusters. Even if the effect influences only one or two individuals with high-intensity behaviors, research shows that decreasing the BSDs of specific individuals frequently results in a generalized decrease of BSDs on the entire unit, especially in designated dementia units [91]. Interventions tailored more specifically to individuals would result in a more efficient use of resources. Once we understand who responds and the characteristics of the behavioral clusters exhibited by individuals who respond, we may be able to tailor and time effective interventions. For example, a nonpharmacological intervention may alter the complexity of BSDs by decreasing the number and intensity of behaviors that occur together, by altering the number of behavioral complexes that contain high-intensity behavior, or by altering the frequency of the behavioral complexes that occur over time. These results can decrease not only staff time and frustration but also the associated costs [92].

The ability to quantify these patterns of behavior and validate these patterns with other biological measures, such as stress hormones and temperature, is key to the development of tailored interventions. Our vision for clinical practice and management is that, by characterizing the patterns of BSD escalation, person-centered interventions [93] will be modified and timed to ameliorate BSDs and to prevent escalation and associated adverse outcomes in both PWDs and staff [78].

9. Conclusions

Results from studies of interventions for reducing and/or eliminating BSDs have had equivocal and somewhat disappointing results. Given the current conceptualization and strategies available for measuring outcomes, however, it is difficult to know if the problem is with the interventions or with the measurement of outcomes. The measures currently used to evaluate treatment efficacy are devised using a single indicator, a dichotomous approach that focuses on the presence or absence of specific high-intensity behaviors such as yelling and intense restlessness. These measurement strategies are based on the belief that behavioral symptoms are separate or that they may occur with one other behavior rather than the notion that behaviors cluster.

Lost in the prevailing measurement approaches is that BSDs are characterized by intensity (troublesomeness) and complexity (variability among co-occurring behaviors) as well as frequency. Temporal patterns of co-occurring behaviors or behavioral clusters are also diminished. Detecting temporal changes in behavioral clusters might be the key to detecting subtle behavior changes that herald an unrecognized treatment response or a response that suggests the need for a different treatment approach. Further information is hidden in analysis techniques that employ aggregation of data or in a priori assumptions about the nature of relationships.

The conceptual and measurement problems in studies of BSDs have been recognized for some time. Most of the currently used behavioral rating instruments were designed for cross-sectional use, and few data are available regarding their usefulness for longitudinal tracking of behaviors or their sensitivity to behavioral changes produced by specific interventions. Therefore, we reconceptualize BSDs not as single events, but as complex patterned clusters of behaviors and suggest that new analysis strategies, such as pattern recognition software, may enhance the detection of BSDs and better enable researchers to evaluate treatment outcomes.

Author Contributions: D.L.W. conceptualized the original article, K.B. completed a literature review and wrote the first drafts of the manuscript. K.B. contributed to the literature review on conceptualizations of BSDs, wrote and revised significant sections of the manuscript, and edited drafts of the article.

Funding: This research received no external funding.

References

1. Woods, D.L.; Rapp, C.G.; Beck, C. Escalation/de-escalation patterns of behavioral symptoms of persons with dementia. *Aging Ment. Health* **2004**, *8*, 126–132. [CrossRef] [PubMed]
2. Kales, H.C.; Gitlin, L.N.; Lyketsos, C.G. Assessment and management of behavioral symptoms of dementia. *BMJ* **2015**, *350*, 369–385. [CrossRef] [PubMed]
3. Kitwood, T.; Bredin, K. Towards a theory of dementia care: Personhood and well-being. *Aging Soc.* **1992**, *12*, 269–287. [CrossRef]
4. Kolanowski, A.; Boltz, M.; Galik, E.; Gitlin, L.; Scerpella, D. Determinants of behavioral and psychological symptoms of dementia: A scoping review. *Nurs. Outlook* **2017**, *65*, 515–529. [CrossRef] [PubMed]
5. Tariot, P.; Blazina, L.; Morris, J. *Handbook of Dementing Illness*; Marcel Dekker: New York, NY, USA, 1993; p. 461.
6. Finkel, S.I.; Costa de Silva, J.; Cohen, G.; Miller, S.; Sartorius, N. Behavioral and psychological signs and symptoms of dementia: A consensus statement on current knowledge and implications for research and treatment. *Int. Psychogeriatr.* **1996**, *8*, 497–500. [CrossRef] [PubMed]
7. Cerejeira, J.; Largarto, L.; Mukaetova-Ladinska, E.B. Behavioral and psychological symptoms of dementia. *Front. Neurol.* **2012**, *3*, 73. [CrossRef] [PubMed]
8. Lawlor, B. Managing behavioral and psychological symptoms in dementia. *Br. J. Psychiatry* **2002**, *181*, 463–465. [CrossRef] [PubMed]
9. Dupuis, S.L.; Wiersma, E.; Loiselle, L. Pathologizing behavior: Meanings of behaviors in dementia care. *J. Aging Stud.* **2012**, *26*, 162–173. [CrossRef]

10. Donnelly, M.L. Behavioral and psychological disturbances in Alzheimer disease: Assessment and treatment. *BC Med. J.* **2005**, *47*, 487–493.

11. Kales, H.C.; Gitlin, L.N.; Lyketsos, C.G. Management of neuropsychiatric symptoms of dementia in clinical settings: Recommendations from a multidisciplinary expert panel. *J. Am. Geriatr. Soc.* **2014**, *62*, 762–769. [CrossRef] [PubMed]

12. Tekin, S.; Mega, M.S.; Masterman, D.M.; Chow, T.; Garakian, J.; Vinters, H.V.; Cummings, J. Orbitofrontal and anterior cingulate cortex neurofibrillary tangle burden is associated with agitation in Alzheimer disease. *Ann. Neurol.* **2001**, *49*, 355–361. [CrossRef] [PubMed]

13. Poulin, S.P.; Dautoff, R.; Morris, J.C.; Barrett, L.F.; Dickerson, B.C. Amygdala atrophy is prominent in early Alzheimer's disease and relates to symptom severity. *Psychiatry Res.* **2011**, *194*, 7–13. [CrossRef] [PubMed]

14. Berlow, Y.A.; Wells, W.M.; Ellison, J.M.; Sung, Y.H.; Renshaw, P.F.; Harper, D.G. Neuropsychiatric correlates of white matter hyperintensities in Alzheimer's disease. *Int. Psychogeriatr.* **2010**, *25*, 780–788. [CrossRef] [PubMed]

15. Borroni, B.; Grassi, M.; Agosti, C.; Costanzi, C.; Archetti, S.; Franzoni, S.; Caltagirone, C.; Di Luca, M.; Caimi, L.; Padovani, A. Genetic correlates of behavioral endophenotypes in alzheimer disease: Role of COMT, 5-HTTLPR and APOE polymorphisms. *Neurobiol. Aging* **2006**, *27*, 1595–1603. [CrossRef] [PubMed]

16. Love, K.; Pinkowitz, J. Dementia Care: The Quality Chasm. National Dementia Initiative (Currently the Dementia Action Alliance). Available online: http://daanow.org/dementia-action-alliance/white-paper (accessed on 1 October 2018).

17. Algase, D.L.; Beck, C.; Kolanowski, A.; Whall, A.; Berent, S.K.; Richards, K.; Beattie, E. Need-driven dementia-compromised behavior: An alternative view of disruptive behavior. *Am. J. Alzheimers Dis. Other Dement.* **1996**, *11*, 10–19. [CrossRef]

18. Hall, G.R.; Buckwalter, K.C. Progressively lowered stress threshold: A conceptual model for care of adults with Alzheimer's disease. *Arch. Psychiatr. Nurs.* **1987**, *1*, 399–406. [PubMed]

19. Cohen-Mansfield, J. Turnover among nursing home staff. A review. *Nurs. Manag.* **1997**, *28*, 59–62, 64. [CrossRef]

20. Kovach, C.R.; Noonan, P.E.; Schlidt, A.M.; Wells, T. A model of consequences of need-driven, dementia-compromised behavior. *J. Nurs. Scholarsh.* **2005**, *37*, 134–140. [CrossRef] [PubMed]

21. Haibo, X.; Shifu, X.; Pin, N.T.; Chao, C.; Guorong, M.; Xuejue, L.; Wenli, F.; Jun, L.; Mingyan, Z.; McCabe, M. Prevalence and severity of behavioral and psychological symptoms of dementia (BPSD) in community dwelling Chinese: Findings from the Shanghai three district study. *Aging Ment. Health* **2013**, *17*, 748–752. [CrossRef] [PubMed]

22. Hodgson, N.; Gitlin, L.N.; Winter, L.N.; Hauck, W.W. Caregiver's perceptions of the relationship of pain to behavioral and psychiatric symptoms in older community residing adults with dementia. *Clin. J. Pain.* **2014**, *30*, 421–427. [CrossRef] [PubMed]

23. Williams, K.N.; Herman, R.E. Linking resident behavior to dementia care communication: Effects of emotional tone. *Behav. Ther.* **2011**, *42*, 42–46. [CrossRef] [PubMed]

24. Algase, D.L.; Moore, D.H.; Vandeweerd, C.; Gavin-Dreschnack, D.J. Mapping the maze of terms and definitions in dementia-related wandering. *Aging Ment. Health* **2007**, *11*, 686–698. [CrossRef] [PubMed]

25. Algase, D.L.; Antonakos, C.; Yao, L.; Beattie, E.; Hong, G.; Beel-Bates, C. Are wandering and physically nonaggressive agitation equivalent? *Am. J. Geriatr. Psychiatry* **2008**, *16*, 293–299. [CrossRef] [PubMed]

26. Whall, A.; Colling, K.; Kolanowski, A.; Kim, H.; Son Hong, G.; DeCicco, B.; Ronnis, D.L.; Richards, K.C.; Algase, D.; Beck, C. Factors associated with aggressive behavior among nursing home residents with dementia. *Gerontologist* **2008**, *48*, 721–731. [CrossRef] [PubMed]

27. Whall, A.; Kim, H.; Colling, K.; Hong, G.R.; DeCicco, B.; Antonakos, C. Measurement of aggressive behaviors in dementia: Comparison of the physical aggression subscales of the Cohen-Mansfield agitation inventory and the Ryden aggression scale. *Res. Gerontol. Nurs.* **2013**, *6*, 171–177. [CrossRef] [PubMed]

28. Beck, C.; Frank, L.; Chumbler, N.R.; O'Sullivan, P.; Vogelpohl, T.S.; Rasin, J.; Walls, R.; Baldwin, B. Correlates of disruptive behavior in severely cognitively impaired nursing home residents. *Gerontologist* **1998**, *38*, 189–198. [CrossRef] [PubMed]

29. Beck, C.; Richards, K.; Lambert, C.; Doan, R.; Landes, R.D.; Whall, A.; Algase, D.; Kolanowski, A.; Feldman, Z. Factors associated with problematic vocalizations in nursing home residents with dementia. *Gerontologist* **2011**, *51*, 389–405. [CrossRef] [PubMed]

30. Moore, D.H.; Algase, D.L.; Powell-Cope, G.; Applegarth, S.; Beattie, E.R. A framework for managing wandering and preventing elopement. *Am. J. Alzheimers Dis. Other Dement.* **2009**, *24*, 208–219. [CrossRef] [PubMed]

31. Song, J.A.; Algase, D. Premorbid characteristics and wandering behavior in persons with dementia. *Arch. Psychiatr. Nurs.* **2008**, *22*, 318–327. [CrossRef] [PubMed]

32. Folstein, M.; Folsten, S.; McHugh, P. Mini-mental state: A practical method for grading the cognitive state of patients for the clinician. *J. Psychiatry Res.* **1975**, *12*, 189–198. [CrossRef]

33. Algase, D.L.; Beattie, E.R.; Therrien, B. Impact of cognitive impairment on wandering behavior. *West. J. Nurs. Res.* **2001**, *23*, 283–295. [CrossRef] [PubMed]

34. Cohen-Mansfield, J.; Billig, N. Agitated behaviors in the elderly: A conceptual review. *J. Am. Geriatr. Soc.* **1986**, *34*, 711–721. [CrossRef] [PubMed]

35. Cohen-Mansfield, J.; Marx, M.S.; Rosenthal, A.S. A description of agitation in a nursing home. *J. Gerontol.* **1989**, *44*, M77–M84. [CrossRef] [PubMed]

36. Emerson, E.; Thompson, S.; Reeves, D.; Henderson, D.; Robertson, J. Descriptive analysis of multiple response topographies of challenging behavior across two settings. *Res. Dev. Disabil.* **1995**, *16*, 301–329. [CrossRef]

37. Ferrari, E.; Fioravanti, M.; Magri, F.; Solerte, S.B. Variability of interactions between neuroendocrine and immunological functions in physiological aging and dementia of the Alzheimer's type. *Ann. N. Y. Acad. Sci.* **2000**, *917*, 582–596. [CrossRef] [PubMed]

38. Kemp, A.S.; Fillmore, P.T.; Lenjavi, M.R.; Lyon, M.; Chicz-Demet, A.; Touchette, P.E.; Sandman, C.A. Temporal patterns of self-injurious behavior correlate with stress hormone levels in the developmentally disabled. *Psychiatry Res.* **2008**, *157*, 181–189. [CrossRef] [PubMed]

39. Souder, E.; Heithoff, K.; O'Sullivan, P.S.; Lancaster, A.E.; Beck, C. Identifying patterns of disruptive behavior in long-term care residents. *J. Am. Geriatr. Soc.* **1999**, *47*, 830–836. [CrossRef] [PubMed]

40. Shin, M.D.; Carter, M.; Masterman, D.; Fairbanks, L.; Cummings, J.L. Neuropsychiatric symptoms and quality of life in Alzheimer disease. *Am. J. Geriatr. Psychiatry* **2005**, *13*, 469–474. [CrossRef] [PubMed]

41. Hsu, T.J.; Tsai, H.T.; Chen, L.Y.; Chen, L.K. Predictors of non-pharmacological intervention effect on cognitive function and behavioral and psychological symptoms of older people with dementia. *Geriatr. Gerontol. Int.* **2017**, *17*, 28–35. [CrossRef] [PubMed]

42. Gerdner, L. Individualized music for dementia: Evolution and application of evidence-based protocol. *World J. Psychiatry* **2012**, *2*, 26–32. [CrossRef] [PubMed]

43. Woods, D.L.; Craven, R.F.; Whitney, J. The effect of therapeutic touch on behavioral symptoms of persons with dementia. *Altern. Ther. Health Med.* **2005**, *11*, 66–74. [CrossRef] [PubMed]

44. Ballard, C.G.; O'Brien, J.T.; Reichelt, K.; Perry, E.K. Aromatherapy as a safe and effective treatment for the management of agitation in severe dementia: The results of a double-blind, placebo-controlled trial with Melissa. *J. Clin. Psychiatry* **2002**, *63*, 553–558. [CrossRef] [PubMed]

45. Snow, L.; Hovanec, L.; Brandt, J. A controlled trial of aromatherapy for agitation in nursing home patients with dementia. *J. Altern. Complement. Med.* **2004**, *10*, 431–437. [CrossRef] [PubMed]

46. Kong, E.H.; Evans, L.K.; Guevara, J.P. Nonpharmacological intervention for agitation in dementia: A systematic review and meta-analysis. *Aging Ment. Health* **2009**, *13*, 512–520. [CrossRef] [PubMed]

47. O'Connor, D.W.; Ames, D.; Gardner, B.; King, M. Psychosocial treatments of psychological symptoms in dementia: A systematic review of reports meeting quality standards. *Int. Psychogeriatr.* **2009**, *21*, 241–251. [CrossRef] [PubMed]

48. Mather, N.; Goldstein, S. Learning disabilities and challenging behaviors: A guide to intervention and classroom management. *J. Am. Geriatr. Soc.* **2001**, *62*, 762–769.

49. Smith, M. *Understanding & Responding to Behavioral Symptoms in Dementia—Revision of Acting Up and Acting Out: Assessment and Management of Aggressive and Acting Out Behaviors*; The John A. Hartford Center of Geriatric Nursing Excellence (HCGNE), College of Nursing, University of Iowa: Iowa City, IA, USA, 2005.

50. Ragneskog, H.; Gerdner, L.; Josefsson, K.; Kihlgren, M. Probable reasons for expressed agitation in persons with dementia. *Clin. Nurs. Res.* **1998**, *7*, 189–206. [CrossRef] [PubMed]

51. Burgio, L.D.; Butler, F.R.; Roth, D.L.; Hardin, J.M.; Hsu, C.C.; Ung, K. Agitation in nursing home residents: The role of gender and social context. *Int. Psychogeriatr.* **2000**, *12*, 495–511. [CrossRef] [PubMed]

52. Kolanowski, A.; Litaker, M.; Buettner, L.; Moeller, J.; Costa, P.T., Jr. A randomized clinical trial of theory-based activities for the behavioral symptoms of dementia in nursing home residents. *J. Am. Geriatr. Soc.* **2011**, *59*, 1032–1041. [CrossRef] [PubMed]

53. Kolanowski, A.; Litaker, M. Social interaction, premorbid personality, and agitation in nursing home residents with dementia. *Arch. Psychiatr. Nurs.* **2006**, *20*, 12–20. [CrossRef] [PubMed]

54. Herman, R.E.; Williams, K.N. Elderspeak's influence on resistiveness to care: Focus on behavioral events. *Am. J. Alzheimers Dis. Other Dement.* **2009**, *24*, 417–423. [CrossRef] [PubMed]

55. Schroeder, S.R.; Oster-Granite, M.L.; Thompson, T. *Self-Injurious Behavior: Gene-Brain-Behavior Relationships*; American Psychological Association: Washington, DC, USA, 2002.

56. Symons, F.J.; Sperry, L.A.; Dropik, P.L.; Bodfish, J.W. The early development of stereotypy and self-injury: A review of research methods. *J. Intellect. Disabil. Res.* **2005**, *49*, 144–158. [CrossRef] [PubMed]

57. van der Linde, R.M.; Dening, T.; Stephan, B.C.M.; Prina, A.M.; Evans, E.; Brayne, C. Longitudinal course of behavioural and psychological symptoms of dementia: Systematic review. *Br. J. Psychiatry* **2016**, *209*, 366–377. [CrossRef] [PubMed]

58. Livingston, G.; Lim, L.S. A systematic review of the clinical effectiveness and cost effectiveness of sensory, psychological, and behavioural interventions for managing agitation in older adults with dementia. *Health Technol. Assess.* **2014**, *18*, 1–226. [CrossRef] [PubMed]

59. von Gunten, A.; Alnawaqil, A.; Abderhalden, C.; Needham, I.; Schupbach, B. Vocally disruptive behavior in the elderly: A systematic review. *Int. Psychogeriatr.* **2008**, *20*, 653–672. [CrossRef] [PubMed]

60. Tible, O.P.; Riese, F.; Savaskan, E.; von Gunten, A. Best practice in the management of behavioural and psychological symptoms of dementia. *Ther. Adv. Neurol. Disord.* **2017**, *10*, 297–309. [CrossRef] [PubMed]

61. Teri, L.; Truax, P.; Logsdon, R.; Uomoto, J.; Zarit, S.; Vitaliano, P.P. Assessment of behavioral problems in dementia: The revised memory and behavior problem checklist. *Psychol. Aging* **1992**, *7*, 622–631. [CrossRef] [PubMed]

62. Davis, L.; Buckwalter, K.; Burgio, L. Measuring problem behaviors in dementia: Developing a methodological agenda. *ANS Adv. Nurs. Sci.* **1997**, *20*, 40–55. [CrossRef] [PubMed]

63. van der Linde, R.M.; Stephan, B.C.; Dening, T.; Brayne, C. Instruments to measure behavioural and psychological symptoms of dementia. *Int. J. Psychiatr. Res.* **2014**, *23*, 69–98. [CrossRef] [PubMed]

64. Skinner, B.F. Behavior modification. *Science* **1974**, *185*, 813. [CrossRef] [PubMed]

65. Cohen-Mansfield, J. Agitated behaviors in the elderly: II. preliminary results in the cognitively deteriorated. *J. Am. Geriatr. Soc.* **1986**, *34*, 722–727. [CrossRef] [PubMed]

66. Boustani, M.; Zimmerman, S.; Williams, C.S.; Gruber-Baldini, A.L.; Watson, L.; Reed, P.S.; Sloane, P.D. Characteristics associated with behavioral symptoms related to dementia in long-term care residents. *Gerontologist* **2005**, *45*, 56–61. [CrossRef] [PubMed]

67. Sloane, P.D.; Davidson, S.; Knight, N.; Tangen, C.; Mitchell, C.M. Severe disruptive vocalizers. *J. Am. Geriatr. Soc.* **1999**, *47*, 439–445. [CrossRef] [PubMed]

68. Reisberg, B.; Borenstein, J.; Salob, S.P.; Ferris, S.H.; Franssen, E.; Georgotas, A. Behavioral symptoms in Alzheimer's disease: Phenomenology and treatment. *J. Clin. Psychiatry* **1987**, *48*, 9–15. [PubMed]

69. Cummings, J. Theories behind existing scales for rating behavior in dementia. *Int. Psychogeriatr.* **1996**, *8*, 293–300. [CrossRef] [PubMed]

70. James, I.A.; McClintock, K.; Reichelt, K.; Ellingford, J. Are staff reliable informants? *Int. J. Geriatr. Psychiatry* **2007**, *22*, 598–600. [CrossRef] [PubMed]

71. Ali, S.; Bokharey, Z. Caregiving in dementia: Emotional and behavioral challenges. *Educ. Gerontol.* **2016**, *42*, 455–464. [CrossRef]

72. Jennings, L.A.; Reuben, D.B.; Everston, L.C.; Serrano, K.S.; Ercoli, L.; Grill, J.; Chodosh, J.; Tan, Z.; Wenger, N.S. Unmet needs of caregivers of patients referred to a dementia care program. *J. Am. Geriatr. Soc.* **2015**, *63*, 282–289. [CrossRef] [PubMed]

73. Martin, J.; Marler, M.; Shochat, T.; Ancoli-Israel, S. Circadian rhythms of agitation in institutionalized patients with Alzheimer's disease. *Chronobiol. Int.* **2000**, *17*, 405–418. [CrossRef] [PubMed]

74. Cohen-Mansfield, J. Temporal patterns of agitation in dementia. *Am. J. Geriatr. Psychiatry* **2007**, *15*, 395–405. [CrossRef] [PubMed]

75. Woods, D.L.; Kim, H.; Yefimova, M. Morning cortisol is associated with behavioral symptoms of nursing home residents with dementia. *Biol. Res. Nurs.* **2010**, *13*, 196–203. [CrossRef] [PubMed]

76. Bliwise, D.L.; Lee, K.A. Development of an agitated behavior rating scale for discrete temporal observations. *J. Nurs. Meas.* **1993**, *1*, 115–124. [PubMed]

77. Woods, D.L.; Dimond, M. The effect of therapeutic touch on agitated behavior and cortisol in persons with Alzheimer's disease. *Biol. Res. Nurs.* **2002**, *4*, 104–114. [CrossRef] [PubMed]

78. Woods, D.L.; Yefimova, M.; Kim, H.; Phillips, L.R. Detecting and characterizing patterns of behavioral symptoms of dementia. In *Discovering Hidden Temporal Patterns in Behavior and Interaction*; Magnusson, M.S., Burgoon, J.K., Cassarrubea, M., Eds.; Springer: New York, NY, USA, 2016.

79. Woods, D.L.; Yefimova, M.; Brecht, M.L. A method for measuring person-centered interventions: Detecting and characterizing complex behavioral symptoms of persons with dementia. *Clin. Gerontol.* **2014**, *37*, 139–150. [CrossRef]

80. Bharucha, A.J.; Rosen, J.; Mulsant, B.H.; Pollock, B.G. Assessment of behavioral and psychological symptoms of dementia. *Prim. Psychiatry* **2002**, *7*, 797–802. [CrossRef]

81. Donaldson, G. Randomized trials for comparative effectiveness: The bronze standard again? In *Advancing Scientific Innovations in Nursing, Proceedings of the Western Institute of Nursing, Communicating Nursing Research Conference, Portland Marriott Downtown Waterfront Hotel, Portland, OR, USA, 14 April 2012*; Western Institute of Nursing: Portland, OR, USA, 2012; pp. 1–17.

82. Sackett, G.P. The lag sequential analysis of contigency and cyclicity in behavioral interaction research. In *Handbook of Infant Development*; Doniger, J., Ed.; John Wiley & Sons: Hoboken, NJ, USA, 1979; pp. 623–649.

83. Marion, S.D.; Touchette, P.E.; Sandman, C.A. Sequential analysis reveals a unique structure for self-injurious behavior. *Am. J. Ment. Retard.* **2003**, *108*, 301–313. [CrossRef]

84. Kovach, C. Editorial. Research in gerontological nursing: How are we doing? *Res. Geron. Nurs.* **2018**, *11*, 227–229. [CrossRef] [PubMed]

85. Woods, N.F.; Ismail, R.; Linder, L.A.; Macpherson, C.F. Midlife women's symptom cluster heuristics: Evaluation of an iPad application for data collection. *Menopause* **2015**, *22*, 1058–1066. [CrossRef] [PubMed]

86. Woods, N.F.; Cray, L.; Mitchell, E.; Farrin, F.; Hertig, J.R. Polymorphisms in estrogen synthesis genes and symptom clusters during the menopausal transition and early postmenopause: Observations from the seattle midlife women's health study. *Biol. Res. Nurs.* **2018**, *20*, 153–160. [CrossRef] [PubMed]

87. Magnusson, M.S. Discovering hidden time patterns in behavior: T-patterns and their detection. *Behav. Res. Methods Instrum. Comput.* **2000**, *32*, 93–110. [CrossRef] [PubMed]

88. Magnusson, M.S. Hidden and real-time patterns in intra and inter-individual behavior: Description and detection. *Eur. J. Psychol. Assess.* **1996**, *12*, 112. [CrossRef]

89. Buckwalter, K.C.; Grey, M.; Bowers, B.; McCarthy, A.M.; Gross, D.; Funk, M.; Beck, C. Intervention research in highly unstable environments. *Res. Nurs. Health* **2009**, *32*, 110–121. [CrossRef] [PubMed]

90. Lawton, M.P. Competence, environmental press and the adaptation of older people. In *Theory Development in Environment and Aging*; Gerontological Society: Washington, DC, USA, 1975; pp. 13–88.

91. Woods, D.L.; Mentes, J.C. Agitated behavior as a prodromal symptom of physical illness: A case of influenza. *J. Am. Geriatr. Soc.* **2006**, *54*, 1953–1954. [CrossRef] [PubMed]

92. Murman, D.L.; Chen, Q.; Powell, M.C.; Kuo, S.B.; Bradley, C.J.; Colenda, C.C. The incremental direct costs associated with behavioral symptoms in AD. *Neurology* **2002**, *59*, 1721–1729. [CrossRef] [PubMed]

93. Fazio, S.; Pace, D.; Flinner, J.; Kallmyer, B. The fundamentals of person-centered care for individuals with dementia. *Gerontologist* **2018**, *58*, S10–S19. [CrossRef] [PubMed]

Permissions

All chapters in this book were first published in HEALTHCARE, by MDPI; hereby published with permission under the Creative Commons Attribution License or equivalent. Every chapter published in this book has been scrutinized by our experts. Their significance has been extensively debated. The topics covered herein carry significant findings which will fuel the growth of the discipline. They may even be implemented as practical applications or may be referred to as a beginning point for another development.

The contributors of this book come from diverse backgrounds, making this book a truly international effort. This book will bring forth new frontiers with its revolutionizing research information and detailed analysis of the nascent developments around the world.

We would like to thank all the contributing authors for lending their expertise to make the book truly unique.

They have played a crucial role in the development of this book. Without their invaluable contributions this book wouldn't have been possible. They have made vital efforts to compile up to date information on the varied aspects of this subject to make this book a valuable addition to the collection of many professionals and students.

This book was conceptualized with the vision of imparting up-to-date information and advanced data in this field. To ensure the same, a matchless editorial board was set up. Every individual on the board went through rigorous rounds of assessment to prove their worth. After which they invested a large part of their time researching and compiling the most relevant data for our readers.

The editorial board has been involved in producing this book since its inception. They have spent rigorous hours researching and exploring the diverse topics which have resulted in the successful publishing of this book. They have passed on their knowledge of decades through this book. To expedite this challenging task, the publisher supported the team at every step. A small team of assistant editors was also appointed to further simplify the editing procedure and attain best results for the readers.

Apart from the editorial board, the designing team has also invested a significant amount of their time in understanding the subject and creating the most relevant covers. They scrutinized every image to scout for the most suitable representation of the subject and create an appropriate cover for the book.

The publishing team has been an ardent support to the editorial, designing and production team. Their endless efforts to recruit the best for this project, has resulted in the accomplishment of this book. They are a veteran in the field of academics and their pool of knowledge is as vast as their experience in printing. Their expertise and guidance has proved useful at every step. Their uncompromising quality standards have made this book an exceptional effort. Their encouragement from time to time has been an inspiration for everyone.

The publisher and the editorial board hope that this book will prove to be a valuable piece of knowledge for researchers, students, practitioners and scholars across the globe.

List of Contributors

Marcus Davidsson
Economist and Independent Researcher

Koji Nonaka, Shin Murata, Kayoko Shiraiwa, Teppei Abiko, Hideki Nakano and Jun Horie
Faculty of Physical Therapy, Department of Health Sciences, Kyoto Tachibana University, Kyoto 607-8175, Japan

Hiroaki Iwase
Faculty of Physical Therapy, Department of Rehabilitation, Kobe International University, Kobe 658-0032, Japan

Koichi Naito
Department of Physical Therapy, Hakuho College, Oji 636-0011, Japan

Shervin Assari
Department of Psychiatry, University of Michigan, Ann Arbor, MI 48109, USA; assari@umich.edu
Center for Research on Ethnicity, Culture and Health, School of Public Health, University of Michigan, Ann Arbor, MI 48109, USA

Birgitta Wallerstedt, Anna Sandgren and Eva Benzein
Center for Collaborative Palliative Care, Department of Health and Caring Sciences, Faculty of Health and Life Sciences, Linnaeus University, SE-351 95 Växjö, Sweden

Lina Behm and Gerd Ahlström
Department of Health Sciences, Faculty of Medicine, Lund University, SE-221 00 Lund, Sweden

Åsa Alftberg
Department of SocialWork, Faculty of Health and Society, Malmö University, SE 205 06 Malmö, Sweden

Per Nilsen
Department of Medical and Health Sciences, Linköping University, SE-581 83 Linköping, Sweden

Judith Ortiz, Yi-ling Lin and Ahmad Khanijahani
College of Health and Public Affairs, University of Central Florida, Orlando, FL 32816, USA

Richard Hofler
College of Business Administration, University of Central Florida, Orlando, FL 32816, USA

Angeline Bushy
College of Nursing, University of Central Florida, Orlando, FL 32816, USA

Andrea Bitney
College of Sciences, University of Central Florida, Orlando, FL 32816, USA

Angela Grocott
The University Hospitals of North Midlands NHS NHS Trust, Newcastle Rd, Stoke-on-Trent ST4 6QG, UK

Wilfred McSherry
The University Hospitals of North Midlands NHS NHS Trust, Newcastle Rd, Stoke-on-Trent ST4 6QG, UK
Department of Nursing, School of Health and Social Care, Staffordshire University, Blackheath Lane, Stafford ST18 0YB, UK
VID vitenskapelige høgskole, Haraldsplass Bergen, Ulriksdal 10, 5009 Bergen, Norway

Chrysi Koliaki
First Department of Propaedeutic Medicine, National Kapodistrian University of Athens, Laiko University Hospital, Athens 11527, Greece

Nicholas Katsilambros
First Department of Propaedeutic Medicine, National Kapodistrian University of Athens, Laiko University Hospital, Athens 11527, Greece
Research Laboratory Christeas Hall, Medical School, National Kapodistrian University of Athens, Athens 11527, Greece

Theodoros Spinos, Marianna Spinou, Maria-Eugenia Brinia and Dimitra Mitsopoulou
Medical School, National Kapodistrian University of Athens, Athens 11527, Greece

Sasha Hernandez, Jessica Oliveira, Leah Jones and Taraneh Shirazian
Saving Mothers, New York, NY 10022, USA

Juan Chumil
Ministerio de Salud Pública y Asistencia Social, Santiago Atitlán, Sololá 07019, Guatemala

Vivek Podder
Department of Internal Medicine, Tairunnessa Memorial Medical College, Gazipur 1704, Bangladesh

Binod Dhakal
Division of Hematology/Oncology, Medical College of Wisconsin, Milwaukee, WI 53226, USA

Gousia Ummae Salma Shaik and Rakesh Biswas
Department of Internal Medicine, Kamineni Institute of Medical Sciences, Narketpally 508254, Indi

Kaushik Sundar
Department of Neurology, Rajagiri Hospital, Chunanangamvely, Aluva 683112, India

Madhava Sai Sivapuram
Department of Internal Medicine, Dr. Pinnamaneni Siddhartha Institute of Medical Sciences and Research Foundation, Chinaoutapalli 521101, India

Vijay Kumar Chattu
Department of Paraclinical Sciences, Faculty of Medical Sciences, The University of theWest Indies

Shervin Assari
Center for Research on Ethnicity, Culture, and Health (CRECH), School of Public Health, University of Michigan, Ann Arbor, MI 48104, USA
Department of Psychiatry, University of Michigan, 4250 Plymouth Rd., Ann Arbor, MI 48109-2700, USA

Paula J Kalksma
Department of Health and Exercise Sciences, School of Health Professions, Rowan University, Glassboro, NJ 08028, USA

Nicole A. Vaughn
Department of Health and Exercise Sciences, School of Health Professions, Rowan University, Glassboro, NJ 08028, USA
Department of Biomedical Sciences, Cooper Medical School of Rowan University, Camden, NJ 08103, USA
Department of Family Medicine, School of Osteopathic Medicine, Rowan University, Stratford, NJ 08084, USA

Darryl Brown
Department of Health Management and Policy, School of Public Health, Drexel University, Philadelphia, PA 19104, USA

Beatriz O. Reyes
Department of Anthropology, Global Health Studies Program, Northwestern University, Evanston, IL 60208, USA;

CrystalWyatt
Ride and Rebuild, LLC, Philadelphia, PA 19151, USA

Kimberly T. Arnold
Department of Health Policy and Management, Bloomberg School of Public Health, Johns Hopkins University, Baltimore, MD 21205, USA

Elizabeth Dalianis
Community College of Philadelphia, Philadelphia, PA 19130, USA

Caryn Roth and Jason Langheier
Zipongo, Inc., San Francisco, CA 94133, USA

Maria Pajil-Battle
AmeriHealth Caritas Partnership, Philadelphia, PA 19113, USA

Meg Grant
Keystone First, Philadelphia, PA 19113, USA

Katharine Aldwell and Margaret Allman-Farinelli
Charles Perkins Centre, University of Sydney, Sydney, NSW 2006, Australia

Corinne Caillaud
Faculty of Health Sciences and Charles Perkins Centre, University of Sydney, Sydney, NSW 2006, Australia

Olivier Galy and Stéphane Frayon
Interdisciplinary Laboratory for Research in Education, EA 7483, School of Education, University of New Caledonia, Nouméa BP R4 98851, New Caledonia

Sherry Shiqian Gao, Kitty Jieyi Chen, Duangporn Duangthip, Edward Chin Man Lo and Chun Hung Chu
Faculty of Dentistry, The University of Hong Kong, Hong Kong, China

Chengwu Yang
Departments of Epidemiology and Health Promotion, College of Dentistry, New York University, New York, NY 10010, USA

Kent E. Vrana
Department of Pharmacology, College of Medicine, The Pennsylvania State University, Hershey, PA 17033, USA

Stephanie R. Partridge
Faculty of Medicine and Health, Westmead Applied Research Centre, The University of Sydney, Westmead, NSW 2145, Australia
Faculty of Medicine and Health, Sydney School of Public Health, Prevention Research Collaboration, Charles Perkins Centre, The University of Sydney, Camperdown, NSW 2006, Australia

Julie Redfern
Faculty of Medicine and Health, Westmead Applied Research Centre, The University of Sydney, Westmead, NSW 2145, Australia

The George Institute for Global Health, The University of New SouthWales, Camperdown, NSW 2006, Australia

Krista Leischner, Lacey Arneson McCormack and Kendra Kattelmann
Health and Nutritional Sciences Department, South Dakota State University, Brookings, SD 57007, USA

Brian C. Britt
Journalism and Mass Communications Department, South Dakota State University, Brookings, SD 57007, USA

Greg Heiberger
Biology and Microbiology, South Dakota State University, Brookings, SD 57007, USA

Alexandra Pereira and Amélia Ferreira
Community Care Unit of Lousada, Rua de Santo Tirso 70, Meinedo, Lousada, 4620-848 Porto, Portugal
Abel Salazar Biomedical Institute, R. Jorge de Viterbo Ferreira 228, 4050-313 Porto, Portugal

José Martins
Nursing School of Coimbra, 3046-841 Coimbra, Portugal

Diana Lynn Woods
School of Nursing, Azusa Pacific University, Azusa, CA 91702, USA

Kathleen Buckwalter
College of Nursing, University of Iowa, Iowa City, IA 52242, USA

Index

www.ingramcontent.com/pod-product-compliance
Lightning Source LLC
Chambersburg PA
CBHW080510200326

41458CB00012B/4154